Studying Brain Activity in Sports Performance

Studying Brain Activity in Sports Performance

Editor

Stéphane Perrey

MDPI • Basel • Beijing • Wuhan • Barcelona • Belgrade • Manchester • Tokyo • Cluj • Tianjin

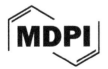

Editor
Stéphane Perrey
Univ. Montpellier
France

Editorial Office
MDPI
St. Alban-Anlage 66
4052 Basel, Switzerland

This is a reprint of articles from the Special Issue published online in the open access journal *Brain Sciences* (ISSN 2076-0825) (available at: https://www.mdpi.com/journal/brainsci/special_issues/brain_sports).

For citation purposes, cite each article independently as indicated on the article page online and as indicated below:

LastName, A.A.; LastName, B.B.; LastName, C.C. Article Title. *Journal Name* **Year**, *Volume Number*, Page Range.

ISBN 978-3-0365-0192-5 (Hbk)
ISBN 978-3-0365-0193-2 (PDF)

Cover image courtesy of Stephane Perrey.

© 2021 by the authors. Articles in this book are Open Access and distributed under the Creative Commons Attribution (CC BY) license, which allows users to download, copy and build upon published articles, as long as the author and publisher are properly credited, which ensures maximum dissemination and a wider impact of our publications.

The book as a whole is distributed by MDPI under the terms and conditions of the Creative Commons license CC BY-NC-ND.

Contents

About the Editor . . . . **vii**

Stéphane Perrey
Exercise: A Gate That Primes the Brain to Perform
Reprinted from: *Brain Sci.* **2020**, *10*, 980, doi:10.3390/brainsci10120980 . . . . **1**

Xuru Wang, Rui Zhu, Chenglin Zhou and Yifan Chen
Distinct Effects of Acute Aerobic Exercise on Declarative Memory and Procedural Memory Formation
Reprinted from: *Brain Sci.* **2020**, *10*, 691, doi:10.3390/brainsci10100691 . . . . **7**

Said Mekari, Meghan Earle, Ricardo Martins, Sara Drisdelle, Melanie Killen, Vicky Bouffard-Levasseur and Olivier Dupuy
Effect of High Intensity Interval Training Compared to Continuous Training on Cognitive Performance in Young Healthy Adults: A Pilot Study
Reprinted from: *Brain Sci.* **2020**, *10*, 81, doi:10.3390/brainsci10020081 . . . . **23**

Jan Wilke, Vanessa Stricker and Susanne Usedly
Free-Weight Resistance Exercise Is More Effective in Enhancing Inhibitory Control than Machine-Based Training: A Randomized, Controlled Trial
Reprinted from: *Brain Sci.* **2020**, *10*, 702, doi:10.3390/brainsci10100702 . . . . **37**

Jan Wilke and Caroline Royé
Exercise Intensity May Not Moderate the Acute Effects of Functional Circuit Training on Cognitive Function: A Randomized Crossover Trial
Reprinted from: *Brain Sci.* **2020**, *10*, 738, doi:10.3390/brainsci10100738 . . . . **47**

Huei-Jhen Wen and Chia-Liang Tsai
Effects of Acute Aerobic Exercise Combined with Resistance Exercise on Neurocognitive Performance in Obese Women
Reprinted from: *Brain Sci.* **2020**, *10*, 767, doi:10.3390/brainsci10110767 . . . . **55**

Jin-Gui Wang, Ke-Long Cai, Zhi-Mei Liu, Fabian Herold, Liye Zou, Li-Na Zhu, Xuan Xiong and Ai-Guo Chen
Effects of Mini-Basketball Training Program on Executive Functions and Core Symptoms among Preschool Children with Autism Spectrum Disorders
Reprinted from: *Brain Sci.* **2020**, *10*, 263, doi:10.3390/brainsci10050263 . . . . **73**

Yi-Kang Chiu, Chien-Yu Pan, Fu-Chen Chen, Yu-Ting Tseng and Chia-Liang Tsai
Behavioral and Cognitive Electrophysiological Differences in the Executive Functions of Taiwanese Basketball Players as a Function of Playing Position
Reprinted from: *Brain Sci.* **2020**, *10*, 387, doi:10.3390/brainsci10060387 . . . . **87**

Cuicui Wang, Yuechuan Zhu, Cheng Dong, Zigui Zhou and Xinyan Zheng
Effects of Various Doses of Caffeine Ingestion on Intermittent Exercise Performance and Cognition
Reprinted from: *Brain Sci.* **2020**, *10*, 595, doi:10.3390/brainsci10090595 . . . . **103**

Cayque Brietzke, Paulo Estevão Franco-Alvarenga, Raul Canestri, Márcio Fagundes Goethel, Ítalo Vínicius, Vitor de Salles Painelli, Tony Meireles Santos, Florentina Johanna Hettinga and Flávio Oliveira Pires
Carbohydrate Mouth Rinse Mitigates Mental Fatigue Effects on Maximal Incremental Test Performance, but Not in Cortical Alterations
Reprinted from: *Brain Sci.* **2020**, *10*, 493, doi:10.3390/brainsci10080493 . . . . **115**

Fabian Herold, Thomas Gronwald, Felix Scholkmann, Hamoon Zohdi, Dominik Wyser, Notger G. Müller and Dennis Hamacher
New Directions in Exercise Prescription: Is There a Role for Brain-Derived Parameters Obtained by Functional Near-Infrared Spectroscopy?
Reprinted from: *Brain Sci.* **2020**, *10*, 342, doi:10.3390/brainsci10060342 . . . . **131**

Katharina Stute, Nicole Hudl, Robert Stojan and Claudia Voelcker-Rehage
Shedding Light on the Effects of Moderate Acute Exercise on Working Memory Performance in Healthy Older Adults: An fNIRS Study
Reprinted from: *Brain Sci.* **2020**, *10*, 813, doi:10.3390/brainsci10110813 . . . . **155**

Kim-Marie Stadler, Wanja Wolff and Julia Schüler
On Your Mark, Get Set, Self-Control, Go: A Differentiated View on the Cortical Hemodynamics of Self-Control during Sprint Start
Reprinted from: *Brain Sci.* **2020**, *10*, 494, doi:10.3390/brainsci10080494 . . . . **179**

Gaoxia Wei, Ruoguang Si, Youfa Li, Ying Yao, Lizhen Chen, Shu Zhang, Tao Huang, Liye Zou, Chunxiao Li and Stephane Perrey
"No Pain No Gain": Evidence from a Parcel-Wise Brain Morphometry Study on the Volitional Quality of Elite Athletes
Reprinted from: *Brain Sci.* **2020**, *10*, 459, doi:10.3390/brainsci10070459 . . . . **195**

Louis-Solal Giboin, Markus Gruber, Julia Schüler and Wanja Wolff
Investigating Performance in a Strenuous Physical Task from the Perspective of Self-Control
Reprinted from: *Brain Sci.* **2019**, *9*, 317, doi:10.3390/brainsci9110317 . . . . **207**

Rouven Kenville, Tom Maudrich, Dennis Maudrich, Arno Villringer and Patrick Ragert
Cerebellar Transcranial Direct Current Stimulation Improves Maximum Isometric Force Production during Isometric Barbell Squats
Reprinted from: *Brain Sci.* **2020**, *10*, 235, doi:10.3390/brainsci10040235 . . . . **223**

Songlin Xiao, Baofeng Wang, Xini Zhang, Junhong Zhou and Weijie Fu
Acute Effects of High-Definition Transcranial Direct Current Stimulation on Foot Muscle Strength, Passive Ankle Kinesthesia, and Static Balance: A Pilot Study
Reprinted from: *Brain Sci.* **2020**, *10*, 246, doi:10.3390/brainsci10040246 . . . . **237**

Pierre Besson, Makii Muthalib, Christophe De Vassoigne, Jonh Rothwell and Stephane Perrey
Effects of Multiple Sessions of Cathodal Priming and Anodal HD-tDCS on Visuo Motor Task Plateau Learning and Retention
Reprinted from: *Brain Sci.* **2020**, *10*, 875, doi:10.3390/brainsci10110875 . . . . **249**

About the Editor

Stéphane Perrey (Ph.D., IUF honorary member, Director of the European Centre for Research and Innovation in the Sciences of Movement) is full professor at the University of Montpellier. He is leading a new Lab named EuroMov Digital Health in Motion (Univ Montpellier, IMT Mines Ales), which involves neuroscientists, physiologists, computer scientists, engineers, and clinicians. His research aims to better understand the relationship between brain plasticity and motor behavior in humans, and to identify optimal procedures to promote brain plasticity and enhance sensorimotor recovery. He is the author and co-author of more than 180 publications in peer-reviewed journals and more than 200 communications in meetings.

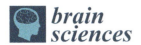

Editorial

Exercise: A Gate That Primes the Brain to Perform

Stéphane Perrey

EuroMov Digital Health in Motion, Univ Montpellier, IMT Mines Ales, 34090 Montpellier, France; stephane.perrey@umontpellier.fr; Tel.: +33-(0)4-34-43-26-23

Received: 3 December 2020; Accepted: 10 December 2020; Published: 14 December 2020

The improvement of exercise performance encountered in sports not only represents the enhancement of physical strength but also includes the development of psychological and cognitive functions. Accumulating evidence has showed that physical exercise is a powerful way to improve a number of aspects of cognition and brain functions at the system and behavioral levels. Yet, several questions remain: what type of exercise program is the most optimal for improving cognitive functions? What are the real effects of some innovative exercise protocols on the relationship between behavior and the brain? To what extent do ergogenic aids boost cognitive functions? What about the efficacy of neuromodulation techniques on behavioral performance? Answers likely require combined insights not only from physiologists and sports scientists, but also from neuroscientists and psychologists. Published manuscripts (sixteen research papers and one perspective article from various academic fields) within this Special Issue "Studying Brain Activity in Sports Performance" did bring novel knowledge and new directions in human exercise-cognition research dealing with performance. Here, we summarize the main insights provided by the contributions and showcase the multiple relationships between cognitive functions, brain activity, and behavioral performance with applications in sports and exercise science.

First, the cognitive benefits of acute and chronic (training) physical exercise need to move beyond simple aerobic activities and resistance training. From a multidisciplinary perspective, this Special Issue proposes some encouraging evidence for other types of physical exercise (more demanding/challenging) or interventions (ergogenic help), improving executive functions for various populations (children to older adults, in healthy and diseased states) that have received far less attention. Following acute endurance exercise of 30 min at constant moderate intensity on a cycle ergometer, Wang et al. [1] observed noticeable facilitation effects on the formation of long-term declarative memory and procedural memory functions that are essential for the development of motor skills, for instance. This study highlights for the first time that traditional endurance-type exercise impacts memory processing by facilitating the encoding period of declarative memory and the consolidation period of procedural memory. Regarding endurance training, it is thought that high-intensity intermittent training consisting of alternating periods of intensive aerobic exercise with periods of recovery may be considerably more effective at improving cognitive function. The effects of such exercise intensity changes on executive functions were examined by Mekari et al. [2]. Their original findings showed that specific executive functions (e.g., flexibility) were more sensitive to high intensity interval training as compared to regular endurance training at moderate intensity in young adults after 6 weeks (3 days/week). Another common exercise modality, resistance exercise (integrated in weight training), is also recognized to improve brain function (see, for a review, [3]). Resistance exercise involves the voluntary activation of specific skeletal muscles against some form of external resistance, provided by body mass, free weights, or a variety of exercise equipment including machines, elastic bands, or manual resistance. The study of Wilke et al. [4] provided new outcomes of interest for such approaches. As compared to machine-based training, the use of free weights appears to be a more effective resistance exercise method to acutely improve cognitive function (i.e., increasing inhibitory control) than the use of conventional training machines in healthy adults [4]. The authors suggested that engagement in free-weight exercise is likely linked to more complex cortical activation patterns when compared to machine-based resistance training or aerobic exercise. While a large body of evidence is available for endurance and resistance training protocols, Wilke and Royé [5] proposed to investigate the beneficial effects of high-intensity functional training that concurrently integrates cardiovascular (endurance) and muscular (resistance) exercises. Through a three-armed randomized crossover trial in healthy adults, exercise intensity did not substantially alter short-term lower-order executive functions, such as attention, working memory, inhibitory control, and cognitive flexibility. However, these preliminary findings indicate that the highest exercise intensities in functional circuit training might be more advantageous to enhance in concert cognitive, cardiovascular, and muscular functions.

Besides healthy adults, a few original articles in this Special Issue were related to other target clinical populations and aimed to test the beneficial effects of novel exercise protocols on cognition. Wen and Tsai [6] investigated the effects of a 30-min bout of supervised moderate-intensity aerobic (dance) combined with resistance exercise on neurophysiological (i.e., behavioral and cognitive electrophysiological) performance in sedentary obese female adults with impaired neurocognitive functions. The authors observed no behavioral (inhibitory control) benefits by the exercise mode but reported improved brain neural processing related to early and late inhibition, captured by brain electrical activity (e.g., event-related potential recording provided by electroencephalography—EEG). In children aged 3–6 years with autism spectrum disorder, Wang et al. [7] showed that implementation of cognitively and/or coordinatively demanding physical exercises (mini-basketball) significantly improved all aspects of executive functions, including working memory and inhibition, following a 12-week training program, as compared to the control group. Beyond these first behavioral outcomes in most of the aforementioned studies, neural correlates (e.g., changes in functional brain activity patterns) of the observed cognitive changes need to be further investigated as carried out by Wen and Tsai [6]. In elite basketball players, Chiu et al. [8] investigated both behavioral responses but also neural correlates that modulated the executive functions as a function of playing positions in basketball. This study showed divergent neural processing efficiency based on EEG recordings related to player position (guards were more efficient than forwards) when performing a cognitive task involving inhibitory control. This suggests that cognitive functioning in open-skilled sports might be dependent on the player's position.

Executive functioning is important for athletic performance and can be affected by ergogenic aids. The ergogenic effect of caffeine might not only enhance physical strength but also the development of cognitive functions during exercise. Wang et al. [9] in a cross-over double-blind study showed that ingestion of a low dose of caffeine had greater positive effects on intermittent exercise (mimicking team sports) and cognitive performance (perceptual-motor speed, executive information processing) than a moderate or high dose of caffeine. In a double-controlled experimental design study, Brietzke et al. [10] showed that a carbohydrate mouth rinse might counteract mental fatigue effects on exercise performance, despite comparable cortical activation assessed by functional near-infrared spectroscopy (fNIRS), an optical neuroimaging method that allows for measuring brain tissue concentration changes in oxygenated and deoxygenated hemoglobin in the cortical layers during exercise [11]. The benefit of applying functional neuroimaging methods, such as fNIRS or EEG, in the field of exercise-cognition research, allows the investigation of to what extent exercise-induced changes in neural processes underlie behavioral outcomes; these methods are presenting a growing interest [10–13]. The study of Brietzke et al. [10] provided an example of a rigorous, well-controlled methodology to assess EEG responses over the prefrontal cortex and primary motor cortex areas at different controlled intensities below 75% of the maximal power output during a maximal incremental cycling test.

Second, after establishing a link between exercise and the outcomes of some specific cognitive function tests, using neuroimaging techniques is required to reveal the electrophysiological (EEG) processes that are associated with some behavioral changes, or evaluate the physiological changes (e.g., increased cerebral blood flow and cerebral metabolism with fNIRS) over the course of the intervention or training program, that have the potential to improve executive functions. In their perspective article, Herold et al. [11] overviewed the most current and suitable portable neuroimaging methods to monitor brain activity during physical exercise. The most common methods used to investigate effects on functional brain activation are fNIRS and EEG. Herold et al. [11] emphasized that brain activity derived from fNIRS measures could be used as valuable and promising indicators of internal load (e.g., cognitive load and fatigue, stress, traits) during physical exercise. Prescribing exercise intensity by using such neurocognitive outcomes sensitive to psychophysiological responses is clearly lacking in sport and exercise sciences and clinical settings. Monitoring cortical hemodynamics opens up a new perspective on exercise–cognition interaction but needs to be further evaluated. The study from Stute et al. [12] advanced knowledge about acute exercise effects from a neurocognitive perspective by assessing cortical hemodynamic activity in the frontal and parietal cortices during cognitive testing before and at three time points post exercise (i.e., 15, 30, and 45 min) in a sample of healthy older adults. The authors concluded that exercise might somewhat influence working memory performance for up to 45 min due to a more heightened executive processing and attention component of working memory in the frontal cortex. Most sports are self-control demanding, such as during a sprint running start. Using fNIRS to monitor cortical hemodynamic changes during a sprint start sequence through a randomized within-subject design in 60 young adults, Stadler et al. [13] provided new support for the involvement of the ventrolateral prefrontal cortex after the set signal, while highlighting gender differences in the processing of sprint start-induced self-control demands. Still, according to a psychological framework, volitional quality as a mental trait for dealing with adverse circumstances is often met in sports. In a parcel-wise brain morphometry study by comparing elite athletes (short track speed skate, national team) with controls, Wei et al. [14] observed that long-term sports training might improve the mental characteristics of volitional qualities. Indeed, they identified specific cortical architecture (e.g., a greater cortical thickness in the left inferior parietal lobule) associated with volitional qualities. Finally, it is now well acknowledged that physical performance is limited by the perception of the effort a task induces and not only by the limits of the physiological systems. Emerging evidence suggests that the maintenance of ongoing physical exercise requires mental effort. Aiming to ascribe a key role to the psychological concept of self-control in the effective regulation of physical performance, Giboin et al. [15] showed according to their experimental design (income manipulation) a more efficient use of resources while performing a strenuous lower-limb isometric task, allowing for a longer time before self-disengagement without a change in psychological (rating of perceived exertion), cortical (lateral prefrontal cortex), or physiological (neuromuscular fatigue) markers of effort. It is possible that some prefrontal-dependent functions are down-regulated to save the mental effort and executive resources that are needed to maintain the physical task.

Third, enabling enhanced physical exercise may benefit from muscle strength and whole-body movement improvements. Within this context, non-invasive brain stimulation (e.g., neuromodulatory techniques such as transcranial direct current stimulation, tDCS) approaches have been employed to uncover strength-related brain–muscle (movement) associations. By applying tDCS over the primary motor cortex and the cerebellum with traditional montages, a randomized counter-balanced sham-controlled double-blinded cross-over design study from Kenville et al. [16] provided novel finding that anodal cerebellar tDCS can improve static force output during whole-body movement production regularly used in resistance training. Two other pilot studies in this Special Issue provided further critical knowledge on the absence of evidence of the effects of high-definition tDCS (HD-tDCS) on functional performance parameters of the foot [17] and wrist [18]. In a randomized double-blinded, self-controlled study, Xiao et al. [17] examined, in young adults, the effects of a single-session anodal HD-tDCS designed to target the sensory-motor regions of the brain with respect to foot muscle strength, passive ankle kinesthesia, and static balance. In a double-blind sham-controlled study, Besson et al. [18] tested the hypothesis that multiple sessions of cathodal priming and anodal tDCS over 3 consecutive days could further enhance motor learning and retention of an already learned visuomotor task compared to anodal tDCS or sham. While both studies observed some positive changes, no significant differences were observed between HD-tDCS and sham stimulation conditions, likely due to ceiling effects in healthy participants.

To conclude, this Special Issue showed that the acute or chronic exercise effects upon cognitive functions are varied and dependent upon exercise duration, intensity, and mode, as well as the type of cognitive tasks assessed. The considerable advancement in wearable neuroimaging methods coupled with neural recording and non-invasive brain stimulation for studying human brain physiology are now enabling the gaining of new insight into the complexities of the behavior–exercise relationship, where the prefrontal cortex as a whole plays a cardinal role in the temporal organization of behavior and cognitive activities. This Special Issue makes the point that exercise and sport sciences are a joint research initiative of exercise scientists, psychologists, neuroscientists, neurophysiologists, and other related disciplines such as neuroimaging.

Funding: This research received no external funding.

Acknowledgments: The author acknowledges all contributors that have made this Special Issue so successful.

Conflicts of Interest: The author declares no conflict of interest.

References

1. Wang, X.; Zhu, R.; Zhou, C.; Chen, Y. Distinct Effects of Acute Aerobic Exercise on Declarative Memory and Procedural Memory Formation. *Brain Sci.* **2020**, *10*, 691. [CrossRef] [PubMed]
2. Mekari, S.; Earle, M.; Martins, R.; Drisdelle, S.; Killen, M.; Bouffard-Levasseur, V.; Dupuy, O. Effect of High Intensity Interval Training Compared to Continuous Training on Cognitive Performance in Young Healthy Adults: A Pilot Study. *Brain Sci.* **2020**, *10*, 81. [CrossRef] [PubMed]
3. Perrey, S. Promoting motor function by exercising the brain. *Brain Sci.* **2013**, *3*, 101–122. [CrossRef] [PubMed]
4. Wilke, J.; Stricker, V.; Usedly, S. Free-Weight Resistance Exercise Is More Effective in Enhancing Inhibitory Control than Machine-Based Training: A Randomized, Controlled Trial. *Brain Sci.* **2020**, *10*, 702. [CrossRef] [PubMed]
5. Wilke, J.; Royé, C. Exercise Intensity May Not Moderate the Acute Effects of Functional Circuit Training on Cognitive Function: A Randomized Crossover Trial. *Brain Sci.* **2020**, *10*, 738. [CrossRef] [PubMed]
6. Wen, H.; Tsai, C. Effects of Acute Aerobic Exercise Combined with Resistance Exercise on Neurocognitive Performance in Obese Women. *Brain Sci.* **2020**, *10*, 767. [CrossRef] [PubMed]
7. Wang, J.; Cai, K.; Liu, Z.; Herold, F.; Zou, L.; Zhu, L.; Xiong, X.; Chen, A. Effects of Mini-Basketball Training Program on Executive Functions and Core Symptoms among Preschool Children with Autism Spectrum Disorders. *Brain Sci.* **2020**, *10*, 263. [CrossRef] [PubMed]
8. Chiu, Y.; Pan, C.; Chen, F.; Tseng, Y.; Tsai, C. Behavioral and Cognitive Electrophysiological Differences in the Executive Functions of Taiwanese Basketball Players as a Function of Playing Position. *Brain Sci.* **2020**, *10*, 387. [CrossRef] [PubMed]
9. Wang, C.; Zhu, Y.; Dong, C.; Zhou, Z.; Zheng, X. Effects of Various Doses of Caffeine Ingestion on Intermittent Exercise Performance and Cognition. *Brain Sci.* **2020**, *10*, 595. [CrossRef] [PubMed]
10. Brietzke, C.; Franco-Alvarenga, P.; Canestri, R.; Goethel, M.; Vínicius, Í.; Painelli, V.; Santos, T.; Hettinga, F.; Pires, F. Carbohydrate Mouth Rinse Mitigates Mental Fatigue Effects on Maximal Incremental Test Performance, but Not in Cortical Alterations. *Brain Sci.* **2020**, *10*, 493. [CrossRef] [PubMed]
11. Herold, F.; Gronwald, T.; Scholkmann, F.; Zohdi, H.; Wyser, D.; Müller, N.; Hamacher, D. New Directions in Exercise Prescription: Is There a Role for Brain-Derived Parameters Obtained by Functional Near-Infrared Spectroscopy? *Brain Sci.* **2020**, *10*, 342. [CrossRef] [PubMed]
12. Stute, K.; Hudl, N.; Stojan, R.; Voelcker-Rehage, C. Shedding Light on the Effects of Moderate Acute Exercise on Working Memory Performance in Healthy Older Adults: An fNIRS Study. *Brain Sci.* **2020**, *10*, 813. [CrossRef]
13. Stadler, K.; Wolff, W.; Schüler, J. On Your Mark, Get Set, Self-Control, Go: A Differentiated View on the Cortical Hemodynamics of Self-Control during Sprint Start. *Brain Sci.* **2020**, *10*, 494. [CrossRef] [PubMed]

14. Wei, G.; Si, R.; Li, Y.; Yao, Y.; Chen, L.; Zhang, S.; Huang, T.; Zou, L.; Li, C.; Perrey, S. "No Pain No Gain": Evidence from a Parcel-Wise Brain Morphometry Study on the Volitional Quality of Elite Athletes. *Brain Sci.* **2020**, *10*, 459. [CrossRef] [PubMed]
15. Giboin, L.; Gruber, M.; Schüler, J.; Wolff, W. Investigating Performance in a Strenuous Physical Task from the Perspective of Self-Control. *Brain Sci.* **2019**, *9*, 317. [CrossRef]
16. Kenville, R.; Maudrich, T.; Maudrich, D.; Villringer, A.; Ragert, P. Cerebellar Transcranial Direct Current Stimulation Improves Maximum Isometric Force Production during Isometric Barbell Squats. *Brain Sci.* **2020**, *10*, 235. [CrossRef] [PubMed]
17. Xiao, S.; Wang, B.; Zhang, X.; Zhou, J.; Fu, W. Acute Effects of High-Definition Transcranial Direct Current Stimulation on Foot Muscle Strength, Passive Ankle Kinesthesia, and Static Balance: A Pilot Study. *Brain Sci.* **2020**, *10*, 246. [CrossRef]
18. Besson, P.; Muthalib, M.; De Vassoigne, C.; Rothwell, J.; Perrey, S. Effects of Multiple Sessions of Cathodal Priming and Anodal HD-tDCS on Visuo Motor Task Plateau Learning and Retention. *Brain Sci.* **2020**, *10*, 875. [CrossRef]

Publisher's Note: MDPI stays neutral with regard to jurisdictional claims in published maps and institutional affiliations.

© 2020 by the author. Licensee MDPI, Basel, Switzerland. This article is an open access article distributed under the terms and conditions of the Creative Commons Attribution (CC BY) license (http://creativecommons.org/licenses/by/4.0/).

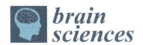

Article

Distinct Effects of Acute Aerobic Exercise on Declarative Memory and Procedural Memory Formation

Xuru Wang, Rui Zhu, Chenglin Zhou and Yifan Chen *

School of Psychology, Shanghai University of Sport, Shanghai 200438, China; 17858950731@163.com (X.W.); lohasmo@163.com (R.Z.); zhouchenglin@sus.edu.cn (C.Z.)
* Correspondence: 1811516012@sus.edu.cn

Received: 20 August 2020; Accepted: 28 September 2020; Published: 30 September 2020

Abstract: *Objective:* To investigate the different effects of acute aerobic exercise on the formation of long-term declarative memory (DM) and procedural memory (PM). *Methods:* Twenty-two young men completed DM and PM tasks under three experimental conditions: pre-acquisition exercise, post-acquisition exercise, and no exercise (control). The DM task encompassed word learning, free recall tests both immediately and 1 h later, and a recognition test conducted 24 h after word learning. A serial reaction time task (SRTT) was utilized to assess exercise effects on PM. The SRTT included a sequence learning phase followed by sequence tests 1 h and 24 h later. The exercise program consisted of 30 min of moderate-intensity aerobic exercise. *Results:* In the DM task, compared to the control condition, pre-acquisition exercise, but not post-acquisition exercise, enhanced free recall performance significantly 1 h and 24 h later. The target word recognition rate and discriminative index (d') of the recognition test were significantly enhanced in both exercise conditions compared to the control condition. In the PM task, we observed significantly reduced (improved) reaction times at the 24-h test in the post-acquisition exercise condition compared to in the control condition. *Conclusion:* Acute aerobic exercise may enhance long-term DM and PM via effects on different processing periods. For DM, exercise had a pronounced effect during the encoding period, whereas for PM, exercise was found to have an enhancing effect during the consolidation period.

Keywords: acute aerobic exercise; declarative memory; procedural memory; coding period; consolidation period

1. Introduction

In recent years, there has been a growing interest in understanding the effects of exercise on cognitive functions. Although much of the literature examining this relationship has focused on chronic exercise paradigms, acute aerobic exercise effects on cognitive functions have been reported [1,2], especially effects on memory [3,4]. A single exercise bout has been shown to induce plasticity-promoting effects on both a molecular and a systems level, and to lead to increases in arousal [2] and cerebral blood flow [5]. Exercise-induced changes in brain structures [6] may potentially facilitate memory and learning processes [7].

Memory encompasses the faculties by which the brain encodes, stores, and retrieves information. Regarding storage duration, information may be held quite briefly, as is the case in sensory processing or may be stored in short-term, intermediate-term, or long-term memory [8]. Importantly, there are distinct types of memory, wherein the information processing system may function explicitly, as in declarative memory (DM), or implicitly, as in procedural memory (PM) [9]. The conscious, intentional recollection of factual information, previous experiences, and concepts is considered to be DM [10]. Generally, DM is established through gradual learning, such as learning through multiple presentations of a stimulus and response. DM can be divided into two categories: episodic memory, which stores specific personal experiences, and semantic memory, which stores factual information [11]. Conversely, PM supports task performance without conscious awareness of one's previous experiences with the task. PM is developed through procedural learning, which is essential for the development of any motor skill or cognitive activity.

Because early explorations of aerobic exercise effects on memory did not distinguish between short- and long-term memory, it was unclear whether aerobic exercise can facilitate long-term memory. Meanwhile, some evidence indicated that acute aerobic exercise failed to improve short-term memory performance, whereas it played a positive role in facilitating long-term memory [3]. In more recent studies, positive impacts of acute aerobic exercise on long-term memory, including DM [12,13] and PM [14,15], have been reported. Moreover, these positive effects have been related to molecular processes during the encoding and consolidation stages of long-term memory [16]. Although acute aerobic exercise has been shown to facilitate long-term memory significantly, it is not yet clear which memory-formation processing period benefits from this facilitative effect.

It is possible that the effects of acute aerobic exercise on different processing periods of long-term memory formation may differ between types of memory. Studies using DM materials (such as stories) have suggested that acute aerobic exercise improved long-term memory performance primarily via a positive influence on encoding [4,17]. Meanwhile, positive effects of acute aerobic exercise on motor sequence learning have been linked mainly to enhanced consolidation [18]. Notably, differing intensity exercise paradigms may differentially affect temporally distinct forms of memory [19,20]. Specifically, it has been suggested that high-intensity exercise performed shortly after memory encoding may not affect long-term memory function [6], whereas moderate-intensity exercise has been widely reported to enhance multiple stages of memory formation [19]. Therefore, because the sorts of memory materials used have been variable across studies and because there is a potential interference caused by different exercise intensities, it has been difficult to make direct comparisons between DM and PM findings. The processing mechanisms by which acute aerobic exercise influences particular types of memory remain to be further explored.

The aim of the present study was to analyze the effects of acute aerobic exercise on DM and PM using the same acute aerobic exercise program, with a consistent intensity, across both settings. Based on previous studies [3,4], a 30-min moderate-intensity acute aerobic exercise program was employed in the present study design. DM was assessed via a word learning task with free recall and recognition tests. PM was assessed with a serial reaction time task (SRTT). Based on previous findings in the literature, we hypothesized that acute aerobic exercise would facilitate the encoding phase of DM recall and would facilitate the consolidation phase of PM.

2. Materials and Methods

2.1. Participants

Twenty-two right-handed students (22 males, mean age = 21.6 ± 3.0; mean body mass index = 22.4 ± 2.1) without intensive athletic experience were recruited randomly from our university. The sample size met the criteria of a power analysis assuming a 3 by 3 repeated-measures design, an alpha of 0.05, a power of 0.9, and an effect size of 0.25. Participants completed the Physical Activity Readiness Questionnaire to determine if it was safe for them to exercise. They also completed the International Physical Activity Questionnaire (Chinese version) to confirm that each had a metabolism of ≥600 metabolic equivalents. The study followed the ethical guidelines of the Declaration of Helsinki and was approved by the Research Ethics Committee at Shanghai University of Sport (approval number 2015003).

2.2. Task and Procedures

2.2.1. Acute Aerobic Exercise

The acute aerobic exercise program consisted of 30 min of moderate-intensity exercise on a cycle ergometer (MONARK 894E, made in Sweden). It began with a 5-min warm-up at a resistance of 0.5 kp. Then, the resistance was adjusted to 1 kp and participants were expected to maintain a rating of perceived exertion (RPE) in the range of 13–15 for 20 min. Finally, the resistance was returned to 0.5 kp for a 5-min cool-down. The target heart rate (HR) across moderate-intensity aerobic exercise was 60~70% maximum HR (maximum HR = 220-age), according to the American College of Sports Medicine guidelines. Participants' HR data were collected via Polar heart rate monitors (RCX3, made in Sweden). HR, ratings of perceived exertion (RPE), and revolutions per minute (RPM) measures were obtained from participants every 3 min during exercise.

2.2.2. DM Task

The DM task consisted of word learning followed by three free recall tests and a recognition test, all of which were administered in Eprime 2.0 (Psychology Software Tools, Pittsburgh, PA, USA). Participants were asked to learn 21 Chinese two-character emotionally neutral words (arousal level of 5.04 ± 0.27 on a 9-point scale) from a pool of 126 words taken from the Emotional Information of Modern Chinese Two-character Word Evaluation Table [21]. These words were randomly assigned to six groups, with 21 words in each group (7 verbs, 7 nouns, and 7 adjectives).

For the word learning phase, first, a black cross was displayed on a white-background computer screen for 500 ms (refresh rate 60 Hz, resolution ratio 1366 × 768). Each learning target word was shown in black (font size 34) at the center of the white screen for 2 s and followed by a 500-ms black screen (Figure 1a). Each participant was presented with 21 Chinese two-character neutral words in a random order without duplication, and participants were asked to memorize as many of the presented words as possible.

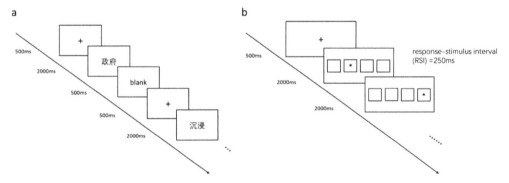

Figure 1. Behavioral task summary. Flow charts of the free recall task (**a**) and serial reaction time task (**b**).

After word learning, participants performed free recall tasks, which required them to write down as many target words as they could within 100 s in any order. After completing the first free recall task, which was conducted immediately after word learning, the participants were reminded not to rehearse the words. Participants completed a 1-h free recall task and 24-h free recall task for the same target words. The numbers of words recalled correctly were recorded for each recall trial.

The recognition test was taken after the last free recall task. It included the 21 target words intermixed randomly with 21 additional distracting words, with no duplications. Participants were asked to press designated buttons (counter-balanced across subjects) to indicate whether they thought each word on the screen had been in the word learning exercise or not.

2.2.3. PM Task

A SRTT was used to assess PM in Eprime 2.0. As shown in Figure 1b, the SRTT began with a black cross being displayed on a white screen for 500 ms. Then, four squares (4 cm × 4 cm) were situated in equidistant positions along a central horizontal line on a white screen. The target stimulus was a black asterisk ("*"; font size 34) at the center of one of aforementioned squares in a set sequence. Participants were asked to press the appropriate keyboard key (d, f, j, or k) designating the position of the target stimulus from left to right in the array. The d, f, j, and k keys were pressed with the left middle finger, left index finger, right index finger, and right middle finger, respectively. The target stimulus was shown for 2000 ms followed by a 250-ms response-to-stimulus interval.

Three 12-stimulus sequences were utilized in the SRTT, which were taken from previous studies [22,23]: sequence 1, 1-2-4-3-1-3-2-1-4-2-3-4; sequence 2, 4-3-2-4-2-3-1-2-1-4-1-3; and sequence 3, 3-4-3-2-1-3-1-4-2-4-1-2. The numbers 1, 2, 3, and 4 represented the four positions on the screen where the target stimuli could appear, from left to right. The SRTT consisted of a sequence learning stage, a 1-h test, and a 24-h test. Ten practice stimuli were delivered prior to the formal experiment. The learning stage was comprised of eight blocks with a 10-s inter-block rest interval. In each block, 76 stimuli were presented. In the first six blocks and the last block, the first 4 stimuli were ordered randomly, and the remaining 72 stimuli included six iterations of one of the above predetermined 12-stimulus sequences. In the seventh block, all 76 stimuli were presented in a random order.

Prior to the experiment, participants were told that the purpose of the PM experiment was to examine reaction time and that they should respond to target stimuli by pressing the corresponding keys as quickly and accurately as possible. After completing all PM experiments, participants were asked if they observed any particular regularity to probe whether selective implicit learning had been achieved.

2.3. Procedure

As summarized in Figure 2, all participants completed the DM task and PM task under three conditions: pre-acquisition exercise, post-acquisition exercise, and no exercise (control). Specifically, in the pre-acquisition exercise condition, participants completed the exercise program before the entire memory task such that the exercise could affect encoding and early consolidation. In the post-acquisition exercise condition, participants completed the exercise program after the first free call task (DM experiment) or sequence learning stage (PM experiment) such that the exercise could influence only consolidation. In the control condition, participants had a rest or read a magazine instead of exercising. These three conditions were ordered randomly in a balanced manner and carried out 1 week apart. Half of the participants first completed the DM task (all three experimental conditions), and the other half first completed the PM task. Participants were asked to not consume caffeine or alcohol and to not engage in strenuous exercise within a 2 h period before the experiment.

Take the DM task (a) as an example. In the pre-acquisition exercise condition, each participant completed a 30-min exercise program and then started the word learning section when his HR had returned to 110% of his resting HR. Immediately after the word learning stage, participants completed the first free recall test and then completed the second free recall test after a 1-h rest. Participants completed the third free recall test and the recognition test 24 h after the learning stage. The protocol for the post-acquisition exercise condition differed from the pre-acquisition exercise condition only in that participants rested prior to word learning and the first free recall test and then completed the same 30-min exercise program exactly as in the pre-acquisition exercise condition, except that it was completed immediately following the first recall test. They then had a 30-min rest prior to completing the 1-h second recall test. In the post-acquisition exercise condition, participants completed the 24-h recall test and recognition test in succession 24 h after the learning stage. In the control condition, participants completed the same learning stage and tests as in the other two conditions but were not engaged in an exercise program at any time.

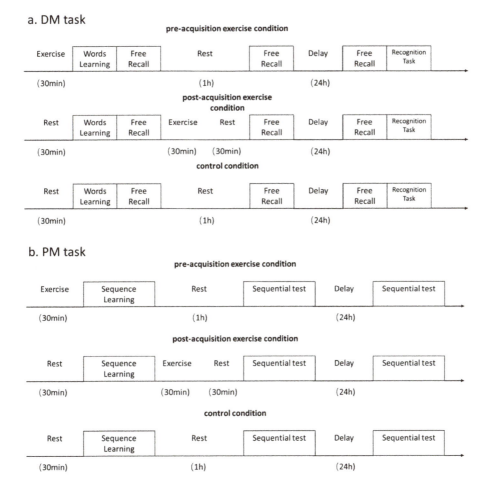

Figure 2. Task flow and experimental conditions for the declarative memory (DM) (**a**) and procedural memory (PM) (**b**) tasks.

2.4. Data Analysis

2.4.1. Behavioral Data Processing

For the PM task, reaction time and accuracy rate were analyzed. As per previous work [24,25], trials containing errors (i.e., an incorrect keystroke response by the subject) and reaction times greater than 1200 ms or less than 200 ms were discarded. For the DM task, the numbers of words recalled correctly in the three free recall tasks and the numbers of correct (e.g., responding "learned" when a learned word was actually present) and incorrect responses (e.g., responding "learned" to a distracting word) in the recognition test were analyzed. The recognition rate was calculated from the difference between separately computed hit rates and false alarm rates. Discrimination index (d′) and response bias (β) values were calculated according to signal detection theory [26].

Data from three participants were discarded due to outlier data falling outside three standard deviations around the mean. Data from one more participant was removed because he reported recognizing the repeating sequence pattern after completing the PM task. Therefore, data from 19 and 18 participants were considered valid for the DM task and PM task, respectively, and thus incorporated in the final statistical analysis.

2.4.2. Statistical Analysis

One-way analyses of variance (ANOVAs) and repeated measures ANOVAs were used to analyze the data in SPSS 23.0 software (SPSS Inc., Chicago, IL, USA) with the Greenhouse Geisser adjustment. The least significant difference method was used for further comparisons. Effect size was represented by partial η^2 values. Mean values for behavioral variables are reported with standard deviations. For all statistical analyses, the alpha significance level was set at 0.05.

To be specific, differences in recall performance across free recall tests conducted at different post-learning delays (immediate, 1 h, 24 h) and under different experimental conditions (pre-acquisition, post-acquisition, control) were assessed with a two-way (time × condition) repeated measures ANOVA. For the recognition test, a one-way repeated measures ANOVA was conducted to compare differences among the three exercise conditions. For the SRTT, differences between exercise conditions and task stages were analyzed with a two-way (stage × condition) repeated measures ANOVA. Additionally, to detect effects of exercise condition and learning sequence within each of two SRTT test time points, two separate two-way 3 (blocks 6–8) × 3 (experimental conditions) repeated measures ANOVAs were employed.

3. Results

3.1. HR, RPE and RPM during Exercise

A two-way 2 (exercise condition: pre- and post-acquisition exercise) × 11 (point-in-time of record) repeated measures ANOVA was applied to analyze HR, RPE, and RPM data from the DM task, and a similarly structured ANOVA was applied to analyze the same variables from the PM task (Table 1). We found that that HR, RPE, and RPM did not differ significantly between the two exercise conditions in either the DM task or the PM task (all $ps > 0.05$; Figure 3).

Table 1. Mean HR, RPE, and RPM (±SD) under pre- and post-acquisition exercise conditions.

Variable	Pre-Acquisition Exercise		Post-Acquisition Exercise	
	DM Task	PM Task	DM Task	PM Task
HR, beats per minute	126.9 ± 6.1	122.9 ± 4.8	127.4 ± 5.3	123.2 ± 5.2
RPM	71.8 ± 1.8	69.5 ± 0.8	71.4 ± 2.6	70.6 ± 0.9
RPE	13.8 ± 0.8	13.6 ± 0.7	13.8 ± 0.8	14.1 ± 0.8
Exercise intensity, percent maximum HR	64.0 ± 3.1%	61.6 ± 2.4%	64.3 ± 2.7%	61.8 ± 2.6%

HR, heart rate; RPM, revolutions per minute; RPE, rating of perceived exertion. DM task, $N = 19$; PM task, $N = 18$.

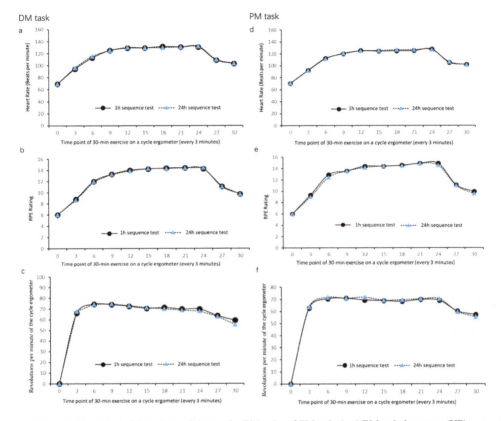

Figure 3. Physiological data obtained during the DM task and PM task. (**a–c**) DM task: heart rate (HR) (**a**); rating of perceived exertion (RPE) (**b**); and revolutions per minute (RPM) (**c**). (**d–f**) PM task: HR (**d**); RPE (**e**); and RPM (**f**). For both tasks, data were collected every 3 min during the exercise bout.

3.2. DM

3.2.1. Free Recall Tests

A two-way 3 (point-in-time of recall) × 3 (experimental conditions) repeated measures ANOVA of the number of words correctly recalled revealed a significant main effect of time ($F_{2,36}$ = 112.8, $p < 0.001$, $\eta_p^2 = 0.9$). As shown in Figure 4a, recall performance showed a significant decreasing trend with increased time between learning and recall (immediate test, 7.1 ± 2.0 words; 1 h test, 4.5 ± 2.2 words; and 24 h test, 3.6 ± 2.0 words). In addition, there was a significant interaction between experimental condition and time ($F_{4,72}$ = 3.3, $p = 0.03$, $\eta_p^2 = 0.16$). As shown in Figure 4b, the number of correctly recalled words was significantly greater in the pre-acquisition exercise condition (5.4 ± 2.1 words) than in the other two conditions (control, 4.1 ± 2.4 words, $p = 0.01$; post-acquisition exercise, 3.9 ± 1.7 words, $p = 0.01$). Furthermore, in 24 h free recall test, the number of words correctly recalled in the pre-acquisition exercise condition (4.3 ± 2.1 words) was significantly greater than in the control condition (3.2 ± 2.0 words, $p = 0.005$).

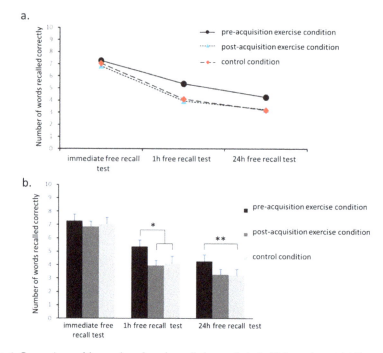

Figure 4. Comparisons of the number of words recalled correctly in the PM experiment. (**a**) Comparisons over time. (**b**) Comparisons between conditions. * $p < 0.05$, ** $p < 0.01$.

3.2.2. Recognition Test

A one-way repeated measures ANOVA of recognition rate across the three experimental conditions revealed a significant main effect of condition on recognition rate ($F_{2,36} = 7.0$, $p = 0.003$, $\eta_p^2 = 0.3$). As shown in Figure 5a, recognition rate in the control condition (25.1% ± 3.1%) was significantly lower than in pre-acquisition exercise (37.9% ± 3.6%, $p = 0.002$) and post-acquisition exercise (38.1% ± 3.9%, $p = 0.007$) conditions, demonstrating that recognition was better in both exercise conditions than in the control condition.

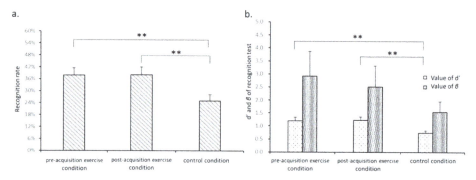

Figure 5. Comparison of word recognition rate (**a**) and of d' and β values (**b**) in the DM experiment across experimental conditions; ** $p < 0.01$.

Meanwhile, a one-way repeated measures ANOVA of d′ also revealed a significant main effect of condition ($F_{2,36} = 8.6$, $p = 0.001$, $\eta_p^2 = 0.3$). As shown in Figure 5b, d′ was significantly greater in the pre-acquisition exercise (1.2 ± 0.6, $p = 0.002$) and post-acquisition exercise (1.2 ± 0.6, $p = 0.002$) conditions than in the control condition (0.7 ± 0.4). No significant main effect of condition on β was found ($p > 0.05$), indicating that the tendency to respond was independent of the experimental condition.

3.3. PM Task

A two-way 3 (experimental condition) × 3 (stage: sequence learning, 1 h sequence test, and 24 h sequence test) repeated measures ANOVA revealed a main effect of stage on reaction time ($F_{2,34} = 62.3$, $p < 0.001$, $\eta_p^2 = 0.8$) in the SRTT. As shown in Figure 6a, there were significant progressive improvements in reaction time across all three stages, from the sequence learning stage (336.8 ± 44.1 ms) to the 1 h sequence test (308.6 ± 29.1 ms) and to the 24 h sequence test (301.8 ± 31.7 ms). In addition, there was a significance interaction between experimental condition and task stage ($F_{4,68} = 2.7$, $p = 0.04$, $\eta_p^2 = 0.1$). Further analysis revealed (Figure 6b) that mean reaction time in the second sequence test was significantly shorter in the post-acquisition exercise condition (296.6 ± 29.9 ms) than in the control condition (311.9 ± 36.5 ms, $p = 0.04$).

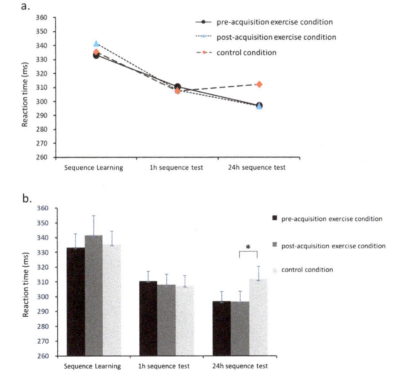

Figure 6. Comparison of reaction times in the serial reaction time task in the PM experiment. (a) Comparisons over time. (b) Comparisons between conditions. * $p < 0.05$.

Accuracy rates did not differ significantly among the three conditions, indicating that there was not an exchange effect of either accuracy or speed between participants' response times and accuracy rates. Thus the analysis based on reaction time can be considered fairly reliable.

A two-way 3 (block: 6, 7 and 8) × 3 (experimental condition) repeated measures ANOVA of reaction time in the 1-h sequence test revealed a significant main effect of block ($F_{2,34} = 16.2, p < 0.001, \eta_p^2 = 0.5$), but not a main effect of exercise condition ($F_{2,34} = 0.3, p = 0.8, \eta_p^2 = 0.02$); moreover, there was no significant block × exercise condition interaction ($F_{4,68} = 0.2, p = 0.9, \eta_p^2 = 0.01$). Further analysis revealed (Figure 7) that reaction time was significantly shorter in block 6 (311.7 ± 29.2 ms) than in block 7 (336.2 ± 36.4 ms, $p < 0.001$) and block 8 (324.0 ± 36.9 ms, $p = 0.004$). Additionally, reaction time was significantly shorter in block 8 than in block 7 ($p = 0.02$).

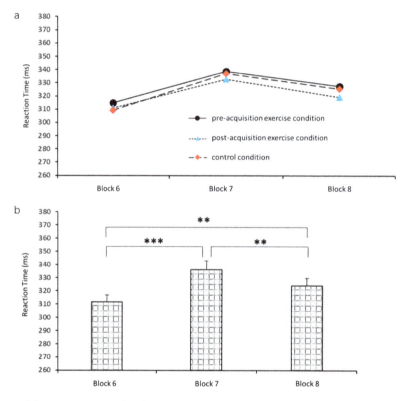

Figure 7. Mean reaction times in the 1-h sequence test by block and by exercise condition. (**a**) Comparison of reaction times among blocks 6, 7, and 8. (**b**) Comparison of reaction times among pre-acquisition exercise, post-acquisition exercise, and control conditions. ** $p < 0.01$, *** $p < 0.001$.

Additionally, a two-way 3 (block) × 3 (exercise condition) repeated measures ANOVA of reaction time in blocks 6, 7, and 8 of the 24-h sequence test revealed a significant main effect of block ($F_{2,34} = 19.1, p < 0.001, \eta_p^2 = 0.5$), but not of exercise condition ($F_{2,34} = 2.0, p = 0.1, \eta_p^2 = 0.1$); and there was not a significant block × exercise condition interaction ($F_{2,34} = 2.4, p = 0.06, \eta_p^2 = 0.1$). Further analysis (Figure 8) revealed that reaction time was significantly shorter in block 6 (304.7 ± 34.3 ms) than in block 7 (332.6 ± 36.6 ms, $p < 0.001$), and reaction time in block 8 (310.6 ± 39.6 ms) was significantly shorter than in block 7 ($p = 0.001$). Reaction times in block 6 and block 8 were statistically similar ($p = 0.1$).

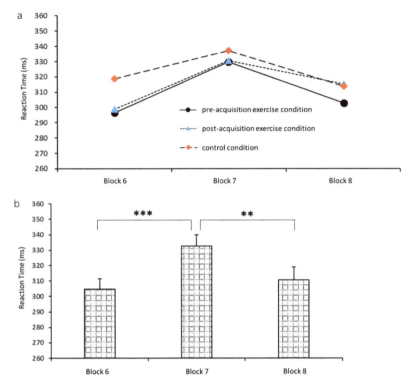

Figure 8. Mean reaction times in the 24-h sequence test by block and by exercise condition. (**a**) Comparison of reaction times among blocks 6, 7, and 8. (**b**) Comparison of reaction times among pre-acquisition exercise, post-acquisition exercise, and control conditions. ** $p < 0.01$, *** $p < 0.001$.

4. Discussion

The current study examined the effects of acute aerobic exercise on DM and PM and showed that acute aerobic exercise enhanced intermediate-term and long-term DM and long-term PM memory via influences on different processing periods. Specifically, acute aerobic exercise appeared to improve DM performance mainly through a positive impact on encoding, but appeared to improve PM performance mainly through facilitation of memory processes during the consolidation period.

HR, RPE, and RPM data in the pre- and post-acquisition exercise condition indicated that all subjects performed moderate-intensity aerobic exercise with RPE values in the range of 13–15. All subjects' HRs remained within the range of 60–70% of maximal HR throughout the exercise session. Furthermore, because exercise intensity levels in the pre- and post- acquisition exercise conditions were similar, differences in free recall, recognition, and SRTT performance cannot be attributed to differences in exercise intensity.

4.1. Acute Aerobic Exercise Enhances Primarily DM Encoding

The DM experiment showed that acute aerobic exercise before, but not after, DM learning had significant positive effects on intermediate-term (1 h) and long-term (24 h) recall test performance. These results are in agreement with previous studies in which subjects showed 1-h and 24-h memory enhancement in response to performing 30 min of moderate intensity acute aerobic exercise prior to memorizing declarative material [4,17]. Exercise completed shortly before the learning stage can potentially affect encoding processes as well as early consolidation processes, and prior studies have reported positive effects of exercise performed after word learning or after the first recall test on long-term memory, which suggests an influence on consolidation [17,27]. However, in this study, we did not obtain significant facilitatory effects of post-acquisition exercise on free recall performance 1 h or 24 h later, suggesting that it was not effective for facilitating long-term memory consolidation.

Contrasting with our free recall test results, our recognition test results showed that either pre- or post-acquisition exercise enhanced word recognition compared to the control (no exercise) condition, which indicates that acute aerobic exercise may enhance both encoding and early consolidation of long-term DM, as has been suggested by previous research. Notably, Hötting et al. examined German-Polish word retention acquired before low- or high-intensity exercise for 30 min and found that only the high-intensity exercise group performed better than the control group in a 24-h recognition test [28]. Etnier et al. also observed an enhancing effect of high-intensity acute aerobic exercise prior to encoding on 24-h recognition test performance [29]. In the present study, subjects' memory performance benefitted from moderate-intensity exercise, suggesting that at least a moderate intensity of acute aerobic exercise near the time of learning may be needed to improve long-term recognition performance 24 h later. Labban did not observe enhanced 24-h recognition test performance with either pre- or post-acquisition exercise [17]. However, Labban's recognition test included only 15 learned words and 15 interference words, which may have been too easy and thus not revealed significant effects. In our study, we observed post-acquisition exercise-associated enhancement of 24-h recognition test performance but not of 1-h or 24-h free recall test performance. It may be that moderate-intensity acute aerobic exercise affects DM consolidation processes, but that the effect size is more pronounced with pre-acquisition exercise than with post-acquisition exercise. The absolute numbers of words recalled were greater in the pre-acquisition exercise condition than in the post-acquisition exercise condition, albeit not significantly so. Importantly, a recognition test, in which one is required only to identify target words, is easier than a free recall test, in which one needs to produce the words, making the recognition test more sensitive to mild enhancing effects.

Altogether, our DM experimental results suggest that acute aerobic exercise may have a pronounced enhancing effect on encoding as well as potentially a mildly enhancing effect on early consolidation of DM. These results thus partially support our hypothesis that acute aerobic exercise enhances the DM encoding processes.

4.2. Acute Aerobic Exercise Enhances Primarily PM Consolidation

Our SRTT results indicated that moderate-intensity acute aerobic exercise enhanced implicit sequence learning performance 24 h after the learning phase. Notably, exercise had a stronger promoting effect when performed after, as opposed to before, the sequential learning phase. Thus, contrasting with our DM experiment findings, an exercise bout prior to the consolidation period enhanced long-term PM, consistent with our hypothesis.

The present PM experiment results fit with findings from a recent study [18], wherein a high-intensity acute aerobic exercise program performed either before or after learning was shown to enhance motor memory learning. The enhancement effects were not significant relative to non-exercise controls at a 1-h test, but they became significant at a 24-h test, with post-learning exercise having a more pronounced enhancing effect at the 24-h test than pre-learning exercise. Moreover, the better PM performance associated with post-learning exercise remained more pronounced than that associated with pre-learning exercise after 7 days. Although the current study did not include a 7-day memory test, it is noteworthy that the PM enhancement in our study was not apparent after 1 h but rather became significant after a 24-h delay. This difference between our 1-h and 24-h PM results is consistent with previous studies. Ostadan et al. examined acute aerobic exercise effects on retention of serial memory 8 h later and found that subjects who engaged in post-acquisition exercise performed better than controls [30]. Similarly, McNerney and Radvansky indicated that serial reaction times remained enhanced relative to controls 7 d after training in subjects who engaged in either pre- or post-acquisition exercise [31]. Together with these prior studies, our results show that acute aerobic exercise can enhance long-term PM, mainly facilitating PM consolidation processes, with a relatively slow facilitatory time course.

Although we balanced exercise conditions and sequence tasks across subjects, because the second experiment had a within-subjects design, it is possible that the enhancement effect of exercise on PM was influenced by a practice effect. In the 1-h sequence test, reaction times in blocks 6 and 8 were significantly shorter than in block 7 (the random sequence block), but reactions times in block 6 were also shorter than those in block 8. Thus, the pattern of results in the 1-h sequence test is consistent with a possible practice effect. In contrast, in the 24-h sequence test, we observed shorter reaction times in blocks 6 and 8 than in block 7 (the random sequence block), but there was no significant difference between blocks 6 and 8. Therefore, further consolidation of implicit learning was more evident at the 24-h sequence test than at the 1-h test, overtaking any practice effect that may have occurred. This finding further suggests that acute aerobic exercise enhancement of PM performance is attributable mainly to enhancement of consolidation over many hours.

In summary, our PM experiment results indicate that acute aerobic exercise can facilitate PM consolidation processes. These consolidation enhancing effects yielded improved long-term PM performance.

4.3. Potential Mechanisms of Distinct Exercise-Induced Effects on Formation of DM and PM

Building upon previous findings, in the present study, we found different effects of acute aerobic exercise on DM and PM. DM is an explicit form of memory that stores information related to facts and events, whereas PM is an implicit form of memory that stores sensorimotor information acquired in motor skill learning [9]. The differential effects of exercise on DM and PM could be related to the fact that these two forms of memory involve different brain areas. DM is highly dependent on superficial temporal lobe structures, especially the hippocampus, whereas PM is dependent on deep subcortical structures, such as the striatum, as well as the cerebellum [32].

The facilitating influence of acute aerobic exercise on DM and PM also differed in relation to time course. Exercise enhanced DM in a manner that was reflected 1 h and 24 h after learning, whereas exercise enhancement of PM became apparent 24 h after learning. It has been hypothesized that acute aerobic exercise effects on cognitive functions may be attributed to exercise induced increases in arousal [33]. If so, exercise induced arousal may facilitate DM encoding processes and PM consolidation processes, thereby improving long-term memory performance. Importantly, some neurochemicals released during acute aerobic exercise, such as brain-derived neurotrophic factor [34], epinephrine [35], and dopamine [36], may respectively facilitating encoding process of DM and consolidation process of PM. Moreover, due to the processing times of encoding and consolidation being inconsistent, the enhancing effect of acute aerobic exercise on DM and PM differed in time as well.

4.4. Limitations

Although we used a widely used maximum HR estimation formula recommended by the American College of Sports Medicine, true maximum HRs differ among individuals. Consequently, exercise at the same HR may differ in actual intensity across individuals. In future studies, we can clarify exercise intensity domains by employing a more flexible graded exercise test. Exercise intensity might also affect experimental results to some extent. Some studies have reported enhancing influences of high-intensity acute aerobic exercise on long-term memory. Thus, to obtain a systematic understanding of the complex relationships among intensity of exercise, time, and particular types of memory, it would be of interest to conduct retention tests at time points that represent a longer delay after the intervention and to examine the effects of different intensities of aerobic exercise. Meanwhile, all of our participants were male college students. Further examination of potential effects of gender and age on the effects of acute aerobic exercise on memory processing, which some evidence has pointed to [37,38], should be studied further. Additionally, the current study provides behavioral evidence of the impacts of exercise on memory processing but does not provide information about the neural mechanisms underlying these effects, which should be examined in future studies.

5. Conclusions

Acute aerobic exercise can enhance long-term DM and PM. Our data indicate that acute aerobic exercise mainly facilitates the encoding period of DM and the consolidation period of PM.

Author Contributions: Writing—original draft preparation, X.W.; writing—review and editing, Y.C.; data curation, R.Z.; funding acquisition, C.Z. All authors have read and agreed to the published version of the manuscript.

Funding: The study was supported by Shanghai Association for Science and Technology (17080503100).

Acknowledgments: We thank the participants for their effort and time.

Conflicts of Interest: The authors declare no conflict of interest. The funders had no role in the design of the study; in the collection, analyses, or interpretation of data; in the writing of the manuscript, or in the decision to publish the results.

References

1. Lambourne, K.; Tomporowski, P.D. The Effect of Exercise-Induced Arousal on Cognitive Task Performance: A Meta-Regression Analysis. *Brain Res.* **2010**, *1341*, 12–24. [CrossRef] [PubMed]
2. Chang, Y.K.; Jeffrey, D.L.; Jennifer, I.G.; Jennifer, L.E. The Effects of Acute Exercise on Cognitive Performance: A Meta-Analysis. *Brain Res.* **2012**, *1453*, 87–101. [CrossRef] [PubMed]
3. Coles, K.; Tomporowski, P.D. Effects of Acute Exercise on Executive Processing, Short-Term and Long-Term Memory. *Sci. Sports.* **2008**, *26*, 333–344. [CrossRef] [PubMed]
4. Labban, J.D.; Jennifer, L.E. Effects of Acute Exercise on Long-Term Memory. *Res. Q. Exerc. Sport* **2011**, *82*, 712–721. [CrossRef] [PubMed]
5. Ogoh, S.; Philip, N.A. Cerebral Blood Flow During Exercise: Mechanisms of Regulation. *J. Appl. Physiol.* **2009**, *107*, 1370–1380. [CrossRef] [PubMed]
6. Loprinzi, P.D. Intensity-Specific Effects of Acute Exercise on Human Memory Function: Considerations for the Timing of Exercise and the Type of Memory. *Health Promot. Perspect.* **2018**, *8*, 255. [CrossRef]
7. McGaugh, J.L. The Amygdala Modulates the Consolidation of Memories of Emotionally Arousing Experiences. *Annu. Rev. Neurosci.* **2004**, *27*, 1–28. [CrossRef]
8. Baddeley, A. *Working Memory, Thought, and Action*; OuP: Oxford, UK, 2007.
9. Stickgold, R. Sleep-Dependent Memory Consolidation. *Nature* **2005**, *437*, 1272–1278. [CrossRef]
10. Ullman, M.T. Contributions of Memory Circuits to Language: The Declarative/Procedural Model. *Cognition* **2004**, *92*, 231–270. [CrossRef]
11. Tulving, E. How Many Memory Systems Are There? *Am. Psychol.* **1985**, *40*, 385–398. [CrossRef]
12. Duncan, M.; Johnson, A. The Effect of Differing Intensities of Acute Cycling on Preadolescent Academic Achievement. *Eur. J. Sport Sci.* **2014**, *14*, 279–286. [CrossRef]
13. Potter, D.; Keeling, D. Effects of Moderate Exercise and Circadian Rhythms on Human Memory. *J. Sport Exerc. Psychol.* **2005**, *27*, 117–125. [CrossRef]
14. Mang, C.S.; Snow, N.J.; Campbell, K.L.; Ross, C.L.; Boyd, L.A. A Single Bout of High-Intensity Aerobic Exercise Facilitates Response to Paired Associative Stimulation and Promotes Sequence-Specific Implicit Motor Learning. *J. Appl. Physiol.* **2014**, *117*, 1325–1336. [CrossRef]
15. Skriver, K.; Roig, M.; Lundbye-Jensen, J.; Pingel, J.; Helge, J.W.; Kiens, B.; Nielsen, J.B. Acute Exercise Improves Motor Memory: Exploring Potential Biomarkers. *Neurobiol. Learn. Men.* **2014**, *116*, 46–58. [CrossRef]
16. Roig, M.; Nordbrandt, S.; Geertsen, S.S.; Nielsen, J.B. The Effects of Cardiovascular Exercise on Human Memory: A Review with Meta-Analysis. *Neurosci. Biobehav. Rev.* **2013**, *37*, 1645–1666. [CrossRef]
17. Labban, J.D. *The Effect of Acute Exercise on the Formation of Long-Term Memory*; The University of North Carolina: Greensboro, NC, USA, 2012.
18. Roig, M.; Skriver, K.; Lundbye-Jensen, J.; Kiens, B.; Nielsen, J.B. A Single Bout of Exercise Improves Motor Memory. *PLoS ONE* **2012**, *7*, e44594. [CrossRef]

19. Wanner, P.; Cheng, F.; Simon, S. Effects of Acute Cardiovascular Exercise on Motor Memory Encoding and Consolidation: A Systematic Review with Meta-Analysis. *Neurosci. Biobehav. Rev.* **2020**, *116*, 365–381. [CrossRef]
20. Wanner, P.; Theresa, M.; Jacopo, C.; Klaus, P.; Simon, S. Exercise Intensity Does Not Modulate the Effect of Acute Exercise on Learning a Complex Whole-Body Task. *Neuroscience* **2020**, *426*, 115–128. [CrossRef]
21. Wang, Y.; Zhou, L.; Luo, Y. The Pilot Establishment and Evaluation of Chinese Affective Words System. *Chin. Ment. Health J.* **2008**, *22*, 608–612.
22. Reber, P.J.; Larry, R.S. Encapsulation of Implicit and Explicit Memory in Sequence Learning. *J. Cogn. Neurosci.* **1998**, *10*, 248–263. [CrossRef]
23. Debarnot, U.; Rémi, N.; Yvette, S.; Elodie, S.; Tadhg, M.; Aymeric, G. Acquisition and Consolidation of Implicit Motor Learning with Physical and Mental Practice across Multiple Days of Anodal Tdcs. *Neurobiol. Learn. Mem.* **2019**, *164*, 107062. [CrossRef]
24. Curran, T. Effects of Aging on Implicit Sequence Learning: Accounting for Sequence Structure and Explicit Knowledge. *Psychol. Res.* **1997**, *60*, 24–41. [CrossRef] [PubMed]
25. Fu, Q.; Bin, G.; Dienes, Z.; Fu, X.; Gao, X. Learning without Consciously Knowing: Evidence from Event-Related Potentials in Sequence Learning. *Conscious Cogn.* **2013**, *22*, 22–34. [CrossRef] [PubMed]
26. Swets, J.A.; Green, D.M. *Applications of Signal Detection Theory*; Springer: New York, NY, USA, 1978.
27. Roig, M.; Thomas, R.; Mang, C.S.; Snow, N.J.; Ostadan, F.; Boyd, L.A.; Lundbye-Jensen, J. Time-Dependent Effects of Cardiovascular Exercise on Memory. *Exerc. Sport Sci. Rev.* **2016**, *44*, 81–88. [CrossRef] [PubMed]
28. Hötting, K.; Schickert, N.; Kaiser, J.; Röder, B.; Schmidt-Kassow, M. The Effects of Acute Physical Exercise on Memory, Peripheral Bdnf, and Cortisol in Young Adults. *Neural Plast.* **2016**, *2016*, 6860573. [CrossRef] [PubMed]
29. Etnier, J.L.; Wideman, L.; Labban, J.D.; Piepmeier, A.T.; Pendleton, D.M.; Dvorak, K.K.; Becofsky, K. The Effects of Acute Exercise on Memory and Brain-Derived Neurotrophic Factor (Bdnf). *J. Sport Exerc. Psychol.* **2016**, *38*, 331–340. [CrossRef]
30. Ostadan, F.; Centeno, C.; Daloze, J.F.; Frenn, M.; Lundbye-Jensen, J.; Roig, M. Changes in Corticospinal Excitability during Consolidation Predict Acute Exercise-Induced Off-Line Gains in Procedural Memory. *Neurobiol. Learn. Mem.* **2016**, *136*, 196–203. [CrossRef]
31. McNerney, M.W.; Radvansky, G.A. Mind Racing: The Influence of Exercise on Long-Term Memory Consolidation. *Memory* **2015**, *23*, 1140–1151. [CrossRef]
32. Squire, L.R. Memory Systems of the Brain: A Brief History and Current Perspective. *Neurobiol. Learn. Mem.* **2004**, *82*, 171–177. [CrossRef] [PubMed]
33. McGaugh, J.L. Make Mild Moments Memorable: Add a Little Arousal. *Trends Cogn. Sci.* **2006**, *10*, 345–347. [CrossRef]
34. Gomez-Pinilla, F.; Shoshanna, V.; Ying, Z. Brain-Derived Neurotrophic Factor Functions as a Metabotrophin to Mediate the Effects of Exercise on Cognition. *Eur. J. Neurosci.* **2008**, *28*, 2278–2287. [CrossRef]
35. Cahill, L.; Michael, T.A. Epinephrine Enhancement of Human Memory Consolidation: Interaction with Arousal at Encoding. *Neurobiol. Learn. Mem.* **2003**, *79*, 194–198. [CrossRef]
36. Chowdhury, R.; Guitart-Masip, M.; Bunzeck, N.; Dolan, R.J.; Düzel, E. Dopamine Modulates Episodic Memory Persistence in Old Age. *J. Neurosci.* **2012**, *32*, 14193–14204. [CrossRef] [PubMed]
37. Maitland, S.B.; Herlitz, A.; Nyberg, L.; Bäckman, L.; Nilsson, L.G. Selective Sex Differences in Declarative Memory. *Mem. Cogn.* **2004**, *32*, 1160–1169. [CrossRef] [PubMed]
38. Ragland, J.D.; Coleman, A.R.; Gur, R.C.; Glahn, D.C.; Gur, R.E. Sex Differences in Brain-Behavior Relationships between Verbal Episodic Memory and Resting Regional Cerebral Blood Flow. *Neuropsychologia* **2000**, *38*, 451–461. [CrossRef]

© 2020 by the authors. Licensee MDPI, Basel, Switzerland. This article is an open access article distributed under the terms and conditions of the Creative Commons Attribution (CC BY) license (http://creativecommons.org/licenses/by/4.0/).

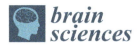

Article

Effect of High Intensity Interval Training Compared to Continuous Training on Cognitive Performance in Young Healthy Adults: A Pilot Study

Said Mekari [1],*, Meghan Earle [1], Ricardo Martins [1], Sara Drisdelle [1], Melanie Killen [1], Vicky Bouffard-Levasseur [2] and Olivier Dupuy [3]

[1] Department of Kinesiology, Acadia University, Wolfville, NS B4P 2R6, Canada; mearle@kinduct.com (M.E.); rs16eg@brocku.ca (R.M.); sajdrisdelle@uwaterloo.ca (S.D.); melanie.n.killen@gmail.com (M.K.)
[2] Sector of Education and Kinesiology, University of Moncton, Edmundston Campus, Edmundston, NB E3V 2S8, Canada; vicky.bouffard-levasseur@umoncton.ca
[3] Laboratory MOVE (EA 6314), Faculty of Sport Sciences, University of Poitiers, 17000 Poitiers, France; olivier.dupuy@univ-poitiers.fr
* Correspondence: said.mekary@acadiau.ca

Received: 7 January 2020; Accepted: 3 February 2020; Published: 4 February 2020

Abstract: To improve cognitive function, moving the body is strongly recommended; however, evidence regarding the proper training modality is still lacking. The purpose of this study was therefore to assess the effects of high intensity interval training (HIIT) compared to moderate intensity continuous exercise (MICE), representing the same total training load, on improving cognitive function in healthy adults. It was hypothesized that after 6 weeks (3 days/week) of stationary bike training, HIIT would improve executive functions more than MICE. Twenty-five participants exercised three times a week for 6 weeks after randomization to the HIIT or MICE training groups. Target intensity was 60% of peak power output (PPO) in the MICE group and 100% PPO in the HIIT group. After training, PPO significantly increased in both the HIIT and MICE groups (9% and 15%, $p < 0.01$). HIIT was mainly associated with a greater improvement in overall reaction time in the executive components of the computerized Stroop task (980.43 ± 135.27 ms vs. 860.04 ± 75.63 ms, $p < 0.01$) and the trail making test (42.35 ± 14.86 s vs. 30.35 ± 4.13 s, $p < 0.01$). T exercise protocol was clearly an important factor in improving executive functions in young adults.

Keywords: exercise physiology; cognition; high intensity interval training; moderate intensity continuous exercise; exercise training

1. Introduction

The positive effects of physical activity (movements carried out by the muscles that require energy) and exercise (planned, structured and intentional movement) [1] on brain function and its metabolism are well known. There is extensive research showing that regular physical activity and exercise can improve cardiorespiratory function and body composition while lowering the risk of chronic disease and mortality [2,3]. It is also well documented that age-related cognitive decline is heterogeneous and several factors modulate the impact of aging on cognition [4]. Exercise intervention studies have supported this and demonstrated that low-intensity aerobic training significantly improves cognitive functions [5]. Interestingly, most studies have documented larger positive impacts of exercise in tasks that involve the prefrontal cortex of the brain [6]. This brain region is involved in many cognitive processes including attention, decision-making, executive function, and working memory [5]. The relationship between aerobic fitness level and attentional control has also been confirmed in a very well-cited meta-analysis of cognitive improvement through aerobic training [7]. Although many aspects of cognitive performance improved significantly after an aerobic training regimen that enhanced cardiorespiratory function, the largest improvement was observed in tasks that implied heavily on executive functions.

The mechanisms related to the beneficial effect of aerobic fitness on brain regions involved with cognitive function are now clearer. Recent findings suggest that an improvement of cardiorespiratory fitness (i.e., $\dot{V}O_2$ max) can induce changes to cellular and molecular pathways that likely initiate changes to the macroscopic properties of the brain and behavior, which in turn can influence cognitive functions in the prefrontal cortex of the brain [8].

Evidence from animal studies also suggests that increasing physical activity can enhance synaptogenesis (i.e., formation of new neuronal synapses), and neurogenesis (i.e., generation of new neurons) via increased production of brain-derived neurotrophic factor, in addition to vascular plasticity [9,10]. Hypotheses proposed to account for the relationship between aerobic fitness and cognition include corresponding increases in vascularization of brain tissue [11]. Several authors reported that fitter subjects displayed better cerebral oxygenation during cognitive tasks, which was associated with better vascularization [12,13].

There is a paucity of information available to determine what type of aerobic exercise training program is most optimal for improving cognitive functions. Several models suggest that replacing aerobic exercise training performed at moderate-intensity (i.e., moderate-intensity continuous exercise (MICE)) with high-intensity intermittent training (HIIT) may be considerably more effective at improving cardiovascular [14,15] and cognitive health [16]. Although first described in the 1950s as a mode of cardiac rehabilitation by the German cardiologist Hans Reindell [17], HIIT has largely been used by elite athletes for aerobic training purposes [18–20]. HIIT consists of alternating periods of intensive aerobic exercise with periods of recovery. It is well established that HIIT training induces a greater increase in cardiac output and stroke volume than MICE training [21–25]. Most importantly, two recent studies demonstrated that HIIT training is both safe and well-tolerated, without evidence of myocardial damage, significant arrhythmias or left ventricular dysfunction [26,27].

Based on previous evidence in which HIIT appeared to be an efficient training method for improving cardiovascular health, a growing research interest concerning the link between intensity training and cognitive function has appeared. A relationship between exercise intensity training and cognitive function seems to be emerging. Using a questionnaire of physical activity level, Van Gelder et al. [28] reported that older adults who exercised at the lowest intensity were more likely to develop dementia 10 years later compared with those who exercised at higher intensity. In this line, Angeraven et al. [29], using the same methodology as a previous report, found that the average intensity of weekly physical activities of middle aged and older adults was positively associated with cognitive performance. More recently, using actigraphy, Brown et al. [30] indicated that intensity rather than quantity of physical activity might be more important in the association between physical activity and cognitive function. Although these results are encouraging, there is no clear evidence that HIIT has a superior effect on cognitive function compared to MICE [16]. Recently, original studies have provided more responses with null [31,32] or positive results [33–37] in animal and human studies. Among the studies that achieved positive results, they only compared HIIT to active controls, and as such, the effects of exercise intensity per se were not examined. Only Kovacevic et al. [34] found that HIIT had a greater impact on cognitive function than MICE in older adults. In younger adults, the evidence that HIIT is the optimal strategy to improve cognitive performance is unclear and the only data available is contradictory.

The aim of this study was to compare a HIIT and MICE program on cognition in young adults and test the hypothesis that HIIT may be a better strategy to improve cognitive function. Based on the evidence that HIIT has a superior impact on cardiorespiratory health, we put forward the hypothesis that cognition was most affected by this form of exercise and executive function was most sensible to this program.

2. Methods

2.1. Participants

In this study, 25 young adults (18 females and 7 males) gave their written informed consent to participate in the study. Their parameters (mean ± SD) were: age (32 ± 8 years), height (1.69 ± 0.02 m), body mass (76 ± 17 kg), body mass index (BMI) (27 ± 6 kg m^{-2}), peak power output (195 ± 44 W) and $\dot{V}O_2$ peak (37 ± 8 mL min^{-1} kg^{-1}). All participants were healthy and had normal-to-corrected vision. None of the participants had a history of neurological or psychiatric disorder, color blindness, surgery with general anesthesia in the past 6 months, involuntary tremors, epilepsy or drug/alcohol problems. The protocol was reviewed and approved by the Institutional Research Ethics Board in the Health Sciences of Acadia University (REB 15-09) and was conducted in accordance with the Declaration of Helsinki.

2.2. Experimental Design

On the first and last visit, participants underwent a complete physical and cognitive evaluation that included measurement of height, weight, cognitive functions, and a maximal continuous graded exercise test. In order to minimize known confounding influences during exercise testing, participants were asked to refrain from consuming caffeine or smoking within 2 h and drinking alcohol within 6 h of any testing, consistent with the exercise testing guidelines from the Canadian Society of Exercise Physiology (CSEP). Participants were also asked to refrain from heavy exercise 24 h prior to any testing. During the six subsequent weeks, participants were randomly assigned to one of the two experimental protocols: MICE (n = 13) or HIIT (n = 12) on a stationary bicycle. We used a stratified randomization procedure to ensure that both groups were balanced at baseline for gender and fitness levels. All trainings were under the supervision of an exercise physiologist. Cycling position, which is known to affect energy expenditure, was standardized by adopting a top bar position. Saddle height was adjusted according to the participant's inseam leg length.

2.3. Maximal Continuous Graded Exercise Test

This test was performed on cycle ergometer (Lode B.V., Groningen, Netherlands). Initial workload was set at 1 W/kg body mass, for example 75 W for an individual with a weight of 75 kg. The workload was increased by 15 W every minute until voluntary exhaustion. Strong verbal encouragement was given throughout the test. The power of the last completed stage was considered as the peak power output (PPO, measured in W). Oxygen uptake ($\dot{V}O_2$ max, in ml min^{-1} kg^{-1}) was determined continuously on a 30 s basis using an automated cardiopulmonary exercise system (Parvo Medics TrueOne 2400, UT, USA). Gas analyzers were calibrated before each test using a gas mixture of known concentration (15% O_2 and 5% CO_2). The turbine was calibrated before each test using a 3-L syringe at several flow rates. The highest $\dot{V}O_2$ max over a 30 s period during the test was considered as the peak oxygen uptake ($\dot{V}O_2$ peak, in ml min^{-1} kg^{-1}).

2.4. Cognitive Testing

2.4.1. Computerized Modified Stroop Task

The computerized modified Stroop task was based on the modified Stroop color test [2]. This test includes four conditions. In the first condition (Congruent), the participant had to read 1 of 4 possible words appearing on the screen; "RED", "BLUE", "YELLOW" or "GREEN". These words were written in the same colour as their meaning. The answers were mapped to the letters "u", "i", "o" and "p" on a keyboard, which participants used to give their answers with the right hand. The mapping remained the same throughout the task. The order was "index finger—red", "middle finger—green", "ring finger—blue", and "little finger—yellow". The second block consisted in a Denomination condition, where participants had to identify the colour of unrelated words, which were "BUT", "FOR",

"WHEN", and "THAN". The third block consisted in a classic Interference task, which requires naming the colour of a colour-word, the meaning of the word being incongruent with the colour itself (e.g., the word BLUE written in green). In these first three blocks, a fixation cross appeared for 500 ms, followed by the word for 3000 ms. The fourth block consisted in a Switching task, which was identical to the Interference task, except that for 25% of the trials a square appeared instead of the fixation cross, and participants were asked to read the colour-word, instead of naming its colour. The reading trials appeared randomly throughout the block. Each of the four blocks contained 60 trials and the screen was blank between the trials. Before each condition, participants completed practice trials; 12 for the Congruent condition, 5 for the Denomination condition, 12 for the Interference condition, and 20 for the Switching condition. During practice and experimental trials a visual feedback ("Error") was given for incorrect responses only. Reaction times and errors were recorded.

2.4.2. Trail Making Test

All participants completed the trail making test part A prior to completing the trail making test part B. The trail making test part A (Trail A) was used to measure an individuals' processing speed. Participants were encouraged to correct their errors and this was included in the total time to complete. The speed at which all the numbers were connected was measured in seconds (s). Part B (Trail B) was used to measure cognitive flexibility or switching ability. In this portion of the test, participants were given the same instructions as Part A but had to alternate between numbers in ascending order and letters in alphabetical order (1-A-2-B-3-C, etc.). The time to complete Part B was also measured in seconds. Prior to the standard administration of this test, participants were given a short practice of each test [38].

2.5. Training

For both training protocols, all sessions were supervised and were conducted 3 days per week (Mondays, Wednesdays and Fridays) for 6-weeks. Eighty percent of the 18 sessions had to be completed to be eligible for post-testing. Training intensities for both groups were determined by percentages of their PPO found during the $\dot{V}O_2$ max test. Resistance was adjusted to maintain a cycling cadence between 50 and 70 revolutions per minute (rpm). For a more precise load monitoring and exercise prescription, we decided to use an external load measurement of intensity (%PPO) instead of an internal load measurement of intensity (% maximal heart rate). Training methodology was based on a recent paper from O'Brien et al. [39].

2.6. Moderate-Intensity Continuous Exercise

The MICE protocol was based on the recommendations of the Canadian Society of Exercise Physiology (CSEP), suggesting that individuals should accumulate at least 150 min of moderate to vigorous physical activity per week. We opted for continuous cycling at 60% PPO for 34 min. Duration was adjusted to match the total calorie expenditure of the HIIT (MICE = 122 kJ vs. HIIT = 120 kJ, for an individual with a PPO of 100 W). To adjust for predicted fitness improvements, the time was increased to 39 min for the remaining four weeks, and during the last two weeks, the intensity was increased by 15 Watts. The participants tapered in the last two training sessions by cycling at the same intensity (initial PPO + 15 Watts) for 30 min. We chose to include the warm up and recovery in the exercise session. The warm-up and cool-down involved 5 min of cycling at 25% PPO.

2.7. High-Intensity Intermittent Training

The HIIT session was based on previous studies that compared the time to exhaustion, participant preference, and time spent near $\dot{V}O_2$ max of various interval protocols [40]. The group performed 15 s intervals at 100% PPO with 15 s of passive recovery between. The intervals were done for two sets of 20 min (40 min total), with five minutes of passive recovery in between. This was performed for the first two weeks and then increased to a total of 45 min for the remaining four weeks. During the last two weeks, the intensity was increased by 15 Watts. The last two training sessions (tapering sessions) were performed at the same intensity for a total of 35 min. The warm up and recovery were equivalent to the MICE protocol of 5 min each at 25% PPO. Training procedures for both the MICE and HIIT are presented in Figure 1.

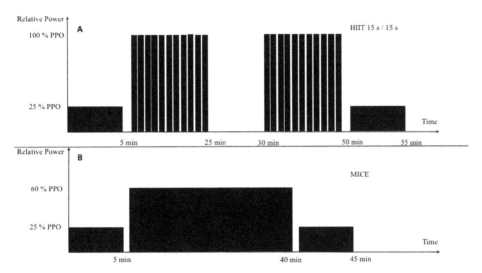

Figure 1. Schematic illustration of our two training modalities. Each training session was preceded by a 5-min standardized warm-up followed by a 5 min passive recovery. HIIT training (**A**) was 15 s at 100% of PPO and 15 s passive recovery (2 × 20-min). MICE training (**B**) was a 34-min exercise at 60% of PPO. Note: *PPO*, peak power output; *HIIT*, high intensity interval training; *MICE*, moderate intensity continuous exercise.

3. Statistical Analysis

Standard statistical methods were used for the calculation of means and standard deviations. Normal Gaussian distribution of the data was verified by the Shapiro–Wilk test and homoscedascticity by a modified Levene Test. The compound symmetry, or sphericity, was checked by the Mauchley test. When the assumption of sphericity was not met, the significance of F-ratios was adjusted according to the Greenhouse–Geisser procedure when the epsilon correction factor was <0.75, or according to the Huyn–Feld procedure when the epsilon correction factor was >0.75. On each physiological measure, an analysis of variance (ANOVA; time × training group) was conducted. For the trail making test, a 2 × 2 ANOVA was conducted to examine (time × training group). For the Stroop test, a 2 × 2 ANOVA was conducted to test (time × training group). All post-hoc tests were Bonferroni corrected for multiple comparisons. The magnitude of the difference between fitness levels was assessed by the Hedges' g (g), as presented elsewhere [41]. The magnitude of the difference was considered either small (0.2 < ES < 0.5), moderate (0.5 < ES < 0.8), or large (ES > 0.8). The significance level was set at $p < 0.05$ for all analyses.

4. Results

4.1. Maximal Continuous Graded Exercise Test

At baseline, there was no significant difference in maximal aerobic power or anthropometrics measured between both groups (Table 1). After the 6 week training protocol, $\dot{V}O_2$ max increased significantly for both the MICE group and the HIIT group (main effect of time $F(1,22) = 15.9$). The MICE group saw a maximal aerobic power increase from 180 ± 41 to 213 ± 43 W ($p < 0.05$) and the HIIT group also saw an increase from 207 ± 44 to 217 ± 42 W ($p < 0.05$).

Table 1. Pre- and post-training participant data values for anthropometric and aerobic exercise measures.

	HIIT PRE	HIIT POST	MICE PRE	MICE POST
Age	29 ± 10.3		35 ± 7.4	
Height (m)	1.7 ± 0.1		1.7 ± 0.1	
Gender	9 F, 3 M		9 F, 4 M	
Weight (kg)	71.3 ± 13.0	70.8 ± 13.4	81.3 ± 13.0	82.4 ± 23.1
BMI	24.6 ± 5.0	24.4 ± 5.1	28.8 ± 8.0	29.2 ± 8.2
$\dot{V}O_2$ max (mL/kg/min)	39.7 ± 8.7	41 ± 8.4	33.8 ± 8.3	35.9 ± 8.6
MAP (W)	207 ± 44.9	217 ± 42.2 [a]	180 ± 41.4	213 ± 43.0 [a]

Note. M, meters; kg, kilograms; BMI, body mass index; MAP, maximal aerobic power; W, Watts; F, Female; M, Male
[a] Statistically different from PRE, $p < 0.05$.

4.2. Cognitive Test

4.2.1. Stroop Task

Concerning the reaction time, the analysis revealed that there was a significant effect of the Stroop Condition ($F(1,22) = 61.87$; $p < 0.05$), with a longer reaction time (RT) in the more Executive compared to Non-Executive conditions (Stroop 1 < 2 < 3 < 4). In addition, we found that time ($F(1,22) = 4.46$; $p < 0.05$) and reaction time were shorter after training than before training. Further analysis (pairwise comparisons) also revealed lower RT in the switching task (executive task), which was selectively associated with only HIIT training ($p < 0.05$). Results for RT as a function of group training are presented in Table 2. Concerning accuracy, the ANOVA revealed a main effect of Task ($F(3,20) = 8.83$; $p < 0.01$) (Stroop 1, 2, 3, are different from 4). No statistical significance was observed between the training protocols.

Table 2. Cognitive Responses to Training Intensity Pre and Post Intervention.

	HIIT PRE	HIIT POST	MICE PRE	MICE POST
Stroop Task (ms)				
Reading	598.83 ± 99.40	574.15 ±106	604.43 ± 89.12	602.58 ± 95.66
Denomination	646.11 ± 93.67	616.33 ± 99.30	646.11 ± 93.67	644.59 ± 92.10
Inhibition	688.65 ± 95.47	680.94 ± 102.20	721.67 ± 110.07	687.41 ± 86.78
Switching	980.43 ± 135.27	860.04 ± 75.63 [a]	1008.45 ± 218.76	987.77 ± 188.20
Trail A (sec)	16.47 ± 4.76	15.44 ± 3.09	16.64 ± 4.21	16.45 ± 3.42
Trail B (sec)	42.35 ± 14.86	30.35 ± 4.13 [ab]	33.15 ± 7.06	34.13 ± 9.91

Note: Values are expressed in mean ± SD; *ms*, milliseconds; *sec*, seconds; *HIIT*, high intensity interval training; *MICE*, moderate intensity continuous exercise. Compared with PRE HIIT training: [a] $p < 0.05$, Compared to MICE training [b] $p < 0.02$.

4.2.2. Trail Making Test

The ANOVA revealed a significant effect of task ($F(1,46) = 89.5$; $p < 0.01$ (Trail A < Trail B)) and time ($F(1,46) = 16.06$; $p < 0.01$ (Pre > Post)). In addition, the analysis revealed an interaction of Task × time ($F(1,46) = 7.83$; $p < 0.001$). The post-hoc revealed that the performance in Trail A did not change before and after training, whereas the performance in Trail B was improved after training. Interestingly, the ANOVA revealed an interaction of Task × time × Group ($F(1,46) = 4.5$; $p < 0.05$). A quicker time for completion of the Trail B test was also selectively associated with only the HIIT training ($p < 0.01$). Results for the trail A and B time as a function of group training are presented in Table 2.

The magnitude of the training effect (Hedes's g) for Stroop and Trail are presented in Figure 2.

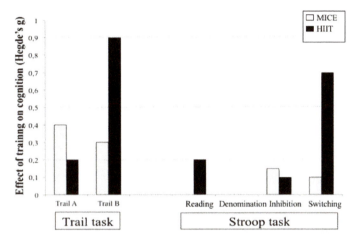

Figure 2. The magnitude of the training effect on cognitive performance for the Trail task and the Stroop task. An increase in effect size corresponds to a decrease in reaction, which means an improvement in cognitive performance.

5. Discussion

The aim of this study was to evaluate the impact of HIIT training compared to continuous training on cognitive performance. The results confirm that selectively executive functions are sensitive to HIIT training. Only subjects from the HIIT group enhanced their flexibility performance as measured by the Stroop task and Trail B.

Our first hypothesis that HIIT training would significantly increase $\dot{V}O_2$ max was not supported. These findings are in contrast to those by Helgerud et al. [25] who found that there was a significantly greater increase in $\dot{V}O_2$ max in HIIT groups compared to MICE groups, where one group used a protocol of 15 s work and 15 s rest, which is similar to the one used in this study. Similarly, a significant increase in $\dot{V}O_2$ max in the HIIT group compared to the MICE group was found after 10 weeks of aerobic exercise training ($p < 0.05$) [42]. Our results are in line with those found by Daussin et al. [24] and Kemmler et al. [43], who found a significant increase in $\dot{V}O_2$ max for both HIIT and MICE training, but no significant difference between the groups' respective increases. Both studies still showed a greater increase in aerobic fitness in the HIIT group compared to the MICE group. However, two recent meta-analyses [44,45] confirmed that the superiority of HIIT on $\dot{V}O_2$ max is not consistent in young populations and our results are in line with these two recent reports.

Increases in performance on the trail test B were found in the HIIT group and are likely to result from the executive portion of the Stroop task, which also showed an increase in executive function in the HIIT group compared to the MICE group. These findings support our second hypothesis that greater improvements in executive functioning will result from HIIT compared to MICE. The results of our study confirm certain results from the literature in children [35], adolescents [33], young adults [37], or the elderly who are healthy [34] or have had a stroke [36]. In addition, our results on the trail making task are consistent with those reported by Pallesen et al. who reported an effect of intermittent high intensity training only on the Trail B and not on the Trail A [36]. In addition, our results on the Stroop 4 (Flexibilty) are consistent with those reported by Jeaon et al. [33] in adolescents. However, all of these studies did not compare high intensity training with moderate intensity training and often used an active control group. It is therefore difficult to conclude what the effect of intensity was. Our study is the only one that has confirmed the superior effect of HIIT training on executive function in young adults. Because this is the first study known to the researcher that examines the effect that exercise protocol may have on executive function in young adults, it can only be speculated as to the mechanisms that underlie this relationship.

It was previously believed that there was a direct correlation between a high aerobic fitness level and increased levels of executive functioning. Many studies have been able to demonstrate, using aerobic training interventions, that an increase in $\dot{V}O_2$ max will elicit improvements in executive functioning. Kramer et al. [6] tested 124 sedentary adults and randomly divided them into aerobic or control groups that trained for 6 months. They found that there was a significant improvement in executive functioning tasks that were correlated with significant improvements in aerobic fitness (5.1% aerobic fitness increase) in the aerobic group only. They concluded that the improvements they found in executive functioning were due to increases in aerobic fitness. Similarly, Colcombe et al. [46] were able to show increases in executive functioning in an aerobic training group that had also improved $\dot{V}O_2$ max by 10.2% over the course of a 6-month training period.

In line with the current study, Smiley-Oyen et al. [47] randomly assigned participants to either a moderate-intensity aerobic training group or a toning/control group for 10 months. Aerobic and cognitive tests were performed before and after the 10-month training period with significant improvements in executive function tests found in the aerobic group but not the control group. There was also no significant difference found between $\dot{V}O_2$ peak between the two groups at the beginning or the cessation of the training period. The results were similar to those found in this study, in that while there was a significant increase in executive function performance, there was no significant increase between intervention groups. Another study was also able to question the link between aerobic fitness interventions and increased cognitive functions. Madden and colleagues [48] were able to show the opposite effect, after randomly placing older adults into either an aerobic training group, yoga group, or non-intervention group. The participants trained for 32 weeks, with the aerobic group training three times per week for 45 min at a moderate intensity of 70% heart rate reserve (HRR). Participants' aerobic fitness and cognition were tested, resulting in a significant ($p < 0.01$) increase in $\dot{V}O_2$ max in the aerobic group but not the yoga or non-intervention group. While there was a significant increase found in aerobic fitness, there was no significant interaction found between exercise and cognitive function. In addition, a meta-analysis of 37 studies conducted by Eitner et al. [49] did not show evidence to support the relationship between cognition and fitness levels. After analyzing correlational studies, they found that aerobic fitness only accounted for 8% of the cognitive variance. These studies offer further evidence to suggest that there might be more to the relationship between aerobic exercise and cognition than just statistically significant improvements in $\dot{V}O_2$ max.

There are two main mechanisms discussed in the literature that may help explain the findings of this study. The first is that exercise may increase the levels of brain-derived neurotrophic factor (BDNF), which could in turn improve cognition. BDNF is a growth factor that encourages neural plasticity and synaptic growth and transmission, and has been shown to enhance cognition due to its up-regulation and role in angiogenesis [9,10,50]. The role of BDNF may be multi-layered, with other enzyme and hormone interactions playing a role on BDNF levels including estrogen, corticosterone, and insulin growth factor-1 (IGF-1) [9]. Even though there are many interactions taking place, exercise has been shown to be the catalyst in BDNF affecting the brain [9]. Indeed, acute exercise is recognized to promote the release of serum BNDF [51] and this release seems to be dependent on exercise intensity [52,53]. For example, Winter and colleagues [54] tested the effect of acute exercise on BDNF serum levels and learning using both HIIT, MICE, and rest interventions. It was found that in the HIIT group, there was an increased level of learning success and this success was related to increased BDNF serum levels ($r = 0.38$; $p = 0.05$). Exercise also increased BDNF levels in serum or plasma, and HIIT seemed a good alternative to MICE as it produced higher levels of BDNF release [54–57]. Because levels remained highest after intense training cessation and also improved cognitive function, it is thought that BDNF may be increasingly elicited by HIIT as opposed to MICE. In contrast, a study by Lou et al. [58] on rats showed an intensity-dependent relationship in which mRNA BDNF levels were significantly lower after 4 weeks of high-intensity running compared to low-intensity running ($p < 0.01$). As there is limited research on humans regarding the effect of intensity on BDNF, we are unable to draw a conclusion based on the literature and this study's results. In saying this, there is evidence suggesting that BDNF plays a key role in cognition, and that BDNF may increase with aerobic exercise training as the chronic production of BDNF seems to mediate improvements in executive function in a long-term intervention [59].

The second mechanism is in regards to increases in cerebral blood flow. Precise mechanisms of the interaction between brain function and exercise are not clearly understood, but cerebral blood flow (CBF) and arterial regulation are thought to play a major role [60]. The cardiovascular hypothesis states that an improvement in cardiovascular function (cardiac output, oxygen transport and metabolism) can lead to improved neurotransmitter function and brain health [61]. Based on the cardiovascular hypothesis, a higher cardiac output typically results in higher cerebral blood flow, implying that the greater cardiovascular adaptation from HIIT should also positively influence cognitive performance. The CBF model is somewhat based on the cardiovascular hypothesis, in that increasing the ability of the heart to pump blood to the body and the brain will thus increase the amount of blood that is being transported to the cerebrum. It has been repeatedly shown that increases in CBF are related to increased cognitive performance and that, as humans age, there is a decline in CBF that is congruent with declines in cognitive function [54]. In a study of 17- to 79-year-old men, Ainslie et al. [60] showed a 17% higher level of CBF in endurance-trained men compared to asymptomatic sedentary men. Recently, Robinson et al. [62] found that the cerebral metabolism was improved only in participants who completed a HIIT training program. These results could explain our cognitive results but further research is needed regarding the relationship between exercise intensity, cerebral metabolism, and cognition.

Limitations

While there were statistically significant results found in the study, there are still some limitations to consider. The training period length was short, and could have resulted in the lack of significant findings regarding $\dot{V}O_2$ max changes. Even though there was an attendance limit of 80%, some participants missed consecutive training sessions, which could have impacted their performance while experiencing detraining effects. In order to control for known physiological influences in exercise (i.e., blood pressure, heart rate, fatigue, hormones, etc.), we attempted to have each participant complete their training sessions early in the morning. Due to prior commitments from the participants, it was difficult for all the participants to complete every session at the same time of day. We also did not keep a record of other activities that the participants were taking part in, such as pre training exercise levels, other workouts or "brain-training" games that could have altered the physical or cognitive results. On other hand, the small sample size could be a limit and these results need to be confirmed by future research. In addition, the authors acknowledged that the cognitive performance in this study was assessed only with the Stroop and trail test and that it is difficult to generalize our findings to cognition in general. A major limitation evident in the study is the lack of measurement regarding potential mechanisms mediating the relationship between exercise protocol and cognition. It would have been beneficial to provide measurements of some of the possible mechanisms, but the positive results of the study imply that a future area of research lies in determining the mechanisms by which exercise influences executive functioning.

6. Conclusions

This study adds to research in favor of HIIT over MICE as a more effective way to improve performance of executive function. To our knowledge, this is the first study to investigate the different protocols of aerobic exercise training on executive function in young adults. These findings may be important in the development of programs that are efficient and effective at combating age-related cognitive decline and increasing levels of cognitive functioning in adults. Considering that HIIT is a safe way to improve fitness in older adults and those with chronic disease, further research is warranted.

Author Contributions: Conceptualization: S.M., M.E., O.D., V.B.-L.; Methodology: S.M., M.E., R.M., S.D., M.K.; Formal Analysis: S.M., V.B.-L., O.D., M.E., M.K.; Original Draft Preparation: S.M., M.E., S.D., R.M., M.K., V.B.-L., O.D.; Writing-Reviewing and Editing: S.M., M.E., S.D., R.M., M.K., V.B.-L., O.D.; Supervision: S.M.; Project Administration: S.M., M.E., M.K. All authors have read and agreed to the published version of the manuscript.

Funding: This research received no external funding.

Conflicts of Interest: The authors declare no conflict of interest

References

1. Budde, H.; Schwarz, R.; Velasques, B.; Ribeiro, P.; Holzweg, M.; Machado, S.; Brazaitis, M.; Staack, F. Wegner M8.The need for differentiating between exercise, physical activity, and training. *Autoimmun. Rev.* **2016**, *15*, 110–111. [CrossRef] [PubMed]
2. Kodama, S.; Saito, K.; Tanaka, S.; Maki, M.; Yachi, Y.; Asumi, M.; Sugawara, A.; Totsuka, K.; Shimano, H.; Ohashi, Y.; et al. Cardiorespiratory fitness as a quantitative predictor of all-cause mortality and cardiovascular events in healthy men and women: A meta-analysis. *JAMA* **2009**, *301*, 2024–2035. [CrossRef] [PubMed]
3. Tremblay, M.S.; Warburton, D.E.; Janssen, I.; Paterson, D.H.; Latimer, A.E.; Rhodes, R.E.; Kho, M.E.; Hicks, A.; Leblanc, A.G.; Zehr, L.; et al. New Canadian physical activity guidelines. *Appl. Physiol. Nutr. Metab.* **2011**, *36*, 47–58. [CrossRef]
4. Bherer, L.; Erickson, K.I.; Liu-Ambrose, T. A review of the effects of physical activity and exercise on cognitive and brain functions in older adults. *J. Aging Res.* **2013**, *2013*, 657508. [CrossRef]
5. Kramer, A.F.; Erickson, K.I.; Colcombe, S.J. Exercise, cognition, and the aging brain. *J. Appl. Physiol. (1985)* **2006**, *101*, 1237–1242. [CrossRef]
6. Kramer, A.F.; Hahn, S.; Cohen, N.J.; Banich, M.T.; McAuley, E.; Harrison, C.R.; Chason, J.; Vakil, E.; Bardell, L.; Boileau, R.A.; et al. Ageing, fitness and neurocognitive function. *Nature* **1999**, *400*, 418–419. [CrossRef]
7. Colcombe, S.; Kramer, A.F. Fitness effects on the cognitive function of older adults: A meta-analytic study. *Psychol. Sci.* **2003**, *14*, 125–130. [CrossRef]
8. Stillman, C.M.; Cohen, J.; Lehman, M.E.; Erickson, K.I. Mediators of Physical Activity on Neurocognitive Function: A Review at Multiple Levels of Analysis. *Front. Hum. Neurosci.* **2016**, *10*, 626. [CrossRef]
9. Cotman, C.W.; Berchtold, N.C. Exercise: A behavioral intervention to enhance brain health and plasticity. *Trends Neurosci.* **2002**, *25*, 295–301. [CrossRef]
10. Cotman, C.W.; Berchtold, N.C.; Christie, L.A. Exercise builds brain health: Key roles of growth factor cascades and inflammation. *Trends Neurosci.* **2007**, *30*, 464–472. [CrossRef]
11. Bullitt, E.; Rahman, F.N.; Smith, J.K.; Kim, E.; Zeng, D.; Katz, L.M.; Marks, B.L. The effect of exercise on the cerebral vasculature of healthy aged subjects as visualized by MR angiography. *AJNR Am. J. Neuroradiol.* **2009**, *30*, 1857–1863. [CrossRef] [PubMed]
12. Dupuy, O.; Gauthier, C.J.; Fraser, S.A.; Desjardins-Crepeau, L.; Desjardins, M.; Mekary, S.; Lesage, F.; Hoge, R.D.; Pouliot, P.; Bherer, L. Higher levels of cardiovascular fitness are associated with better executive function and prefrontal oxygenation in younger and older women. *Front. Hum. Neurosci.* **2015**, *9*, 66. [CrossRef] [PubMed]
13. Mekari, S.; Dupuy, O.; Martins, R.; Evans, K.; Kimmerly, D.S.; Fraser, S.; Neyedli, H.F. The effects of cardiorespiratory fitness on executive function and prefrontal oxygenation in older adults. *Geroscience* **2019**, *41*, 681–690. [CrossRef] [PubMed]
14. Cao, M.; Quan, M.; Zhuang, J. Effect of High-Intensity Interval Training versus Moderate-Intensity Continuous Training on Cardiorespiratory Fitness in Children and Adolescents: A Meta-Analysis. *Int. J. Environ. Res. Public Health* **2019**, *16*. [CrossRef] [PubMed]
15. Ito, S. High-intensity interval training for health benefits and care of cardiac diseases—The key to an efficient exercise protocol. *World J. Cardiol.* **2019**, *11*, 171–188. [CrossRef] [PubMed]
16. Lucas, S.J.; Cotter, J.D.; Brassard, P.; Bailey, D.M. High-intensity interval exercise and cerebrovascular health: Curiosity, cause, and consequence. *J. Cereb. Blood Flow Metab.* **2015**, *35*, 902–911. [CrossRef]
17. Reindell, H.; Roskamm, H. Ein Beitrag zu den physiologischen Grundlagen des Intervall training unter besonderer Berück- sichtigung des Kreilaufes. *Schweiz Z Sportmed* **1959**, *7*, 1–8.

18. Billat, V.L. Interval training for performance: A scientific and empirical practice. Special recommendations for middle and long distance running. Part II: Anaerobic interval training. *Sports Med.* **2001**, *31*, 75–90. [CrossRef]
19. Billat, V.L. Interval training for performance: A scientific and empirical practice. Special recommendations for middle and long distance running. Part I: Aerobic interval training. *Sports Med.* **2001**, *31*, 13–31. [CrossRef]
20. Daniels, J.T.; Scardina, N. Interval training and performance. *Sports Med.* **1984**, *1*, 327–334. [CrossRef]
21. Gaitanos, G.C.; Williams, C.; Boobis, L.H.; Brooks, S. Human muscle metabolism during intermittent maximal exercise. *J. Appl. Physiol.* **1993**, *75*, 712–719. [CrossRef] [PubMed]
22. Laursen, P.B.; Jenkins, D.G. The scientific basis for high intensity interval training: Optimising training programmes and maximising performance in highly trained endurance athletes. *Sports Med.* **2002**, *32*, 53–73. [CrossRef] [PubMed]
23. Daussin, F.N.; Ponsot, E.; Dufour, S.P.; Lonsdorfer-Wolf, E.; Doutreleau, S.; Geny, B.; Piquard, F.; Richard, R. Improvement of VO2max by cardiac output and oxygen extraction adaptation during intermittent versus continuous endurance training. *Eur. J. Appl. Physiol.* **2007**, *101*, 377–383. [CrossRef] [PubMed]
24. Daussin, F.N.; Zoll, J.; Dufour, S.P.; Ponsot, E.; Lonsdorfer-Wolf, E.; Doutreleau, S.; Mettauer, B.; Piquard, F.; Geny, B.; Richard, R. Effect of interval versus continuous training on cardiorespiratory and mitochondrial functions: Relationship to aerobic performance improvements in sedentary. *Am. J. Physiol.* **2008**. [CrossRef]
25. Helgerud, J.; Hoydal, K.; Wang, E.; Karlsen, T.; Berg, P.; Bjerkaas, M.; Simonsen, T.; Helgesen, C.; Hjorth, N.; Bach, R.; et al. Aerobic high-intensity intervals improve VO2max more than moderate training. *Med. Sci. Sports Exerc.* **2007**, *39*, 665–671. [CrossRef]
26. Juneau, M.; Roy, N.; Nigam, A.; Tardif, J.C.; Larivee, L. Exercise above the ischemic threshold and serum markers of myocardial injury. *Can. J. Cardiol.* **2009**, *25*, e338–e341. [CrossRef]
27. Noël, M.; Jobin, J.; Marcoux, A.; Poirier, P.; Dagenais, G.; Bogaty, P. Can prolonged exercise-induced myocardial ischaemia be innocuous? *Eur. Heart J.* **2007**, *28*, 1559–1565. [CrossRef]
28. van Gelder, B.M.; Tijhuis, M.A.; Kalmijn, S.; Giampaoli, S.; Nissinen, A.; Kromhout, D. Physical activity in relation to cognitive decline in elderly men: The FINE Study. *Neurology* **2004**, *63*, 2316–2321. [CrossRef]
29. Angevaren, M.; Vanhees, L.; Wendel-Vos, W.; Verhaar, H.J.; Aufdemkampe, G.; Aleman, A.; Verschuren, W.M. Intensity, but not duration, of physical activities is related to cognitive function. *Eur. J. Cardiovasc. Prev. Rehabil.* **2007**, *14*, 825–830. [CrossRef]
30. Brown, B.M.; Peiffer, J.J.; Sohrabi, H.R.; Mondal, A.; Gupta, V.B.; Rainey-Smith, S.R.; Taddei, K.; Burnham, S.; Ellis, K.A.; Szoeke, C.; et al. Intense physical activity is associated with cognitive performance in the elderly. *Transl. Psychiatry* **2012**, *2*, e191. [CrossRef]
31. Freitas, D.A.; Rocha-Vieira, E.; De Sousa, R.A.L.; Soares, B.A.; Rocha-Gomes, A.; Chaves Garcia, B.C.; Cassilhas, R.C.; Mendonca, V.A.; Camargos, A.C.R.; De Gregorio, J.A.M.; et al. High-intensity interval training improves cerebellar antioxidant capacity without affecting cognitive functions in rats. *Behav. Brain Res.* **2019**, *376*, 112181. [CrossRef] [PubMed]
32. Nicolini, C.; Toepp, S.; Harasym, D.; Michalski, B.; Fahnestock, M.; Gibala, M.J.; Nelson, A.J. No changes in corticospinal excitability, biochemical markers, and working memory after 6 weeks of high-intensity interval training in sedentary males. *Physiol. Rep.* **2019**, *7*, e14140. [CrossRef] [PubMed]
33. Jeon, Y.K.; Ha, C.H. The effect of exercise intensity on brain derived neurotrophic factor and memory in adolescents. *Environ. Health Prev. Med.* **2017**, *22*, 27. [CrossRef] [PubMed]
34. Kovacevic, A.; Fenesi, B.; Paolucci, E.; Heisz, J.J. The effects of aerobic exercise intensity on memory in older adults. *Appl. Physiol. Nutr. Metab.* **2019**. [CrossRef]
35. Moreau, D.; Kirk, I.J.; Waldie, K.E. High-intensity training enhances executive function in children in a randomized, placebo-controlled trial. *Elife* **2017**, *6*. [CrossRef]
36. Pallesen, H.; Bjerk, M.; Pedersen, A.R.; Nielsen, J.F.; Evald, L. The Effects of High-Intensity Aerobic Exercise on Cognitive Performance After Stroke: A Pilot Randomised Controlled Trial. *J. Cent. Nerv. Syst. Dis.* **2019**, *11*. [CrossRef]
37. Venckunas, T.; Snieckus, A.; Trinkunas, E.; Baranauskiene, N.; Solianik, R.; Juodsnukis, A.; Streckis, V.; Kamandulis, S. Interval Running Training Improves Cognitive Flexibility and Aerobic Power of Young Healthy Adults. *J. Strength Cond. Res.* **2016**, *30*, 2114–2121. [CrossRef]
38. Bowie, C.R.; Harvey, P.D. Administration and interpretation of the Trail Making Test. *Nat. Protoc.* **2006**, *1*, 2277–2281. [CrossRef]

39. O'Brien, M.W.; Johns, J.A.; Robinson, S.A.; Bungay, A.; Mekary, S.; Kimmerly, D.S. Impact of HIIT, MICT, and Resistance Training on Endothelial Function in Older Adults. *Med. Sci. Sports Exerc.* **2019**. [CrossRef]
40. Guiraud, T.; Juneau, M.; Nigam, A.; Gayda, M.; Meyer, P.; Mekary, S.; Paillard, F.; Bosquet, L. Optimization of high intensity interval exercise in coronary heart disease. *Eur. J. Appl. Physiol.* **2010**, *108*, 733–740. [CrossRef]
41. Dupuy, O.; Lussier, M.; Fraser, S.; Bherer, L.; Audiffren, M.; Bosquet, L. Effect of overreaching on cognitive performance and related cardiac autonomic control. *Scand. J. Med. Sci. Sports* **2014**, *24*, 234–242. [CrossRef] [PubMed]
42. Rognmo, O.; Hetland, E.; Helgerud, J.; Hoff, J.; Slordahl, S.A. High intensity aerobic interval exercise is superior to moderate intensity exercise for increasing aerobic capacity in patients with coronary artery disease. *Eur. J. Cardiovasc. Prev. Rehabil.* **2004**, *11*, 216–222. [CrossRef] [PubMed]
43. Kemmler, W.; Scharf, M.; Lell, M.; Petrasek, C.; von Stengel, S. High versus moderate intensity running exercise to impact cardiometabolic risk factors: The randomized controlled RUSH-study. *Biomed. Res. Int.* **2014**, *2014*, 843095. [CrossRef] [PubMed]
44. Bacon, A.P.; Carter, R.E.; Ogle, E.A.; Joyner, M.J. VO2max trainability and high intensity interval training in humans: A meta-analysis. *PLoS ONE* **2013**, *8*, e73182. [CrossRef] [PubMed]
45. Scribbans, T.D.; Vecsey, S.; Hankinson, P.B.; Foster, W.S.; Gurd, B.J. The Effect of Training Intensity on VO2max in Young Healthy Adults: A Meta-Regression and Meta-Analysis. *Int. J. Exerc. Sci.* **2016**, *9*, 230–247. [PubMed]
46. Colcombe, S.J.; Kramer, A.F.; Erickson, K.I.; Scalf, P.; McAuley, E.; Cohen, N.J.; Webb, A.; Jerome, G.J.; Marquez, D.X.; Elavsky, S. Cardiovascular fitness, cortical plasticity, and aging. *Proc. Natl. Acad. Sci. USA* **2004**, *101*, 3316–3321. [CrossRef] [PubMed]
47. Smiley-Oyen, A.L.; Lowry, K.A.; Francois, S.J.; Kohut, M.L.; Ekkekakis, P. Exercise, fitness, and neurocognitive function in older adults: The "selective improvement" and "cardiovascular fitness" hypotheses. *Ann. Behav. Med.* **2008**, *36*, 280–291. [CrossRef]
48. Madden, D.J.; Blumenthal, J.A.; Allen, P.A.; Emery, C.F. Improving aerobic capacity in healthy older adults does not necessarily lead to improved cognitive performance. *Psychol. Aging* **1989**, *4*, 307–320. [CrossRef]
49. Etnier, J.L.; Nowell, P.M.; Landers, D.M.; Sibley, B.A. A meta-regression to examine the relationship between aerobic fitness and cognitive performance. *Brain Res. Rev.* **2006**, *52*, 119–130. [CrossRef]
50. Best, J.R. Effects of Physical Activity on Children's Executive Function: Contributions of Experimental Research on Aerobic Exercise. *Dev. Rev.* **2010**, *30*, 331–551. [CrossRef]
51. Piepmeier, A.T.; Etnier, J.L. Brain-derived neurotrophic factor (BDNF) as a potential mechanism of the effects of acute exercise on cognitive performance. *J. Sport Health Sci.* **2015**, *4*, 14–23. [CrossRef]
52. Piepmeier, A.T.; Etnier, J.L.; Wideman, L.; Berry, N.T.; Kincaid, Z.; Weaver, M.A. A preliminary investigation of acute exercise intensity on memory and BDNF isoform concentrations. *Eur. J. Sport Sci.* **2019**. [CrossRef] [PubMed]
53. Schmolesky, M.T.; Webb, D.L.; Hansen, R.A. The effects of aerobic exercise intensity and duration on levels of brain-derived neurotrophic factor in healthy men. *J. Sports Sci. Med.* **2013**, *12*, 502–511. [PubMed]
54. Winter, B.; Breitenstein, C.; Mooren, F.C.; Voelker, K.; Fobker, M.; Lechtermann, A.; Krueger, K.; Fromme, A.; Korsukewitz, C.; Floel, A.; et al. High impact running improves learning. *Neurobiol. Learn. Mem.* **2007**, *87*, 597–609. [CrossRef]
55. Enette, L.; Vogel, T.; Fanon, J.L.; Lang, P.O. Effect of Interval and Continuous Aerobic Training on Basal Serum and Plasma Brain-Derived Neurotrophic Factor Values in Seniors: A Systematic Review of Intervention Studies. *Rejuvenation Res.* **2017**, *20*, 473–483. [CrossRef]
56. Jimenez-Maldonado, A.; Renteria, I.; Garcia-Suarez, P.C.; Moncada-Jimenez, J.; Freire-Royes, L.F. The Impact of High-Intensity Interval Training on Brain Derived Neurotrophic Factor in Brain: A Mini-Review. *Front. Neurosci.* **2018**, *12*, 839. [CrossRef]
57. Saucedo Marquez, C.M.; Vanaudenaerde, B.; Troosters, T.; Wenderoth, N. High-intensity interval training evokes larger serum BDNF levels compared with intense continuous exercise. *J. Appl. Physiol. (1985)* **2015**, *119*, 1363–1373. [CrossRef]
58. Lou, S.J.; Liu, J.Y.; Chang, H.; Chen, P.J. Hippocampal neurogenesis and gene expression depend on exercise intensity in juvenile rats. *Brain Res.* **2008**, *1210*, 48–55. [CrossRef]

59. Freitas, D.A.; Rocha-Vieira, E.; Soares, B.A.; Nonato, L.F.; Fonseca, S.R.; Martins, J.B.; Mendonca, V.A.; Lacerda, A.C.; Massensini, A.R.; Poortamns, J.R.; et al. High intensity interval training modulates hippocampal oxidative stress, BDNF and inflammatory mediators in rats. *Physiol. Behav.* **2018**, *184*, 6–11. [CrossRef]
60. Ainslie, P.N.; Cotter, J.D.; George, K.P.; Lucas, S.; Murrell, C.; Shave, R.; Thomas, K.N.; Williams, M.J.; Atkinson, G. Elevation in cerebral blood flow velocity with aerobic fitness throughout healthy human ageing. *J. Physiol.* **2008**, *586*, 4005–4010. [CrossRef]
61. Dustman, R.E.; Emmerson, R.Y.; Ruhling, R.O.; Shearer, D.E.; Steinhaus, L.A.; Johnson, S.C.; Bonekat, H.W.; Shigeoka, J.W. Age and fitness effects on EEG, ERPs, visual sensitivity, and cognition. *Neurobiol. Aging* **1990**, *11*, 193–200. [CrossRef]
62. Robinson, M.M.; Lowe, V.J.; Nair, K.S. Increased Brain Glucose Uptake After 12 Weeks of Aerobic High-Intensity Interval Training in Young and Older Adults. *J. Clin. Endocrinol. Metab.* **2018**, *103*, 221–227. [CrossRef] [PubMed]

© 2020 by the authors. Licensee MDPI, Basel, Switzerland. This article is an open access article distributed under the terms and conditions of the Creative Commons Attribution (CC BY) license (http://creativecommons.org/licenses/by/4.0/).

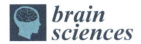

Article

Free-Weight Resistance Exercise Is More Effective in Enhancing Inhibitory Control than Machine-Based Training: A Randomized, Controlled Trial

Jan Wilke *, Vanessa Stricker and Susanne Usedly

Department of Sports Medicine, Goethe University, Ginnheimer Landstraße 39, 60487 Frankfurt am Main, Germany; vanessastricker@aol.com (V.S.); s.usedly@t-online.de (S.U.)
* Correspondence: wilke@sport.uni-frankfurt.de; Tel.: +49-69-798-24588

Received: 10 September 2020; Accepted: 28 September 2020; Published: 3 October 2020

Abstract: Resistance exercise has been demonstrated to improve brain function. However, the optimal workout characteristics are a matter of debate. This randomized, controlled trial aimed to elucidate differences between free-weight (RE_{free}) and machine-based (RE_{mach}) training with regard to their ability to acutely enhance cognitive performance (CP). A total of n = 46 healthy individuals (27 ± 4 years, 26 men) performed a 45-min bout of RE_{free} (military press, barbell squat, bench press) or RE_{mach} (shoulder press, leg press, chest press). Pre- and post-intervention, CP was examined using the Stroop test, Trail Making Test and Digit Span test. Mann–Whitney U tests did not reveal between-group differences for performance in the Digit Span test, Trail Making test and the color and word conditions of the Stroop test (p > 0.05). However, RE_{free} was superior to RE_{mach} in the Stroop color-word condition (+6.3%, p = 0.02, R = 0.35). Additionally, RE_{free} elicited pre-post changes in all parameters except for the Digit Span test and the word condition of the Stroop test while RE_{mach} only improved cognitive performance in part A of the Trail Making test. Using free weights seems to be the more effective RE method to acutely improve cognitive function (i.e., inhibitory control). The mechanisms of this finding merit further investigation.

Keywords: resistance training; cognition; barbell training; strength training

1. Introduction

For millennia, resistance exercise (RE) has represented an essential type of physical training, evoking manifold benefits in a plethora of populations and conditions [1–5]. For instance, RE has been shown to counteract age-related sarcopenia [1], reduce arterial blood pressure [2], improve recovery from musculoskeletal disorders [3] and increase sports-related motor performance [4,5]. Most studies examining the effects of RE predominantly focused on peripheral adaptations in the soft tissue, i.e., the cross-sectional area of the skeletal muscles. However, beyond this, RE also appears to impact brain function. Pooling the results from 12 trials, a recent multilevel meta-analysis concluded that a single training bout acutely increases specific sub-domains such as inhibitory control and cognitive flexibility [6].

Despite the established knowledge about the general interaction between RE and brain function, the moderators driving the changes in cognitive performance (CP) are a matter of debate. Studies addressing this issue have yielded heterogeneous results and a high level of uncertainty regarding the influence of modifiable (e.g., intensity, duration) and non-modifiable (e.g., age) factors [6]. Besides these quantitative variables, Pesce [7] suggested to focus on qualitative characteristics. In fact, studies using electroencephalography or near-infrared spectroscopy have revealed that cortical activations patterns and hemodynamics vary as a function of task complexity (e.g., stable repetitive monotonous vs. variable or alternating, coordinatively challenging activities; [8–11]). The question arises if changes such as higher perfusion and/or a facilitation of specific sensorimotor cortices could be beneficial for cognitive performance.

Some researchers investigated the impact of varying task complexity on brain function. In adolescents attending an elite performance school, Budde et al. [12] found a 10-min, coordinatively challenging exercise session (e.g., bouncing one or two balls, alternatingly and/or simultaneously, concurrently passing balls with foot and hand) to acutely enhance executive function to a greater degree than a traditional intervention of identical duration (general moderate-intensity exercise without major coordinative demands). Gallotta et al. [13] made opposite findings. They instructed primary school children (8–11 years) to either participate in a normal school lesson lacking physical activity, a regular non-enriched physical education session (e.g., walking, running, skipping) or a coordinatively enriched physical education session (e.g., basketball mini-games with varying rules fostering decision-making). Interestingly, the coordinatively challenging session was least effective.

Hitherto, no study has examined the cognitive effects of task complexity in RE. However, in a pioneering trial, Carraro et al. [14] found free-weights training to more strongly increase arousal (a psychological state of being attentive) than machine-based training. As exercise-induced gains in arousal are linked to better CP [15], the objective of the present study was to test the hypothesis that free-weight RE would enhance cognition more effectively than a quantitatively matched intervention with machines.

2. Materials and Methods

2.1. Ethical Standards and Study Design

The study is nested within the COINS (COgnition and INjury in Sports) network project. A two-armed, randomized, controlled trial was performed. It was prospectively registered at the German Register of Clinical Trials (DRKS00022281) and conducted in accordance with the Declaration of Helsinki including its recent modification of Fortaleza (2013). Ethical approval (ref. 2020-39) was obtained on 7 June 2020 from the ethics committee of the Faculty of Psychology and Sports Sciences of Goethe University Frankfurt, and each volunteer provided written informed consent.

Participants were randomly allocated to two groups: (1) resistance training with free weights (RE_{free}) or (2) resistance training with machines (RE_{mach}). Prior to and after the intervention, cognitive performance was assessed. All participants visited the laboratory twice with 5 to 7 days in-between. While the first session served for familiarization with the tests and the training equipment, the actual intervention was performed on the second appointment. Randomization was performed using the software package "BiAS for Windows", version 9.05 (Goethe University, Frankfurt, Germany).

2.2. Participants

Healthy adults (n = 46, 27 ± 4 years, 26 men) were recruited between June and August 2020 by means of personal contact and poster advertising at the local university campus. They had to engage in a minimum of five sporting hours per week. Exclusion criteria were (a) severe orthopedic, cardiovascular, pulmonary, neurological, psychiatric or inflammatory rheumatic diseases; (b) pregnancy or nursing period; (c) analgesic intake during the trial or in the 48 h prior to study enrollment; (d) impairments in color vision and (e) history of surgery or trauma in the lower extremity.

2.3. Intervention

The interventions and related procedures have been validated in a previous trial assessing the impact of RE on arousal [14]. When allocated to RE_{mach}, the participants completed a resistance training session using conventional training machines (shoulder press, leg press and chest press). Exercises for individuals in RE_{free} (military press, back squat, bench press) were executed with a barbell. Repetition numbers, set durations and relative intensities were identical in both groups. Participants performed four sets with the descending pyramid system (six, eight, ten, and twelve repetitions, weight progressively decreasing from set to set). To standardize movement velocity, the concentric phases lasted one second and the eccentric phases two seconds. Rest duration between-sets was 115 s. Weights were determined according to the individual 6-repetition maximums (6RM) of the respective exercises, which was determined during the familiarization session [14]. Prior to testing, participants performed two warm-up sets at 25% and 50% of the anticipated 1RM [16]. These sets, together with previous training records, were used to determine the starting weight. In the actual measurements, weight was increased once six correct repetitions had been performed. The interval between sets was 180 s [17]. Only assessments with a maximum of 5 attempts were considered valid [18]. In our sample, most participants required 1–3 sets (range 1–4 sets). All workouts were monitored by investigators holding an academic degree in Sports Sciences. Verbal feedback was continuously given if errors in movement execution were observed.

2.4. Outcomes

Immediately before and after the intervention, markers of CP were measured. To prevent practice effects, three strategies were used [19]. Firstly, in the familiarization session, all participants completed three repetitions of each test. Secondly, prior to initiating the actual assessments, one warm-up trial was performed. Finally, no identical tests forms (different color/number orders) were applied. Testing order was randomized and the delay between the end of the experimental condition and the start of the post-measurements was standardized amounting to 60 s.

Assessments included three tests. The *Stroop task* has three parts. In the first and second which both capture attention, the participants were required to name words written (S_w) or colors (S_c) displayed on a sheet as quickly as possible. The third section, a measure of inhibition control (S_{cw}), consisted of color words presented incongruently (e.g., "green" written in red or "blue written in yellow). Here, the participants needed to name the color of the word while ignoring the letters. In all three parts, time until task completion was documented. The Stroop test exhibits high reliability (ICC: 0.82) and internal consistency (Cronbach's alpha: 0.93 to 0.97) [20].

The *Trail Making test* (TMT) has two parts. In part A, the participants were required to connect successive numbers using a pen at maximal possible speed (e.g., 1–4). In part B, numbers and letters (e.g., 1 to a to 2 to b) were to be linked in an alternating manner. Similar to the Stroop test, time needed for completion was recorded. The results are suggested to represent a measure of visual screening/attention (TMT-A) and cognitive flexibility/working memory (TMT-B). High reliability (ICC: 0.81 to 0.86) and construct validity of the TMT have been demonstrated [21,22].

In the *Digit Span* (DS) test, two conditions were performed. In the first, the participants had to recall and repeat increasing amounts of numbers read to them. Initially, four numbers were to be memorized. In case of success, five numbers were named. For each step, two repetitions were performed and one or zero points awarded depending on recall success. The test ends if both trials were failed. The second condition was identical to the first, but the numbers had to be repeated in reversed order (e.g., 2,4,7,9 becomes 9,7,4,2). Both test parts and the composite score were linked to short-term and working memory [23]. The DS test is reliable for repeated measurements ($r = 0.73$; [24]).

Prior to starting outcome assessments, subjective arousal (Likert scale from "0—not activated" to "6—highly activated"), concentration (10 cm Visual Analogue Scale, 0 = not concentrated at all to 10 = highly concentrated) and heart rate (heart rate monitor) were assessed. Additionally, after the interventions, the participants stated their rate of perceived exertion (6–20 RPE scale [25]) as well as enjoyment of the intervention (Likert scale from "0—not fun at all" to "6—most possible fun").

2.5. Data Processing and Statistics

Kolmogorov–Smirnov analyses revealed violations of the normalcy assumption. To identify relative pre-post changes of CP within groups, we constructed parameter-free 95% confidence intervals [26] while between-group differences were detected by means of the Mann–Whitney U test. With regard to the latter, in case of significance, effect sizes ($R = Z/\sqrt{n}$) were computed according to Rosenthal [27] and interpreted as small (R = 0.1), moderate (R = 0.3), large (R = 0.5) or very large (R > 0.7). To reveal potential moderators of the intervention effect (age, sex, BMI, physical activity volume, arousal, exercise enjoyment, subjective exertion during exercise), we used Kendall's tau correlation. *p*-values < 0.05 were considered to be significant in all calculations, the software used was "BiAS for Windows", version 9.05 (Goethe University, Frankfurt, Germany).

3. Results

Both groups showed comparable cognitive performance at baseline and were not different regarding age, sex, BMI, physical activity and pre-exercise arousal (*p* > 0.05, Table 1). All participants completed the disposed interventions without the occurrence of adverse effects.

Table 1. Characteristics of the two groups measured pre- and post-intervention.

	RE_{mach}		RE_{free}		Total Pre	Total Post
	Pre	Post	Pre	Post		
Age (yrs.)	27.0 ± 4.3		27.3 ± 4.4		27.2 ± 4.3	
Sex	12♂, 11♀		14♂, 9♀		26♂, 20♀	
Physical Activity (hrs./week)	8.2 ± 3.8		7.8 ± 3.6		8.0 ± 3.7	
BMI	22.7 ± 2.5		23.8 ± 3.1		23.3 ± 2.8	
Arousal (0–10)	6.2 ± 1.6	7.1 ± 1.4	6.5 ± 1.5	7.0 ± 1.7	6.3 ± 1.5	7.1 ± 1.6
Heart rate (bpm)	79.2 ± 15.5	103.4 ± 17.6	77.3 ± 9.7	104.9 ± 18.4	78.2 ± 12.8	104.1 ± 17.8
Enjoyment (0–10)		6.8 ± 2.1		7.6 ± 2.0		7.2 ± 2.0
Subjective exertion (6–20)		15.2 ± 2.1		15.1 ± 2.2		15.2 ± 2.1

Table shows means and standard deviations. RE_{mach} = machine-based resistance training, RE_{free} = free-weights resistance training, yrs= years, hrs= hours, bpm = beats per minute.

3.1. Exercise Effects on Cognitive Performance

No differences between groups were found for DS, TMT as well as S_c and S_w (*p* < 0.05, Table 2). However, analysis of the confidence intervals revealed that RE_{free} increased TMT-A (+34.6%), TMT-B (+24.3%), S_w (+2.9%) and S_c (+4.2%) performance relative to baseline, while RE_{mach} only improved TMT-A (+23.5%, Figures 1 and 2). Additionally, RE_{free} improved S_{cw} both pre to post according to the confidence intervals (+9.6%) and in comparison to RE_{mach} (+6.3%, *p* = 0.02, R = 0.35; moderate effect size, Figure 2).

Table 2. Cognitive performance measured pre- and post-intervention in both groups.

	RE_{mach}		RE_{free}	
	Pre	Post	Pre	Post
Stroop word (s)	25.9 (24.6–28.1)	25.9 (24.2–28.5)	27.2 (24.0–30.6)	25.7 (24.4–29.7)
Stroop color (s)	31.2 (28.9–35.5)	29.3 (26.8–33.1)	33.1 (28.3–35.7)	30.2 (27.5–34.9) *
Stroop color-word (s)	45.9 (42.2–52.3)	44.7 (40.9–48.1)	49.7 (42.6–56.1)	43.9 (38.3–49.0) *#
TMT-A (s)	25.5 (21.2–34.3)	19.5 (16.3–25.2) *	28.3 (24.7–32.6)	18.5 (16.6–23.2) *
TMT-B (s)	34.3 (28.7–39.1)	30.3 (23.5–38.6)	33.7 (27.4–41.7)	25.5 (21.7–38.1) *
Digit Span (pts.)	11 (10–13)	11 (8–12)	13 (8–14)	12 (10–14)

Table shows medians and (interquartile ranges). RE_{mach} = machine-based resistance training, RE_{free} = free-weights resistance training, s = seconds, pts = points, * = difference to pre-intervention value according to 95% confidence intervals, # = significant difference of pre-post change when compared to the other group.

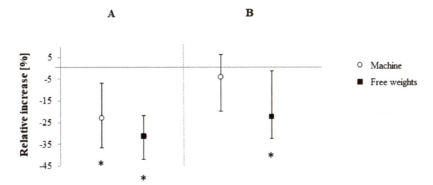

Figure 1. Relative changes in the two parts (**A**,**B**) of the Trail Making test (TMT) following free-weight and machine-based resistance exercise. Displayed are medians and parameter-free 95% confidence intervals. * = difference to pre-intervention value according to 95% confidence intervals

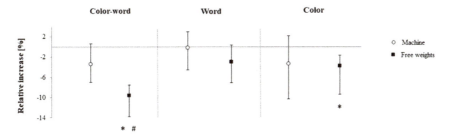

Figure 2. Relative changes in the three conditions of the Stroop test following free-weight and machine-based resistance exercise. Displayed are medians and parameter-free 95% confidence intervals. * = difference to pre-intervention value according to 95% confidence intervals, # = significant difference of pre-post change when compared to the other group.

3.2. Potential Moderators

Exhaustion, enjoyment as well as changes in arousal and heart rate were not different between groups ($p < 0.05$). Additionally, none of these variables correlated with changes in cognitive performance ($p < 0.05$).

4. Discussion

A wealth of evidence supports the beneficial short-term impact of resistance exercise on cognitive performance [6]. However, so far, research on the moderators of this effect predominantly focused on training intensity [28–32] while the relevance of exercise characteristics, i.e., the type of RE, had been scarcely examined. In detail, available studies mostly investigated machined-based (e.g., [33–36]) or a combination of machined-based and free-weight RE (e.g., [37–42]) but none provided a direct comparison of different regimes. The present trial reveals that the magnitude of exercise-induced CP improvements following free-weight RE is substantially larger when compared to machine-based training.

Several mechanisms potentially mediating short-term CP changes following RE have been discussed. A previous study demonstrated free-weight exercise to induce higher arousal levels when compared to machine-based training [14]. However, this finding could not be replicated in our trial as arousal was not different between groups. A potential reason for this could be that we used a 10-point Likert scale, while Carraro and colleagues had applied the Felt Arousal Scale with six points. Irrespectively, the impact of arousal as an effect trigger in different RE types requires further examination. Cerebral blood flow represents another factor suspected to explain activity-induced CP improvements. Experiments using aerobic exercise showed an intensity-dependent increase of brain perfusion until the ventilatory threshold [43]. Only few studies examined this association for RE, but initial evidence points towards the existence of blood flow fluctuations during exercise which may facilitate CP [43,44]. Together with or in absence of perfusion changes, altered cortical activation patterns may be triggered by RE. In both, younger adults and individuals with mild cognitive impairment, increased P3 amplitudes (linked to activity and cognitive functioning) were detected immediately following an exercise bout [45,46]. Finally, exercise generally modulates the production of cortisol and moderately elevated concentrations of the stress hormone can enhance working memory [47]. Evidence, however, is ambiguous for RE and both acute decreases [38] and increases [48] have been reported. While all these findings are intriguing, none of the mechanistic studies particularly addressed the question as to whether the magnitude of the metabolic, circulatory and electrophysiological changes is dependent on the RE characteristics (i.e., RE with free weights vs. RE with machines). Based on the available evidence showing an association of task complexity and cortical activation [8–10] and our data, we speculate that training with free weights may require higher levels of concentration, sensory processing and motor coordination and with this, higher or more complex brain activation levels than similar interventions using training machines.

RE with free-weights, in contrast to machine-based RE, improved S_c and TMT-B performance but no significant between-group differences were found. Some uncertainty therefore remains regarding a higher effectiveness of free-weight exercise in enhancing simple cognitive functions such as attention, processing speed, reaction time and visual scanning. Contrarily, a moderate effect indicating superiority of RE with free weights was found for inhibitory control (S_{cw}). This finding seems plausible as exercising with a barbell requires constant fine and gross motor adaptations and corrections of the ongoing movement. Improvements of inhibitory control may be of relevance in a variety of contexts. Previous studies found that poor performance during response inhibition tasks is associated with the risk of future falls in community-dwelling older adults and individuals with neurological diseases [49–52]. Health professionals may hence consider incorporating free-weight exercises when designing exercise programs for seniors or patients. Beyond this, using free- or bodyweight resistance exercise could also be of value as a warm-up for athletes from both an injury-preventive and a performance-related perspective. Giesche et al. [53] examined the relation between inhibitory control and dynamic postural control during unplanned single-leg landings in healthy active individuals. Participants with low S_{cw} values had higher center of pressure path lengths, which is indicative of a possible stability deficit. With regard to sporting success, several studies [54,55] have shown an association between inhibitory control and game performance sports.

Although machine-based paradigms are frequently used in studies examining the effects of RE on CP, R_{mach} did only improve TMT-A performance but, as said, had no effects on measures of executive function (TMT-B, S_{cw}) or other tests capturing lower order cognitive skills. Compared to S_c and S_w, the TMT-A places higher demands to visual search [56], and hence, it may be speculated that RE_{mach} rather improves this skill than processing speed and reaction time in general.

Our results call for further research. (1) From a general point of view, gaining insight into the mechanisms explaining the higher effectiveness of R_{free} in increasing CP should be a paramount objective of future trials. (2) In detail, we found a superiority of R_{free} in inhibitory control, which is typically classified as a higher-order cognitive function. As the analysis of the confidence intervals also revealed pre-post improvements in lower-order functions (e.g., processing speed and visual scanning), which did not occur following machine-based training but failed statistical significance in the group comparison, we recommend follow-up experiments focusing on this area. Finally, it would be of interest to compare the traditional RE methods studied here with newer approaches such as high-intensity functional training, which mixes characteristics of endurance and resistance exercise.

Some limitations need to be discussed. Analysis of our data showed that it was non-normally distributed. As the choice of the sample size had been based on a biometric calculation for parametric testing and as non-parametric testing is more conservative, our trial may have had a slight lack of power preventing the detection of small-magnitude differences. When considering the confidence intervals, this, e.g., may relate to performance in the Trail Making test. Two other issues relate to the comparability of the interventions. Firstly, although we matched training intensity relative to individual maximal strength, exercising with free weights is known to achieve higher muscle activations [57]. Secondly, we did not use a linear encoder to control movement velocity. Minor differences may hence have occurred between the training regimes.

5. Conclusions

Resistance exercise performed with free weights is more effective in acutely increasing inhibitory control than the use of conventional training machines. It may hence be of interest for both, elderly individuals aiming to prevent falls or athletes seeking to improve performance.

Author Contributions: J.W.; data curation, J.W., V.S., S.U.; formal analysis, J.W.; investigation, J.W., V.S., S.U.; methodology, J.W.; project administration, J.W.; supervision, J.W.; visualization, J.W.; writing—original draft, J.W.; writing—review and editing, J.W., V.S., S.U. All authors have read and agreed to the published version of the manuscript.

Funding: This research received no external funding.

Conflicts of Interest: The authors declare no conflict of interest.

References

1. Beckwée, D.; Delaere, A.; Aelbrecht, S.; Baert, V.; Beaudart, C.; Bruyère, O.; De Saint-Hubert, M.; Bautmans, I. Exercise Interventions for the Prevention and Treatment of Sarcopenia. A Systematic Umbrella Review. *J. Nutr. Health Aging* **2019**, *23*, 494–502. [CrossRef]
2. Cornelissen, V.; Fagard, R.H.; Coeckelberghs, E.; Vanhees, L. Impact of Resistance Training on Blood Pressure and Other Cardiovascular Risk Factors. *Hypertension* **2011**, *58*, 950–958. [CrossRef] [PubMed]
3. Kristensen, J.; Franklyn-Miller, A. Resistance training in musculoskeletal rehabilitation: A systematic review. *Br. J. Sports Med.* **2011**, *46*, 719–726. [CrossRef] [PubMed]
4. Young, W.B. Transfer of Strength and Power Training to Sports Performance. *Int. J. Sports Physiol. Perform.* **2006**, *1*, 74–83. [CrossRef] [PubMed]
5. Harries, S.K.; Lubans, D.R.; Callister, R. Resistance training to improve power and sports performance in adolescent athletes: A systematic review and meta-analysis. *J. Sci. Med. Sport* **2012**, *15*, 532–540. [CrossRef]
6. Wilke, J.; Giesche, F.; Klier, K.; Vogt, L.; Herrmann, E.; Banzer, W. Acute Effects of Resistance Exercise on Cognitive Function in Healthy Adults: A Systematic Review with Multilevel Meta-Analysis. *Sports Med.* **2019**, *49*, 905–916. [CrossRef] [PubMed]
7. Pesce, C. Shifting the Focus from Quantitative to Qualitative Exercise Characteristics in Exercise and Cognition Research. *J. Sport Exerc. Psychol.* **2012**, *34*, 766–786. [CrossRef] [PubMed]
8. Jäncke, L.; Himmelbach, M.; Shah, N.J.; Zilles, K. The Effect of Switching between Sequential and Repetitive Movements on Cortical Activation. *NeuroImage* **2000**, *12*, 528–537. [CrossRef]
9. Verstynen, T.V.; Diedrichsen, J.; Albert, N.; Aparicio, P.; Ivry, R.B. Ipsilateral Motor Cortex Activity During Unimanual Hand Movements Relates to Task Complexity. *J. Neurophysiol.* **2005**, *93*, 1209–1222. [CrossRef]
10. Holper, L.; Biallas, M.; Wolf, M. Task complexity relates to activation of cortical motor areas during uni- and bimanual performance: A functional NIRS study. *NeuroImage* **2009**, *46*, 1105–1113. [CrossRef]
11. Leff, D.R.; Orihuela-Espina, F.; Elwell, C.; Athanasiou, T.; Delpy, D.T.; Darzi, A.W.; Yang, G.Z. Assessment of the cerebral cortex during motor task behaviours in adults: A systematic review of functional near infrared spectroscopy (fNIRS) studies. *NeuroImage* **2011**, *54*, 2922–2936. [CrossRef] [PubMed]
12. Budde, H.; Voelcker-Rehage, C.; Pietraßyk-Kendziorra, S.; Ribeiro, P.; Tidow, G. Acute coordinative exercise improves attentional performance in adolescents. *Neurosci. Lett.* **2008**, *441*, 219–223. [CrossRef] [PubMed]

13. Gallotta, M.C.; Guidetti, L.; Franciosi, E.; Emerenziani, G.P.; Bonavolontà, V.; Baldari, C. Effects of Varying Type of Exertion on Children's Attention Capacity. *Med. Sci. Sports Exerc.* **2012**, *44*, 550–555. [CrossRef] [PubMed]
14. Carraro, A.; Paoli, A.; Gobbi, E. Affective response to acute resistance exercise: A comparison among machines and free weights. *Sport Sci. Health* **2018**, *14*, 283–288. [CrossRef]
15. Lambourne, K.; Tomporowski, P. The effect of exercise-induced arousal on cognitive task performance: A meta-regression analysis. *Brain Res.* **2010**, *1341*, 12–24. [CrossRef] [PubMed]
16. Saeterbakken, A.H.; Fimland, M.S. Electromyographic Activity and 6RM Strength in Bench Press on Stable and Unstable Surfaces. *J. Strength Cond. Res.* **2013**, *27*, 1101–1107. [CrossRef] [PubMed]
17. Drinkwater, E.J.; Lawton, T.W.; Lindsell, R.P.; Pyne, D.B.; Hunt, P.H.; McKenna, M.J. Training leading to repetition failure enhances bench press strength gains in elite junior athletes. *J. Strength Cond. Res.* **2005**, *19*, 382–388.
18. Wilke, J.; Kaiser, S.; Niederer, D.; Kalo, K.; Engeroff, T.; Morath, C.; Vogt, L.; Banzer, W. Effects of high-intensity functional circuit training on motor function and sport motivation in healthy, inactive adults. *Scand. J. Med. Sci. Sports* **2018**, *29*, 144–153. [CrossRef]
19. Hausknecht, J.P.; Halpert, J.A.; Di Paolo, N.T.; Gerrard, M.O.M. Retesting in selection: A meta-analysis of coaching and practice effects for tests of cognitive ability. *J. Appl. Psychol.* **2007**, *92*, 373–385. [CrossRef]
20. Wöstmann, N.M.; Aichert, D.S.; Costa, A.; Rubia, K.; Möller, H.-J.; Ettinger, U. Reliability and plasticity of response inhibition and interference control. *Brain Cogn.* **2013**, *81*, 82–94. [CrossRef]
21. Wagner, S.; Helmreich, I.; Dahmen, N.; Lieb, K.; Tadic, A. Reliability of Three Alternate Forms of the Trail Making Tests A and B. *Arch. Clin. Neuropsychol.* **2011**, *26*, 314–321. [CrossRef] [PubMed]
22. Sánchez-Cubillo, I.; A Periañez, J.; Adrover-Roig, D.; Rodríguez-Sánchez, J.; Rios-Lago, M.; Tirapu, J.; Barcelo, F. Construct validity of the Trail Making Test: Role of task-switching, working memory, inhibition/interference control, and visuomotor abilities. *J. Int. Neuropsychol. Soc.* **2009**, *15*, 438–450. [CrossRef] [PubMed]
23. Unsworth, N.; Engle, R. On the division of short-term and working memory: An examination of simple and complex span and their relation to higher order abilities. *Psychol. Bull.* **2007**, *133*, 1038–1066. [CrossRef] [PubMed]
24. Youngjohn, J.R.; Larrabee, G.J.; Crook, T.H. Test-retest reliability of computerized, everyday memory measures and traditional memory tests. *Clin. Neuropsychol.* **1992**, *6*, 276–286. [CrossRef]
25. Chen, M.; Fan, X.; Moe, S.T. Criterion-related validity of the Borg ratings of perceived exertion scale in healthy individuals: A meta-analysis. *J. Sports Sci.* **2002**, *20*, 873–899. [CrossRef]
26. Sachs, L. *Angewandte Statistik: Anwendung Statistischer Methoden*, 10th ed.; Springer-Verlag GmbH: Heidelberg, Germany, 2002; p. 893. (In German)
27. Rosenthal, R. Applied Social Research Methods Series. In *Meta-Analytic Procedures for Social Research, Rev. ed.*; SAGE Publications, Inc.: Thousand Oaks, CA, USA, 1991; Volume 6.
28. Brisswalter, J.; Collardeau, M.; René, A. Effects of Acute Physical Exercise Characteristics on Cognitive Performance. *Sports Med.* **2002**, *32*, 555–566. [CrossRef]
29. McMorris, T.; Sproule, J.; Turner, A.; Hale, B.J. Acute, intermediate intensity exercise, and speed and accuracy in working memory tasks: A meta-analytical comparison of effects. *Physiol. Behav.* **2011**, *102*, 421–428. [CrossRef]
30. Chang, Y.; Labban, J.; Gapin, J.; Etnier, J. The effects of acute exercise on cognitive performance: A meta-analysis. *Brain Res.* **2012**, *1453*, 87–101. [CrossRef]
31. Loprinzi, P.D. Intensity-specific effects of acute exercise on human memory function: Considerations for the timing of exercise and the type of memory. *Heal. Promot. Perspect.* **2018**, *8*, 255–262. [CrossRef]
32. Moreau, D.; Chou, E. The Acute Effect of High-Intensity Exercise on Executive Function: A Meta-Analysis. *Perspect. Psychol. Sci.* **2019**, *14*, 734–764. [CrossRef]
33. Pontifex, M.B.; Hillman, C.H.; Fernhall, B.; Thompson, K.M.; Valentini, T.A. The Effect of Acute Aerobic and Resistance Exercise on Working Memory. *Med. Sci. Sports Exerc.* **2009**, *41*, 927–934. [CrossRef] [PubMed]
34. Hsieh, S.-S.; Chang, Y.-K.; Hung, T.-M.; Fang, C.-L. The effects of acute resistance exercise on young and older males' working memory. *Psychol. Sport Exerc.* **2016**, *22*, 286–293. [CrossRef]

35. Tsukamoto, H.; Suga, T.; Takenaka, S.; Takeuchi, T.; Tanaka, D.; Hamaoka, T.; Hashimoto, T.; Isaka, T. An acute bout of localized resistance exercise can rapidly improve inhibitory control. *PLoS ONE* **2017**, *12*, e0184075. [CrossRef] [PubMed]
36. Dunsky, A.; Abu-Rukun, M.; Tsuk, S.; Dwolatzky, T.; Carasso, R.; Netz, Y. The effects of a resistance vs. an aerobic single session on attention and executive functioning in adults. *PLoS ONE* **2017**, *12*, e0176092. [CrossRef] [PubMed]
37. Alves, C.R.R.; Gualano, B.; Takao, P.P.; Avakian, P.; Fernandes, R.M.; Morine, D.; Takito, M.Y. Effects of Acute Physical Exercise on Executive Functions: A Comparison Between Aerobic and Strength Exercise. *J. Sport Exerc. Psychol.* **2012**, *34*, 539–549. [CrossRef]
38. Tsai, C.-L.; Wang, C.-H.; Pan, C.-Y.; Chen, F.-C.; Huang, T.-H.; Chou, F.-Y. Executive function and endocrinological responses to acute resistance exercise. *Front. Behav. Neurosci.* **2014**, *8*, 262. [CrossRef]
39. Chang, H.; Kim, K.; Jung, Y.-J.; Kato, M. Effects of acute high-Intensity resistance exercise on cognitive function and oxygenation in prefrontal cortex. *J. Exerc. Nutr. Biochem.* **2017**, *21*, 1–8. [CrossRef]
40. Chang, Y.-K.; Ku, P.-W.; Tomporowski, P.D.; Chen, F.-T.; Huang, C.-C. Effects of Acute Resistance Exercise on Late-Middle-Age Adults' Goal Planning. *Med. Sci. Sports Exerc.* **2012**, *44*, 1773–1779. [CrossRef]
41. Chang, Y.-K.; Tsai, C.-L.; Huang, C.-C.; Wang, C.-C.; Chu, I.-H. Effects of acute resistance exercise on cognition in late middle-aged adults: General or specific cognitive improvement? *J. Sci. Med. Sport* **2014**, *17*, 51–55. [CrossRef]
42. Johnson, L.; Addamo, P.K.; Raj, I.S.; Borkoles, E.; Wyckelsma, V.L.; Cyarto, E.; Polman, R. An Acute Bout of Exercise Improves the Cognitive Performance of Older Adults. *J. Aging Phys. Act.* **2016**, *24*, 591–598. [CrossRef]
43. Smith, K.J.; Ainslie, P.-N. Regulation of cerebral blood flow and metabolism during exercise. *Exper. Physiol.* **2017**, *102*, 1356–1371. [CrossRef] [PubMed]
44. Edwards, M.R.; Martin, D.H.; Hughson, R.L. Cerebral hemodynamics and resistance exercise. *Med. Sci. Sports Exerc.* **2002**, *34*, 1207–1211. [CrossRef]
45. Pedroso, R.V.; Fraga, F.J.; Pérez, C.A.; Carral, J.C.; Scarpari, L.; Santos-Galduróz, R.F. Effects of physical activity on the P300 component in elderly people: A systematic review. *Psychogeriatrics* **2017**, *17*, 479–487. [CrossRef]
46. Herold, F.; Törpel, A.; Schega, L.; Mueller, N. Functional and/or structural brain changes in response to resistance exercises and resistance training lead to cognitive improvements—A systematic review. *Eur. Rev. Aging Phys. Act.* **2019**, *16*, 10. [CrossRef] [PubMed]
47. Basso, J.C.; Suzuki, W.A. The Effects of Acute Exercise on Mood, Cognition, Neurophysiology, and Neurochemical Pathways: A Review. *Brain Plast.* **2017**, *2*, 127–152. [CrossRef]
48. Arent, S.M.; Landers, D.M.; Matt, K.S.; Etnier, J.L. Dose-Response and Mechanistic Issues in the Resistance Training and Affect Relationship. *J. Sport Exerc. Psychol.* **2005**, *27*, 92–110. [CrossRef]
49. Chen, T.Y.; Peronto, C.L.; Edwards, J.D. Cognitive function as a prospective predictor of falls. *J. Gerontol.* **2012**, *67*, 720–728. [CrossRef]
50. Mirelman, A.; Herman, T.; Brozgol, M.; Dorfman, M.; Sprecher, E.; Schweiger, A.; Giladi, N.; Hausdorff, J.M. Executive Function and Falls in Older Adults: New Findings from a Five-Year Prospective Study Link Fall Risk to Cognition. *PLoS ONE* **2012**, *7*, e40297. [CrossRef]
51. Nagamatsu, L.S.; Kam, J.W.Y.; Liu-Ambrose, T.; Chan, A.; Handy, T.C. Mind-wandering and falls risk in older adults. *Psychol. Aging* **2013**, *28*, 685–691. [CrossRef]
52. Saverino, A.; Waller, D.; Rantell, K.; Parry, R.; Moriarty, E.; Playford, E.D. The Role of Cognitive Factors in Predicting Balance and Fall Risk in a Neuro-Rehabilitation Setting. *PLoS ONE* **2016**. [CrossRef]
53. Giesche, F.; Wilke, J.; Engeroff, T.; Niederer, D.; Hohmann, H.; Vogt, L.; Banzer, W. Are biomechanical stability deficits during unplanned single-leg landings related to specific markers of cognitive function? *J. Sci. Med. Sport* **2020**, *23*, 82–88. [CrossRef] [PubMed]
54. Verburgh, L.; Scherder, E.J.A.; Van Lange, P.A.M.; Oosterlaan, J. Executive Functioning in Highly Talented Soccer Players. *PLoS ONE* **2014**, *9*, e91254. [CrossRef] [PubMed]
55. Huijgen, B.C.H.; Leemhuis, S.; Kok, N.M.; Verburgh, L.; Oosterlaan, J.; Elferink-Gemser, M.T.; Visscher, C. Cognitive Functions in Elite and Sub-Elite Youth Soccer Players Aged 13 to 17 Years. *PLoS ONE* **2015**, *10*, e0144580. [CrossRef] [PubMed]

56. Crowe, S.F. The differential contribution of mental tracking, cognitive flexibility, visual search, and motor speed to performance on parts A and B of the trail making test. *J. Clin. Psychol.* **1998**, *54*, 585–591. [CrossRef]
57. Schick, E.E.; Coburn, J.W.; Brown, L.E.; Judelson, D.A.; Khamoui, A.V.; Tran, T.T.; Uribe, B.P. A comparison of muscle activation between a Smith Machine and free weight bench press. *J. Strength Cond. Res.* **2010**, *24*, 779–784. [CrossRef]

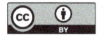

© 2020 by the authors. Licensee MDPI, Basel, Switzerland. This article is an open access article distributed under the terms and conditions of the Creative Commons Attribution (CC BY) license (http://creativecommons.org/licenses/by/4.0/).

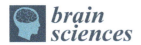

Communication

Exercise Intensity May Not Moderate the Acute Effects of Functional Circuit Training on Cognitive Function: A Randomized Crossover Trial

Jan Wilke * and Caroline Royé

Department of Sports Medicine, Goethe University Frankfurt, 60488 Frankfurt am Main, Germany; carolineroye@yahoo.de
* Correspondence: wilke@sport.uni-frankfurt.de; Tel.: +49-(0)69-798-24588; Fax: +49-(0)69-798-24582

Received: 18 September 2020; Accepted: 12 October 2020; Published: 14 October 2020

Abstract: Functional circuit training (FCT) has been demonstrated to acutely enhance cognitive performance (CP). However, the moderators of this observation are unknown. This study aimed to elucidate the role of exercise intensity. According to an a priori sample size calculation, $n = 24$ healthy participants (26 ± 3 years, 13 females), in randomized order, performed a single 15-min bout of FCT with low (20–39% of the heart rate reserve/HRR), moderate (40–59% HRR) or high intensity (maximal effort). Immediately pre- and post-workout, CP was measured by use of the Digit Span test, Stroop test and Trail Making test. Non-parametric data analyses did not reveal significant differences between conditions ($p > 0.05$) although parameter-free 95% confidence intervals showed pre-post improvements in some outcomes at moderate and high intensity only. The effort level does not seem to be a major effect modifier regarding short-term increases in CP following HCT in young active adults.

Keywords: HIFT; cognition; neurocognition; effort; exertion

---

1. Introduction

Many studies have established the beneficial effects of physical exercise on cognitive performance (CP, [1–8]). According to the available literature, chronic interventions (e.g., aerobic or resistance training), performed over weeks to months, enhance a variety of higher and lower order brain functions [5–8], which may be attributed to factors, such as enhanced cerebrovascular regulation, reduced systemic inflammation, improved insulin sensitivity or cortical neurogenesis [9–11]. Interestingly, also a single exercise bout can trigger improvements in specific domains, such as attention, working memory, inhibitory control and cognitive flexibility [1–4]. Acute increases in CP could be of interest in a variety of settings, including preparation for sporting activity or learning at schools and universities. However, the biological mechanisms and, even more, the optimal training parameters underpinning short-term gains in CP are obscure.

Aside from non-modifiable factors (e.g., age) which may also affect the effect magnitude [2,3,12], it has been proposed that exercise intensity represents a modifiable prime candidate driving immediate changes. Recent systematic reviews, however, differ in their conclusions. While some authors found light intensities most beneficial [2] others reported the largest effects at moderate [13], moderate to vigorous [4,5] exertion. Most studies examining the effects of exercise on CP focused on aerobic-type or resistance exercise. High-intensity functional training (HIFT) is a highly popular training method, which ranks among the top fitness trends worldwide [14] and aims to concurrently integrate cardiovascular and muscular efforts. Related workouts are based on the repeated execution of complex movement patterns (e.g., squats, lunges, push-ups) with minimal breaks in-between [15]. Data from intervention studies suggest that HIFT can acutely increase endurance capacity and muscle function [16], but beyond this, it also seems to enhance cognition. Following a 15-min bout of all-out circuit training, healthy individuals displayed improved short-term memory and inhibitory control [17]. This is of interest because the intensity spectrum for CP increases, so far, included light and moderate to vigorous but not maximal intensities [2,4,5,13]. The objective of the present trial, therefore, was to examine if changes in brain function following all-out HIFT, in fact, represent an outlier regarding previous knowledge or if functional circuit training performed at lower intensities would be comparably or even more effective.

2. Materials and Methods

2.1. Ethical Standards and Study Design

A three-armed, randomized, crossover trial, following the CONSORT (Consolidated Standards of Reporting Trials) guidelines [18] was performed in July 2020. It was prospectively registered at the German Register of Clinical Trials (DRKS00022285) and conducted in compliance with the Declaration of Helsinki. Ethics approval was granted by the local review board (2020-41, 14 July 2020, Ethics committee of the Faculty of Psychology and Sports Sciences, Goethe University, Frankfurt). Each participant signed informed consent. Enrolled individuals, in random order, completed three conditions: (1) functional circuit training at high-intensity (FCT-H), (2) functional circuit training at moderate intensity (FCT-M) or (3) functional circuit training at low intensity (FCT-L). Prior to and after the intervention, outcomes of CP were assessed. All participants visited the laboratory four times with seven-day intervals between the appointments. While the second to fourth visit included the actual experiments, the first was a familiarization session. Besides being introduced to the cognitive tests applied, participants received a demonstration of the functional circuit training workout.

2.2. Participants

Healthy adults (n = 24, 26 ± 4 years, 13 females) (Table 1) were recruited by means of personal addressing and poster advertising. All were physically active students engaging in 5 ± 2 sporting hours per week. The most performed types of exercise were fitness training in the gym and running. Exclusion criteria included (a) severe orthopaedic, cardiovascular, pulmonary, neurological, psychiatric or inflammatory rheumatic diseases, (b) pregnancy or nursing period, (c) analgesic intake during the trial or in the 48 h prior to study enrollment, (d) impairments in color vision, and (e) history of surgery or trauma in the lower extremity. Participants were asked to refrain from alcohol, caffeine, sugary drinks and strenuous physical activity during the 24 h preceding the three exercise sessions. To prevent influences of circadian rhythm, daytimes were kept constant within participants. Appointments were scheduled between 10 am and 2 pm (at least three hours after habitual wake-up time) as well as between 4 pm and 10 pm, as these intervals have been shown to be optimal for healthy individuals [19].

Table 1. Sample data.

Parameter	Value
Weight (kg)	70 ± 11
Height (cm)	174 ± 10
BMI	23 ± 2
Resting heart rate (bpm)	67 ± 9
Maximal heart rate (bpm)	189 ± 3
Perceived exertion during exercise (RPE scale)	L: 9 ± 2, M: 12 ± 2, H: 16 ± 2

kg = kilogram, cm = centimeters, bpm = beats per minute, RPE = rate of perceived exertion (6: no exertion to 20: maximal exertion), L = light intensity, M = moderate intensity, H = high intensity.

2.3. Intervention

The functional training intervention, performed at high intensity, has been shown to acutely enhance cognitive performance in a previous trial [17]. It consisted of 15 functional whole-body exercises performed in a circuit format with repeated 20s training bouts and 10s rest periods. At a total duration of 15 min, one workout thus had 30 exercise cycles. The selection of the exercises was based on two main goals: a) the concurrent activation of multiple major muscle groups to increase absolute oxygen consumption and b) the involvement of fundamental movement patterns mimicking activities of daily life (e.g., Squat, Lunge, Push-Up). Prior to the workout, a short general warm-up (rope skipping) was conducted.

The three exercise sessions differed with regard to exercise intensity. In FCT-H, the participants were encouraged to attain maximum workload (rather by increasing repetitions per bout than by increasing weights) while maintaining high movement quality. To facilitate the achievement of maximal workout intensity, music (140–160 beats per minute) was played [15].

In FCT-L and FCT-M, the participants performed an identical bout of functional circuit training but with light (20–39% of the heart rate reserve/HRR) and moderate (40–59% HRR) intensity, respectively [20]. To obtain HRR ($HR_{max} - HR_{rest}$), we estimated HR_{max} by means of equation 208 (0.7 × age) [21] and measured HR_{rest} using electrical heart rate monitors (Beurer PM80, Beurer GmbH, Ulm, Germany) after being inactively seated for five minutes. Appropriate intensities were met by means of (a) reducing movement velocity and (b) offering modifications of the exercises (e.g., push-up on knees, use of lighter/heavier weights, such as medicine balls or rubber bands). Additionally, in these two conditions, music was played and constant feedback regarding exercise execution was provided to create an identical environment compared to the high-intensity workout. All interventions were supervised by a trained investigator with an academic degree in Sports Science. Session order was randomized by an investigator not involved in data collection using the software package "BiAS for Windows", version 9.05 (Goethe-University Frankfurt, Frankfurt am Main, Germany).

2.4. Outcomes

Guided by the choice of tests in a previous study demonstrating CP improvements following FCT-H, we performed three assessments. The Stroop test measures aspects of attention and inhibitory control. In the word condition (S_w), participants had to read black-inked words as fast as possible. In the color condition (S_c), the same applied to naming colors. In the incongruent condition (S_{cw}), words are presented in false colors (e.g., "green" written in red or "blue" written in yellow). Here, the participants had to name the color of the word while ignoring the letters. In all three parts, time until task completion was documented. The Stroop test has been demonstrated to display high reliability (Intraclass Correlation Coefficient/ICC: 0.82) and internal consistency (Cronbach's alpha: 0.93 to 0.97) [22].

The Trail Making test (TMT) assesses attention, visual search and cognitive flexibility/working memory. In part A, disordered numbers have to be connected in ascending order using pen and paper (1 to 2 to 3 etc.). In part B, numbers and letters (e.g., 1 to a to 2 to b) were to be linked alternatingly. Similar to the Stroop test, time needed for completion was recorded. High reliability (ICC: 0.81 to 0.86) and construct validity of the TMT have been shown [23,24].

The Digit Span test has two conditions, which both measure short-term/working memory [25]. In the first, the participants need to memorize and repeat increasing amounts of numbers read to them. At the beginning, four numbers are to be recalled. In case of successful memorization, five numbers are named. For each step, two repetitions are performed, and one or zero points are awarded depending on recall success. The test ends if both trials are failed. The second condition is identical to the first, but numbers need to be repeated in reversed order (e.g., 2,4,7,9 becomes 9,7,4,2). The Digit Span test is reliable for repeated measurements (r = 0.73) [26].

Repeated assessments of cognitive function have been shown to be associated with practice effects [27]. We used two strategies to counteract this: 1) In the familiarization session, all individuals performed a series of tests until no further performance increments were noted; 2) different versions were used for each of the tests (two before and after each of the three sessions; six in total), which hence were never identical [27].

Besides cognitive performance, subjective arousal (Likert scale from "0—not activated" to "6—highly activated") and concentration (10 cm Visual Analogue Scale, 0—not concentrated at all to 10—highly concentrated) were assessed. After the interventions, the participants furthermore reported perceived exertion (6–20 RPE scale [28]) and exercise enjoyment (Likert scale from "0—not fun at all" to "6—most imaginable fun").

2.5. Data Processing and Statistics

The recruitment of the 24 participants was based on an a priori sample size calculation for a repeated measures ANOVA (F = 0.3, p = 0.05, power: 80%, drop-out 20%). Checks of sphericity (Mauchly's test) and normal distribution (Kolmogorov–Smirnov test) revealed violations of the testing assumptions and hence, data were analyzed by means of non-parametric methods. We used the Friedman test to detect differences between conditions (FCT-L vs. FCT-M vs. FCT-H). For the detection of potential pre-post changes within the respective conditions (e.g., Δ FCT-L baseline to FCT-L post), parameter-free 95% confidence intervals (CIs) were constructed. While classical CIs are based on the mean value, parameter-free CIs use the sample median and do not depend on data distribution. Their interpretation, however, is identical [29]. Calculations were made with "SPSS Statistics", version 24 (IBM, SPSS Inc., Chicago, IL, USA) and "BiAS for Windows", version 9.05 (Goethe-University Frankfurt, Germany).

3. Results

All individuals completed the study without the occurrence of dropouts. No baseline differences were found for arousal, concentration and cognitive baseline performance (p < 0.05; Table 2).

Table 2. Pre-intervention values of cognitive performance prior to the three sessions.

	Light	Moderate	High	p Value
Stroop Word (t)	25.1 (21.1/31.5)	25.8 (19.3/30.8)	25.7 (19.5/33.5)	0.72
Stroop Color (t)	36.3 (25.5/46.1)	34.6 (24.5/44.3)	35.6 (26.2/52.3)	0.13
Stroop Interference (t)	55.1 (36.9/60.2)	52.0 (39.1/65.4)	54.5 (36.7/70.7)	0.25
Trail Making Test A (t)	22.1 (15.0/44.5)	21.6 (13.0/44.5)	22.9 (13.9/60.6)	0.10
Trail Making Test B (t)	24.5 (11.1/44.8)	21.8 (12.6/47.2)	21.5 (12.5/48.2)	0.42
Digit Span Score (pts)	11.5 (5/19)	11.5 (5/20)	11.0 (5/22)	0.95

Table shows medians and range (minimum/maximum). t = time in seconds, pts = points.

Friedman tests did not reveal significant differences between the three exercise conditions (p < 0.05, Table 3). However, analysis of the 95% CIs suggested that both FCT-M (TMT-B: −11.59%, S_w: −5.8%) and FCT-H (S_c: −4.64%, S_{cw}: −11.01%), contrarily to FCT-L, increased CP from pre to post in some outcomes (Figures 1 and 2).

Table 3. Absolute pre-post differences in cognitive measures as a function of exercise.

	Light	Moderate	High
Stroop Word (t)	−0.51 (−1.57 to 0.18)	−1.22 (−2.66 to 0.05)	−1.35 (−3.9 to 4.39)
Stroop Color (t)	−1.17 (−2.87 to 0.16)	−0.28 (−2.0 to 0.78)	−1.65 (−2.81 to −0.22)
Stroop Interference (t)	−0.15 (−3.78 to 0.65)	−0.71 (−4.21 to 1.49)	−3.72 (−6.31 to −0.38)
Trail Making Test A (t)	0.11 (−4.05 to 6.09)	2.64 (−3.05 to 6.48)	−1.46 (−8.43 to 4.36)
Trail Making Test B (t)	−2.71 (−5.78 to 1.87)	−2.56 (−6.75 to −0.93)	−1.80 (−8.44 to 3.13)
Digit Span Score (pts)	0 (−2 to 1.75)	0 (−4 to 5)	−0.5 (−1 to 1.75)

Table shows medians and interquartile range. t = time in seconds, pts = points.

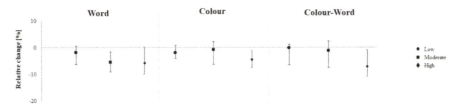

Figure 1. Pre-post differences in the Trail Making test as a function of exercise intensity. Figure shows medians and parameter-free 95% confidence intervals.

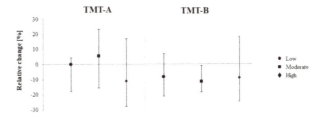

Figure 2. Pre-post differences in the Stroop test as a function of exercise intensity. Figure shows medians and parameter-free 95% confidence intervals.

4. Discussion

During the last few decades, the role of exercise intensity has been a controversial topic in studies examining the acute cognitive effects of physical activity interventions [2,4]. While a large body of evidence is available for classical regimes, such as aerobic and resistance training, our trial is the first to address this issue in FCT. Contrary to our assumptions, no between-group differences were detected for the three tested effort levels. Therefore, we suggest that exercise intensity may be central for the achievement of motor function improvements [16], but does not seem to substantially drive CP changes.

If intensity would not represent a decisive effect modifier, the question arises which factors, in addition to the often-proposed quantitative variables (e.g., intensity, training duration) are intervening [30]. In a recent trial [31], we investigated the relevance of task complexity in resistance exercise. Interestingly, participants performing free-weight training, which requires higher levels of concentration and sensory motor coordination when compared to machine-based training, achieved larger improvements in executive function. Exercises performed in functional circuit training are very similar or sometimes, although performed with smaller or no weight, even identical to those in free weight training (e.g., squats, lunges, deadlifts [15]). We therefore suggest that the improvements following HIFT may be due to the complex nature of the exercises. Experiments using functional near-infrared spectroscopy and electroencephalography support this assumption. It has been demonstrated that complex motor activities lead to stronger cortical activations and larger oxygenation changes than simple tasks [32–35]. Against this background, future studies should test the hypothesis that the engagement in HIFT or free-weight exercise is linked to more complex cortical activation patterns when compared to simple or rather monotonous activities such as machine-based resistance training or aerobic exercise (e.g., cycling).

The present study has two major clinical implications. Firstly, as mentioned, exercise professionals should tie the selection FCT intensity to the goals of the intervention. If metabolic conditioning is targeted, the probable best solution is aiming to achieve high effort levels [16]. In contrast, if cognitive improvements are wanted, intensity may be sacrificed in favor of the introduction of complex exercises requiring high attentional demand and sensorimotor control. Nevertheless, secondly, if considering the acute CP effects of FCT in isolation, moderate or high intensity levels may still be preferable over light intensities. Although we failed to reveal differences between the three disposed conditions, analysis of the 95% confidence intervals suggested that only the two higher intensities induced CP improvements.

Our study has some limitations. The small-magnitude difference between effort levels could not be detected, possibly owing to the use of non-parametric data analyses exhibiting slightly lower power than parametric methods. Furthermore, we decided not to recruit a control group because the general effectiveness of FCT-H in increasing CP had already been demonstrated and our focus was to compare different exercise intensities. As a result, it cannot be ruled out that the observed pre-post changes were practice effects originating from repeated testing, although we made a strong effort to prevent them. Finally, another issue relates to the cognitive assessments itself. Our tests mainly captured lower-order executive functions, such as inhibitory control, cognitive flexibility or working memory. It can hence not be judged if different intensities in FCT would more strongly moderate changes in higher-order executive functions, such as problem solving or planning. Future studies may therefore consider expanding or modifying the choice of tests. Another call for further research relates to the target population. We examined young active individuals. Although exercise intensity does not seem to represent a major effect modifier for CP improvements following functional circuit training here, this may be different in elderly persons or sedentary participants.

5. Conclusions

In young and active adults, exercise intensity does not affect the magnitude of CP improvements following FCT to a major degree, although moderate and high exertions may be most beneficial. Additional research further delineating the dominant factors modifying CP—i.e., brain activation patterns—is warranted.

Author Contributions: Conceptualization, J.W.; Formal analysis, J.W.; Investigation, J.W. and C.R.; Methodology, J.W.; Supervision, J.W.; Visualization, J.W.; Writing—original draft, J.W.; Writing—review & editing, J.W. and C.R. All authors have read and agreed to the published version of the manuscript.

Funding: There was no external funding.

Conflicts of Interest: The authors declare no conflict of interest.

Data Availability Statement: Data will be made available on request.

References

1. Basso, J.C.; Suzuki, W.A. The effects of acute exercise on mood, cognition, neurophysiology, and neurochemical pathways: A review. *Brain Plast.* **2017**, *2*, 127–152. [CrossRef]
2. Chang, Y.K.; Labban, J.D.; Gapin, J.I.; Etnier, J.L. The effects of acute exercise on cognitive performance: A meta-analysis. *Brain Res.* **2012**, *1453*, 87–101. [CrossRef]
3. Wilke, J.; Giesche, F.; Klier, K.; Vogt, L.; Herrmann, E.; Banzer, W. Acute effects of resistance exercise on cognitive function in healthy adults: A systematic review with multilevel meta-analysis. *Sports Med.* **2019**, *49*, 905–916. [CrossRef]
4. Brisswalter, J.; Collardeau, M.; René, A. Effects of acute physical exercise characteristics on cognitive performance. *Sports Med.* **2002**, *32*, 555–566. [CrossRef] [PubMed]
5. Northey, J.M.; Cherbuin, N.; Pumpa, K.L.; Smee, D.J.; Rattray, B. Exercise interventions for cognitive function in adults older than 50: A systematic review with meta-analysis. *Br. J. Sports Med.* **2018**, *52*, 154–160. [CrossRef]
6. Loprinzi, P.D.; Blough, J.; Crawford, L.; Ryu, S.; Zou, L.; Li, H. The Temporal Effects of Acute Exercise on Episodic Memory Function: Systematic Review with Meta-Analysis. *Brain Sci.* **2019**, *9*, 87. [CrossRef]
7. Etnier, J.L.; Salazar, W.; Landers, D.M.; Petruzzello, S.J.; Han, M.; Nowell, P. The influence of physical fitness and exercise upon cognitive functioning: A meta-analysis. *J Sport Exerc. Psychol.* **1997**, *19*, 249–277. [CrossRef]
8. Landrigan, J.; Bell, T.; Crowe, M.; Clay, O.J.; Mirman, D. Lifting cognition: A meta-analysis of effects of resistance exercise on cognition. *Psychol. Res.* **2020**, *84*, 1167–1183. [CrossRef]

9. Guadagni, V.; Drogos, L.L.; Tyndall, A.V.; Davenport, M.H.; Anderson, T.J.; Eskes, G.A.; Lognman, R.; Hill, M.D.; Hogan, D.B.; Poulin, M.J. Aerobic exercise improves cognition andcerebrovascular regulation in older adults. *Neurology* **2020**, *94*, e2245–e2257. [CrossRef]
10. Van Praag, H. Neurogenesis and exercise: Past and future directions. *Neuromol. Med.* **2008**, *10*, 128–140. [CrossRef]
11. Kennedy, G.; Hardman, R.J.; Macpherson, H.; Scholey, A.B.; Pigingas, A. How does exercise reduce the rate of age-associated cognitive decline? A review of potential mechanism. *J. Alzheimer Dis.* **2016**, *55*, 1–18. [CrossRef] [PubMed]
12. Oberste, M.; Javelle, F.; Sharma, S.; Joisten, N.; Walzik, D.; Bloch, W.; Zimmer, P. Effects and Moderators of Acute Aerobic Exercise on Subsequent Interference Control: A Systematic Review and Meta-Analysis. *Front. Psychol.* **2019**. [CrossRef]
13. McMorris, T.; Hale, B.J. Differential effects of differing intensities of acute exercise on speed and accuracy of cognition: A meta-analytical investigation. *Brain Cogn.* **2012**, *80*, 338–351. [CrossRef]
14. Thompson, W.R. worldwide survey of fitness trends for 2019. *Acsm's Health Fit. J.* **2018**, *22*, 10–17. [CrossRef]
15. Feito, Y.; Heinrich, K.M.; Butcher, S.J.; Poston, W.S.C. High-intensity functional training (HIFT): Definition and research implications for improved fitness. *Sports* **2018**, *6*, 76. [CrossRef]
16. Wilke, J.; Mohr, L. Chronic effects of high-intensity functional training on motor function: A systematic review with multilevel meta-analysis. *Sci. Rep.* **2020**. under review.
17. Wilke, J. Functional high-intensity exercise is more effective in acutely increasing working memory than aerobic walking: An exploratory randomized, controlled trial. *Sci. Rep.* **2020**, *10*. [CrossRef]
18. Schulz, K.F.; Altman, D.G.; Moher, D. CONSORT 2010 Statement: Updated guidelines for reporting parallel group randomised trials. *BMC Med.* **2010**, *8*, 18. [CrossRef] [PubMed]
19. Valdez, P.; Ramírez, C.; García, A. Circadian rhythms in cognitive performance: Implications for neuropsychological assessment. *Chronophysiol. Ther.* **2012**, *2*, 81–92. [CrossRef]
20. *ACSM's Guidelines for Exercise Testing and Prescription*, 9th ed.; Pescatello, L.S. (Ed.) Wolters Kluwer/Lippincott Williams & Wilkins: Philadelphia, PA, USA, 2014; ISBN 978-1-60913-605-5.
21. Tanaka, H.; Monahan, K.D.; Seals, D.R. Age-predicted maximal heart rate revisited. *J. Am. Coll. Cardiol.* **2001**, *37*, 153–156. [CrossRef]
22. Wöstmann, N.M.; Aichert, D.S.; Costa, A.; Rubia, K.; Möller, H.-J.; Ettinger, U. Reliability and plasticity of response inhibition and interference control. *Brain Cogn.* **2013**, *81*, 82–94. [CrossRef]
23. Wagner, S.; Helmreich, I.; Dahmen, N.; Lieb, K.; Tadic, A. Reliability of three alternate forms of the trail making tests a and B. *Arch. Clin. Neuropsychol.* **2011**, *26*, 314–321. [CrossRef]
24. Sánchez-Cubillo, I.; Periáñez, J.A.; Adrover-Roig, D.; Rodríguez-Sánchez, J.M.; Ríos-Lago, M.; Tirapu, J.; Barceló, F. Construct validity of the trail making test: Role of task-switching, working memory, inhibition/interference control, and visuomotor abilities. *J. Int. Neuropsychol. Soc.* **2009**, *15*, 438–450. [CrossRef]
25. Unsworth, N.; Engle, R.W. On the division of short-term and working memory: An examination of simple and complex span and their relation to higher order abilities. *Psychol. Bull.* **2007**, *133*, 1038–1066. [CrossRef]
26. Youngjohn, J.R.; Larrabee, G.J.; Crook, T.H. Test-retest reliability of computerized, everyday memory measures and traditional memory tests. *Clin. Neuropsychol.* **1992**, *6*, 276–286. [CrossRef]
27. Hausknecht, J.P.; Halpert, J.A.; Di Paolo, N.T.; Gerrard, M.O.M. Retesting in selection: A meta-analysis of coaching and practice effects for tests of cognitive ability. *J. Appl. Psychol.* **2007**, *92*, 373–385. [CrossRef]
28. Chen, M.J.; Fan, X.; Moe, S.T. Criterion-related validity of the Borg ratings of perceived exertion scale in healthy individuals: A meta-analysis. *J. Sports Sci.* **2002**, *20*, 873–899. [CrossRef]
29. Woodruff, R.S. Confidence Intervals for Medians and Other Position Measures. *J. Am. Stat. Ass.* **1952**, *47*, 635–646. [CrossRef]
30. Pesce, C. Shifting the focus from quantitative to qualitative exercise characteristics in exercise and cognition research. *J. Sport Exerc. Psychol.* **2012**, *34*, 766–786. [CrossRef]
31. Wilke, J.; Stricker, V.; Usedly, S. Free-weight resistance exercise is more effective in enhancing inhibitory control than machine-based training: A randomized, controlled trial. *Brain Sci.* **2020**, *10*, 702. [CrossRef]
32. Leff, D.R.; Orihuela-Espina, F.; Elwell, C.E.; Athanasiou, T.; Delpy, D.T.; Darzi, A.W.; Yang, G.-Z. Assessment of the cerebral cortex during motor task behaviours in adults: A systematic review of functional near infrared spectroscopy (fNIRS) studies. *Neuroimage* **2011**, *54*, 2922–2936. [CrossRef]

33. Holper, L.; Biallas, M.; Wolf, M. Task complexity relates to activation of cortical motor areas during uni- and bimanual performance: A functional NIRS study. *Neuroimage* **2009**, *46*, 1105–1113. [CrossRef]
34. Verstynen, T.; Diedrichsen, J.; Albert, N.; Aparicio, P.; Ivry, R.B. Ipsilateral motor cortex activity during unimanual hand movements relates to task complexity. *J. Neurophysiol.* **2005**, *93*, 1209–1222. [CrossRef]
35. Jäncke, L.; Himmelbach, M.; Shah, N.J.; Zilles, K. The effect of switching between sequential and repetitive movements on cortical activation. *Neuroimage* **2000**, *12*, 528–537. [CrossRef] [PubMed]

Publisher's Note: MDPI stays neutral with regard to jurisdictional claims in published maps and institutional affiliations.

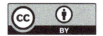

© 2020 by the authors. Licensee MDPI, Basel, Switzerland. This article is an open access article distributed under the terms and conditions of the Creative Commons Attribution (CC BY) license (http://creativecommons.org/licenses/by/4.0/).

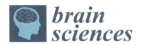

Article

Effects of Acute Aerobic Exercise Combined with Resistance Exercise on Neurocognitive Performance in Obese Women

Huei-Jhen Wen [1,2,*] and Chia-Liang Tsai [3,*]

[1] Physical Education Center, College of Education and Communication, Tzu Chi University, Hualien 97004, Taiwan
[2] Sports Medicine Center, Tzu Chi Hospital, Hualien 97004, Taiwan
[3] Institution of Physical Education, Health and Leisure Studies, National Cheng Kung University, Tainan 70101, Taiwan
* Correspondence: win@gms.tcu.edu.tw (H.-J.W.); andytsai@mail.ncku.edu.tw (C.-L.T.); Tel.: +886-3-8565-301 (ext. 1217) (H.-J.W.); +886-6-2757-575 (ext. 81809) (C.-L.T.)

Received: 7 October 2020; Accepted: 19 October 2020; Published: 22 October 2020

Abstract: To the best of the author's knowledge, there have been no previous studies conducted on the effects of a combination of acute aerobic and resistance exercise on deficit of inhibitory control in obese individuals. The aim of this study was, thus, to examine the effect of a single bout of such an exercise mode on behavioral and cognitive electrophysiological performance involving cognitive interference inhibition in obese women. After the estimated VO_2max and percentage fat (measured with dual-energy X-ray absorptiometry (Hologic, Bedford, MA, USA) were assessed, 32 sedentary obese female adults were randomly assigned to an exercise group (EG) and a control group (CG), with their behavioral performance being recorded with concomitant electrophysiological signals when performing a Stroop task. Then, the EG engaged in 30 min of moderate-intensity aerobic exercise combined with resistance exercise, and the CG rested for a similar duration of time without engaging in any type of exercise. After the interventions, the neurocognitive performance was measured again in the two groups. The results revealed that although acute exercise did not enhance the behavioral indices (e.g., accuracy rates (ARs) and reaction times (RTs)), cognitive electrophysiological signals were improved (e.g., shorter N2 and P3 latencies, smaller N2 amplitudes, and greater P3 amplitudes) in the Stroop task after the exercise intervention in the EG. The findings indicated that a combination of acute moderate-intensity aerobic and resistance exercise may improve the neurophysiological inhibitory control performance of obese women.

Keywords: obesity; inhibitory control; event-related potential; aerobic exercise; resistance exercise

1. Introduction

Obesity is considered to be an immunodeficient, chronic inflammation state, which may contribute to an increased risk of premature death [1]. This chronic disease has been associated not only with increases in non-communicative diseases (e.g., type II diabetes, hypertension), but also with reduced brain volume (e.g., frontal cortex and anterior cingulate cortex) and impaired neurocognitive outcomes (e.g., frontal-lobe-based executive functions) [2]. In particular, attentional inhibition and inhibitory control are cognitive domains that are affected negatively by obesity [3–5], reflecting a deficit in the neural networks within the anterior cingulate or prefrontal cortex [6,7].

Acute exercise is defined as a single bout of exercise lasting from a few seconds to as long as several hours [8]. Acute exercise can enhance a wide range of cognitive performance, including basic information processing, attention, crystallized intelligence, and executive functions [9,10].

Acute exercise has also been shown to be associated with improvements in the inhibition process [11], a subcomponent of executive functions modulated by the dorsolateral prefrontal cortex, which is known to be particularly affected by exercise [12] in healthy children and adults [13,14].

In addition, a comparison of lean individuals with obese individuals indicated that acute exercise leads to decreased neural responses to food cues compared with non-food cues, suggesting different effects of exercise on the neural processing of food cues based on weight status [15]. Quintero et al. (2018) also found that, compared to an acute bout of progressive resistance exercise (PRE), both acute high-intensity aerobic interval exercise (HIIE) and PRE + HIIE interventions significantly enhance behavioral performance on cognitive inhibition and attention capacity in overweight inactive male adults when performing the Stroop test and d2 test of attention [16]. However, by contrast, Tomporowski et al. (2008) reported that a 23-min bout of treadmill walking did not influence error rates and global switch cost scores in overweight children when performing a task-switching task [17]. Also, one study found no reliable improvements in executive functions (e.g., Stroop and Go/nogo tasks) after a 30-min bout of moderate-intensity aerobic exercise among adults with co-morbid overweight/obesity and type 2 diabetes [18]. However, female participants and those who were more physically active showed reduced Stroop interference scores following moderate exercise [18]. Accordingly, the effects of acute exercise on cognitive performance are still inconsistent in overweight/obese event-related potential (ERP), and age- and gender-related differences may exist in this population [16–18]. Additionally, although a previous study reported the beneficial effects of acute aerobic exercise on behavioral cognitive control in overweight inactive male adults [16], whether acute exercise affects behavior and, especially, neurophysiological (e.g., ERP) signals involving attentional and inhibitory control in obese female adults is still worthy of further investigation.

Electroencephalographic signals can provide insights into the effects of exercise on cognition [19,20]. The ERP components of the brain have been demonstrated to be selective in terms of differentiating cognitive electrophysiological performance in obese and normal-weight individuals [5]. Previous studies have reported deviant behavioral (e.g., slower reaction times (RTs)) and ERP performance (e.g., longer N2 and P3 latencies and smaller P3 amplitudes) in obese individuals when they are performing various cognitive tasks involving attentional inhibition and inhibitory control [3–5]. Since the Stroop task involves a complex cognitive interference inhibition process, and female adults suffering from obesity show deficits in such underlying neural systems [5], this type of cognitive task was used to assess the effects of an acute exercise intervention on inhibitory control [5,19] in obese female adults in the present study.

According to the American College of Sports Medicine (ACSM), appropriate physical activity intervention strategies for weight loss are recommended for a minimum of 150 min per week comprising moderate-intensity aerobic exercise combined with resistance exercise for overweight and obese adults to improve their health [21]. Accumulating evidence supports the positive influence of acute aerobic exercise on attentional control/inhibitory control in healthy individuals [12–14,22,23]. In addition, some studies have proven that neurocognitive performance can be enhanced via acute and chronic resistance exercise [10,24–26]. A combination of aerobic and resistance exercise has also been proven to be beneficial to cognitive functions in patients with stroke [27] and dementia [28], as well as in overweight inactive adult men [16]. This type of exercise mode has even been found to have stronger effects on executive functions (i.e., inhibition, impulse control, planning, and set-shifting) in in adolescents [29], in healthy sedentary adults [30], and older adults [31] as compared to an aerobic exercise program alone since a combined aerobic and resistance exercise program can simultaneously positively increase the levels of brain-derived neurotrophic factors [14,23,25,32] and insulin-like growth factor-1 [10,25,26,32]. In addition, resistance exercise may improve cognitive functions specifically through lowering the levels of neurotoxic homocysteine [26,31]. Therefore, moderate-intensity aerobic exercise combined with resistance exercise may be a potential effective exercise mode, as suggested by the ACSM that can be used to improve neurocognitive problems related to inhibitory control in obese individuals.

Obesity is caused by a number of multidimensional factors [33] and results in deficits in neural circuits related to inhibitory control [4,7,22,34]. Obese adults have been shown to obtain advantages related to neurocognitive performance through engaging in regular exercise as compared to obese individuals with a sedentary lifestyle [35], suggesting that obesity does not preclude benefits derived from physical exercise and cardiorespiratory fitness to cognitive functions and neural networks. Although a number of studies have reported that a combination of aerobic and resistance exercise mode may effectively improve cognitive behavioral performance in overweight inactive male adults [16] and in patients with stroke [27] and dementia [28], thus far, a paucity of data exist on the possible additive effects of an acute bout combining these two exercise modes on behavioral and cognitive electrophysiological performance involving inhibitory control in obese female individuals. Therefore, the purpose of the current study was to investigate the potential effects of acute aerobic exercise coupled with resistance exercise on neurocognitive performance related to cognitive interference inhibition in sedentary obese women when performing the Stroop task. Based on the previous findings mentioned above, we hypothesized that an acute bout of a program combining aerobic exercise and resistance exercise is a feasible and effective intervention that can improve cognitive deficits in obese female individuals.

2. Materials and Methods

2.1. Ethical Approval

This research meets the standards set by terms of the Declaration of Helsinki. All protocols in this study were approved by the Research Ethics Committee at Hualien Tzu Chi Hospital, Hualien, Taiwan (IRB105-61-A). The participants were freely to withdraw their consent at any time during the course of the study without any reason.

2.2. Participants

An experiment procedure of the Consolidated Standards of Reporting Trials (CONSORT) outlining the number of participants for the present study is shown in Figure 1. This study was broadcasted on a local radio station and also advertised in a local newspaper in Hualien County, Taiwan. Based on the criteria for obesity established by the Western Pacific Regional Office of the World Health Organization for Asian populations according to related mortality and morbidity risks [36,37], females with body mass index (BMI) > 25.0 kg/m^2 were recruited as participants in the present study. Additional inclusion standards were (a) right-handed, as assessed by the Edinburgh Handedness Inventory using the arbitrary cut-off points between 0 to ±60 [38,39], (b) non-smokers, (c) normal or corrected-to-normal vision, (d) no symptoms of depression as measured by the Beck depression inventory II (BDI-II; all scored below 13) [40], (e) cognitive integrity measured by the Mini-Mental State Examination (MMSE; all scored above 24) [41].

According to these criteria, and after determining a priori power for a repeated measures analysis of variance (RM-ANOVA) using G-Power 3.1, the minimum sample size of ~16 participants for each group was required to reach a power of 80% and moderate effect sizes [42]. Fifty women from the community in Hualien City were interested in participating in the study. Eighteen were excluded because of not meeting the criteria or declined to participate after hearing a detailed explanation of the protocol. Eligible participants were self-reported to be free of metabolic or cardiovascular diseases, neurological, or psychiatric disorders and professed to be free of a history of brain injury, or medication intake that would influence central nervous system (CNS) functioning. Thirty-two eligible healthy women with obesity were then randomized to an exercise group (EG) or a control group (CG). The demographic characteristics data for the two groups are provided in Table 1.

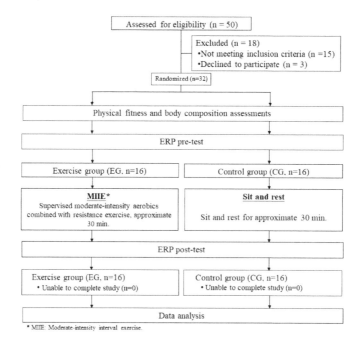

Figure 1. Schematic representation of experimental procedure.

Table 1. Demographic characteristics of the obese participants.

Characteristics	Exercise Group (*n* = 16)	Control Group (*n* = 16)	*t*	*p* Value
Age (years)	33.13 ± 6.27	32.92 ± 7.17	0.09	0.930
Height (cm)	160.72 ± 4.21	159.21 ± 5.69	0.86	0.400
Weight (kg)	79.82 ± 11.57	79.14 ± 18.10	0.13	0.900
BMI (kg/m^2)	30.83 ± 3.61	31.07 ± 6.08	−0.14	0.891
SBP (mmHg)	116.73 ± 11.37	110.19 ± 14.46	1.40	0.174
DBP (mmHg)	77.20 ± 8.11	73.50 ± 9.99	1.13	0.269
Resting HR (bpm)	74.53 ± 8.67	75.69 ± 6.03	−0.43	0.668
Estimated VO$_2$max	24.53 ± 4.88	24.66 ± 4.74	−0.07	0.943
Strength of leg extension (kg)	33.21 ± 9.74	35.81 ± 8.65	−0.79	0.438
BDI-II	6.25 ± 2.83	6.88 ± 2.94	−0.61	0.545
MMSE	29.44 ± 0.89	29.13 ± 0.83	0.98	0.336
PA energy expenditure (MET/day)	36.02 ± 13.18	32.34 ± 7.74	0.96	0.356
PA energy expenditure (kcal/day)	2522.19 ± 695.04	2652.49 ± 706.39	−0.49	0.631
Dietary (kcal/day)	2081.59 ± 579.98	1905.10 ± 558.73	0.82	0.420
Circumference				
Waist (cm)	91.81 ± 11.28	92.52 ± 17.19	−0.14	0.893
Abdominal (cm)	100.35 ± 11.85	102.84 ± 18.45	−0.45	0.660
Hip (cm)	113.64 ± 6.75	113.14 ± 14.59	0.12	0.905
Waist-Hip Ratio	0.81 ± 0.06	0.81 ± 0.06	−0.40	0.693
Percentage fat				
Whole body (%)	41.43 ± 3.89	44.12 ± 4.34	−1.85	0.075
Upper limbs (%)	48.71 ± 5.51	45.56 ± 3.92	1.86	0.073
Trunk (%)	42.23 ± 4.51	45.24 ± 5.38	−1.72	0.097
Lower limb (%)	41.40 ± 4.54	42.12 ± 4.25	−0.46	0.649

BMI, body mass index; SBP: systolic blood pressure; DBP: diastolic blood pressure; HR: heart rate; bpm: beat per minute; BDI, Beck Depression Inventory; MMSE, Mini-Mental State Examination; and PA, physical activity. Values are means ± SD.

2.3. Experimental Procedure

All participants visited the study site twice. At the first visit, dual-energy X-ray absorptiometry (DXA) and physical fitness tests (2 km walk test and submaximal leg extension strength test) were scheduled to respectively assess the body composition and cardiovascular/muscular fitness of the participants at Tzu Chi Hospital (Hualien, Taiwan) and the cognitive neurophysiology laboratory at Tzu Chi University (Hualien, Taiwan).

Each participant had a 2nd visit at approximately 7:50–08:30 AM in the same week. All participants were asked to refrain from caffeine or alcohol intake and strenuous exercise for 24 h. The research assistant explained the experimental procedure to each participant and then asked her to complete an informed consent form, a medical history, a handedness inventory, a demographic questionnaire, the MMSE, and the BDI-II. After completing all of the questionnaires, each participant sat comfortably 80 cm in front of a laptop screen in a semi-dark room. An electrocap and electro-oculographic (EOG) electrodes were then attached to the scalp and face of each participant prior to the cognitive tests. After some practice trials, a simultaneous formal cognitive task test with concomitant electrophysiological recording was performed. Then, the participants in the EG performed a single 30-min bout comprising a combination of moderate-intensity physical exercises (please see the detailed protocols in Section 2.4.). After engaging in acute exercise and after the participants' heart rate (HR) had returned to within 10% of pre-exercise levels (mean 28.4 ± 10.8 min), they completed the cognitive task along with ERP recording again. In the CG, the participants were instructed to sit quietly for 30 min, after which they took the cognitive task test again.

2.4. Exercise Intervention

The participants in the EG were taught to determine their target exercise HR, and HR was monitored throughout the exercise session using a telemetry HR monitor (S810, Polar, Kempele, Finland).

Target exercise HR = [(220−age)−HR rest] × 50% + HR rest

The exercise was held in the laboratory. The exercise program (see Figure 2) consisted of a 3–5 min warm-up session, 30-min of supervised moderate-intensity aerobic dance (i.e., corresponding to 55% of the individual target HR reserve (HRR) alternately combined with dumbbell resistance exercises specifically designed for this study, followed by a 3–5 min cool-down session.

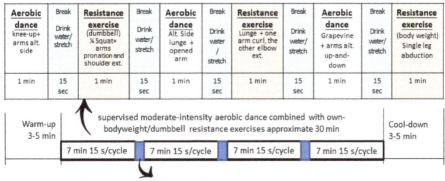

The next cycle would be started from a break between cycles when the HR arrived 50% HRR of individual's target HR.

Figure 2. A single bout of exercise intervention.

The exercises involved 4 cycles accompanied with music at 126 beats per min. The next cycle was started after a break between cycles when the HR reached the 50% HRR of the individual's target HR. There were 6 sets of aerobic dance and resistance exercises alternating in each cycle in 1 min sets following a 15 s break to drink water and stretch. Approximately 12–16 repetitions per set of six dumbbell/bodyweight resistance exercises targeting the major muscle groups were carried out at moderate intensity [43]. The repetition velocity of each resistance training movement was set to: shoulder extension with arm pronation (8.4 s of slow motion to 2.1 s of normal pace), arm curl (4.2 s of slow motion to 2.1 s of normal pace), and elbow extension (8.4 of slow motion to 2.1 s seconds of normal pace). One set in each session was supervised and led by a trained instructor. The instructor led participants through a full range of motion for each movement, which expended between 350 and 500 kcal according to the participant's weight. The investigator provided verbal encouragement throughout the exercise period. The average intensity of all participants in the EG was 60.05 ± 3.57% HRR when they performed the aerobic exercise.

2.5. Whole and Regional Body Composition

Body composition was measured using DXA (Discovery Wi, Hologic Inc., Bedford, MA, USA). The measurement was performed by a certified technician according to the standard operating procedure. The scanning instructions and procedures were standardized for all participants. The trunk region included the area from the bottom of the neckline to the top of the pelvis, excluding the arms. The mass output from the DXA scanner was expressed in grams. Each testing day, the accuracy of the densitometer was calibrated using the manufacturer's spine phantom with a known hydroxyapatite density.

2.6. Cognitive Task- Stroop Task

A two-choice Stroop task inducing inhibitory control effects of executive functions in both young and older adults [44] programmed using E-prime (Psychology Software Tools, Sharpsburg, PA, USA) was adopted in the current study. Because semantics interferes significantly with the naming of colors [45], and color interferes very little with reading words [46,47], the color-naming condition was used to investigate the effect of acute exercise on neurocognitive functioning associated with cognitive interference inhibition in obese women. The stimuli, two color names in Chinese presented as 4.5 × 4.5 cm letters in "紅" (red) and "綠" (green), were displayed in the center of a 21-in. cathode-ray tube against a black background at viewing distance of 80-cm. In the congruent condition, the meaning of the word matched its color, whereas the color of the word was different from its word meaning in the congruent condition. A single test block consisted of an equal number of both incongruent and congruent trials in a randomized order. A total of 240 trials were divided into two blocks of 120 trials, with a rest period of 2 min between blocks. Each stimulus appeared on the screen until the participant responded, and the next stimulus appeared 1.5 to 2 s after the response. The participants were asked to press the computer keyboard as accurately and quickly as possible in response to the color while ignoring the word meaning. The stimulus response pairs were counterbalanced across participants. All participants performed the Stroop task along with simultaneous cognitive electrophysiological recording. After a practice block of 10 trials to ensure that the participants understood the task rules, the formal test was administered to allow for data collection of neurocognitive performance.

2.7. Event-Related Potential (ERP) Recording and Analysis

Brain electrical activity was recorded using the eegoTM amplifier system (ANT Neuro, EE-211, revision Nr 1.2, Berlin, Germany) from 64 scalp sites (10–10 system) with Ag/AgCl electrodes mounted in an elastic cap. The raw electroencephalography (EEG) signal was acquired at an A/D rate of 500 Hz/channel using a 60-Hz notch filter and a 0.1–50 Hz band-pass filter. All inter-electrode impedance was kept below 5 KΩ. Prior to averaging the ERP components, an offline electrooculographic correction was applied to the individual trials. All trials with artefacts (i.e., electromyogram and electrooculogram readings exceeding ± 100 µV) and response errors were eliminated. The remaining effective ERP data in the Stroop task were separately averaged offline and constructed from congruent and incongruent conditions over a 1000 ms epoch beginning 200 ms before the onset of the target stimulus. The mean latencies and amplitudes of the P2, N2, and P3 components were measured for the Fz and Cz electrodes [48]. The time windows for detection of the P2, N2, and P3 components were 150–275 ms, 200–400 ms [49], and 300–800 ms [50,51], respectively. Latency was defined as the time at which the peak amplitude was reached within the latency window for every participant and was calculated as the time in milliseconds.

2.8. Data Processing and Statistical Analyses

The behavioral performance in the Stroop task was assessed with the accuracy rates (ARs) (%) and RTs (milliseconds) to each target presentation automatically calculated by the E-prime software (Psychology software tool, Pittsburgh, PA, USA). Responses later than 1500 ms and sooner than 200 ms after target onset were excluded in both the congruent and incongruent conditions.

Descriptive statistics are presented for the basic demographic characteristics of the participants. For the behavioral analyses (i.e., ARs and RTs) and cognitive electrophysiological (i.e., P2, N2, and P3 latencies and amplitudes), all of the independent variables were analyzed with a two-way repeated measures analysis of variance (RM-ANOVA) (i.e., **Group** (EG vs. CG) × **Time** (pre- vs. post-test) × **Condition** (congruent vs. incongruent) × **Electrode** (Fz vs. Cz)). If the assumption of sphericity was violated, analyses employing the Greenhouse–Geisser correction with three or more within-subject levels were conducted. Where a significant difference occurred, Bonferroni *post-hoc* analyses were performed. Partial Eta squared (η_p^2) was used to calculate the effect sizes of significant main effects and interactions, with the following standard used to determine the magnitude: <0.08 (small effect size), between 0.08 and 0.14 (medium effect size), and >0.14 (large effect size). A *p*-value < 0.05 was accepted as statistically significant.

3. Results

3.1. Demographic Data

As shown in Table 1, there were no significant between-group differences in the weight and circumference measures (e.g., BMI, waist girth, abdominal girth, and hip girth), body composition status, estimated VO_2max, and blood pressure (e.g., systolic blood pressure (SBP) and diastolic blood pressure (DBP)). In addition, no significant differences were found in the values for the other demographic measures.

3.2. Behavioral Performance of Stroop Task

The pre- and post-test behavioral performance of the EG and CG groups are shown in Figure 3.

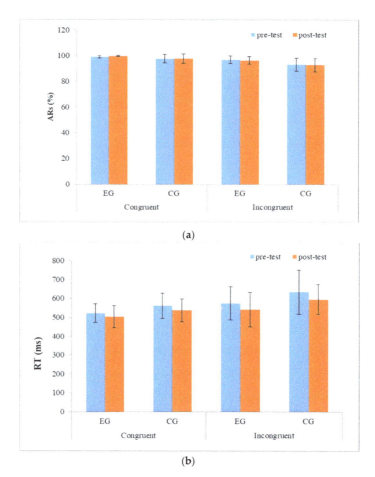

Figure 3. Behavioral performance (**a**) accuracy rates (ARs) (%) and (**b**) reaction times (RTs, ms) on the Stroop task in the exercise group (EG) and control group (CG) pre- and post-test.

- Accuracy rate (AR)

The RM-ANOVA for the ARs showed significant main effects of ***Group*** [$F_{(1,30)}$ = 7.17, p = 0.013, η_p^2 = 0.22] and ***Condition*** [$F_{(1,30)}$ = 57.38, p < 0.001, η_p^2 = 0.69], with the ARs in the EG (98.06 ± 1.45%) being significantly higher than those in the CG (95.31 ± 3.78%) across two time points and two electrodes, and with the ARs being significantly higher in the congruent condition (98.70 ± 2.04%) as compared to those in the incongruent condition (95.07 ± 4.18%). Neither a significant main effect of ***Time***, nor significant interactions between ***Time***, ***Group***, and ***Condition*** were found.

- Reaction time (RT)

The RM-ANOVA for the RTs showed significant main effects of ***Time*** [$F_{(1,30)}$ = 12.30, p = 0.002, η_p^2 = 0.31] and ***Condition*** [$F_{(1,30)}$ = 40.80, p < 0.001, η_p^2 = 0.59], with the RTs being significantly faster in the post-test (543.04 ± 72.49 ms) than in the pre-test (571.40 ± 80.90 ms) across both groups and two conditions, with the RTs being significantly faster in the congruent condition (530.05 ± 56.38 ms) as compared to in the incongruent condition (584.40 ± 93.72 ms). Neither a significant main effect of ***Group*** nor significant interactions between ***Time***, ***Group***, and ***Condition*** were found.

3.3. Electrophysiological Performance

Figure 4 displays the grand-average ERP waveforms for the two midline electrodes pre- and post-test in the two groups when performing the Stroop task.

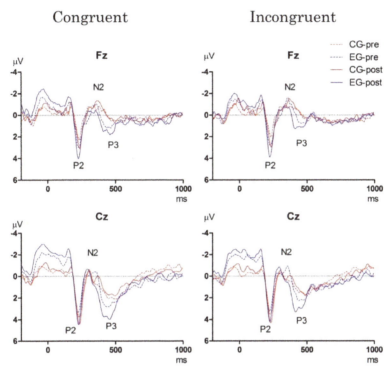

Figure 4. Grand averaged event-related potentials (ERPs) of P2, N2, and P3 waveforms in the congruent and incongruent conditions in two electrodes (Fz and Cz) for the exercise group (EG) and control group (CG) pre- and post-test when performing the Stroop task.

- P2 component

The RM-ANOVA for the P2 latency revealed neither main effects of *Time* and *Group* nor significant interactions among *Group*, *Time*, *Condition*, or *Electrode*.

The RM-ANOVA for the P2 amplitude showed that there was a significant main effect of *Time* [$F_{(1,30)} = 47.71$, $p < 0.001$, $\eta_p^2 = 0.61$], with the P2 amplitude being significantly greater in the post-test (3.91 ± 0.68 µV) than in the pre-test (2.97 ± 0.52 µV) across both groups for two conditions and two electrodes. No significant interactions of *Group*, *Time*, *Condition*, or *Electrode* were found.

- N2 component

The RM-ANOVA for the N2 latency showed significant main effects of *Time* [$F_{(1,30)} = 8.26$, $p = 0.007$, $\eta_p^2 = 0.22$] and *Condition* [$F_{(1,30)} = 14.94$, $p = 0.001$, $\eta_p^2 = 0.33$], where the N2 latency in post-test (260.09 ± 68.69 ms) was shorter than in the pre-test (269.78 ± 72.69 ms) across both groups for two conditions and two electrodes, and where the N2 latency in the congruent condition (264.08 ± 69.23 ms) was shorter than that in the incongruent condition (265.80 ± 69.86 ms) across both groups, two time points, and two electrodes. These main effects were superseded by significant interactions of *Group* × *Time* [$F_{(1,30)} = 26.65$, $p < 0.001$, $\eta_p^2 = 0.47$] and *Group* × *Time* × *Condition* [$F_{(1,30)} = 7.19$, $p = 0.012$, $\eta_p^2 = 0.19$]. The *post-hoc* analyses revealed that, when compared to the pre-test, the N2 latency in the EG was significantly shorter post-test in both the congruent (pre- vs.

post-test: 277.19 ± 78.97 ms vs. 249.25 ± 64.51 ms, $p < 0.001$) and incongruent (pre- vs. post-test: 278.84 ± 79.36 ms vs. 253.94 ± 67.47 ms, $p < 0.001$) conditions. In contrast, the N2 latency was significantly longer post-test relative to pre-test in the CG in the congruent condition (pre- vs. post-test: 260.25 ± 66.86 ms vs. 268.13 ± 72.45 ms, $p = 0.025$).

In terms of N2 amplitude, there was a significant main effect of **Condition** [$F_{(1,30)} = 33.14$, $p < 0.001$, $\eta_p^2 = 0.53$], with the N2 amplitude being significantly smaller in the incongruent condition (−0.94 ± 0.23 μV) as compared to in the congruent condition (−0.72 ± 0.16 μV) across two time points, two groups, and two electrodes. These main effects were superseded by significant interactions of **Group × Time** [$F_{(1,30)} = 96.18$, $p < 0.001$, $\eta_p^2 = 0.76$] and **Group × Time × Condition** [$F_{(1,30)} = 5.92$, $p = 0.021$, $\eta_p^2 = 0.17$]. The *post-hoc* analyses revealed that, when compared to the pre-test, the N2 amplitude in the EG was significantly smaller post-test in both the congruent (pre- vs. post-test: −0.72 ± 0.16 μV vs. −0.52 ± 0.09 μV, $p < 0.001$) and incongruent (pre- vs. post-test: −1.26 ± 0.26 μV vs. −0.90 ± 0.25 μV, $p < 0.001$) conditions. No change was found in the CG for either condition pre- and post-test.

- P3 component

The RM-ANOVA for the P3 latency revealed a significant main effect of **Condition** [$F_{(1,30)} = 9.23$, $p = 0.005$, $\eta_p^2 = 0.24$], with the P3 latency being significantly shorter in the congruent condition (450.39 ± 133.59 ms) as compared to in the incongruent condition (463.67 ± 133.45 ms, $p = 0.019$) across the two time points, the two groups, and two electrodes. The interaction of **Group × Time** [$F_{(1,30)} = 8.55$, $p = 0.007$, $\eta_p^2 = 0.22$] was also significant. The *post-hoc* analyses revealed that the P3 latency was significantly shorter post-test compared to in the pre-test only in the EG (pre- vs. post-test: 445.31 ± 128.27 ms vs. 421.88 ± 126.59 ms, $p = 0.002$) across two conditions and two electrodes.

The RM-ANOVA for the P3 amplitude revealed significant main effects of **Time** [$F_{(1,30)} = 14.32$, $p = 0.001$, $\eta_p^2 = 0.32$], **Group** [$F_{(1,30)} = 58.08$, $p < 0.001$, $\eta_p^2 = 0.66$], **Condition** [$F_{(1,30)} = 45.12$, $p < 0.001$, $\eta_p^2 = 0.60$], and **Electrode** [$F_{(1,30)} = 543.94$, $p < 0.001$, $\eta_p^2 = 0.95$], with the P3 amplitude being significantly greater in the post-test (1.79 ± 0.89 μV) than in the pre-test (1.51 ± 0.40 μV) across both groups, two conditions, and two electrodes, with the P3 amplitude being significantly greater in the EG (1.78 ± 0.32 μV) than in the CG (1.25 ± 0.28 μV) across two time points, two conditions, and two electrodes, with greater P3 amplitudes shown in the congruent condition (1.83 ± 0.69 μV) than in incongruent condition (1.48 ± 0.57 μV) across the two groups, two time points, and two electrodes, and with greater P3 amplitudes being observed at the Cz site (2.24 ± 0.57 μV) than at the Fz site (0.79 ± 0.38 μV) across the two groups, two time points, and two conditions. The interaction of **Group × Time** [$F_{(1,30)} = 37.63$, $p < 0.001$, $\eta_p^2 = 0.63$] was also significant. The *post-hoc* analyses revealed that the P3 amplitude was significantly larger at post-test as compared to pre-test in the EG (pre- vs. post-test: 1.78 ± 0.32 μV vs. 2.51 ± 0.64 μV, $p < 0.001$) across two conditions and two electrodes.

4. Discussion

To the best of our knowledge, this is the first study to investigate the effects of an acute intervention combining aerobic exercise and resistance exercise on behavioral and cognitive electrophysiological performance related to inhibitory control deficits in female adults with obesity. The main findings indicated that, although a single bout of acute aerobic-and-resistance exercise did not improve behavioral performance (e.g., ARs and RTs) in the obese women when performing the Stroop task, beneficial effects on the cognitive electrophysiological signals (e.g., shorter N2 and P3 latencies, smaller N2 amplitudes, and greater P3 amplitudes) were induced through this exercise mode intervention in the EG. In contrast, after a 30-min sitting rest, significantly slower N2 latency in the congruent condition was observed in the CG.

4.1. Behavior Performance

In the present study, acute aerobic-and-resistance exercise did not produce a significant behavioral (e.g., ARs and RTs) improvement in the Stroop test performance in the obese women, suggesting that the acute exercise intervention did not facilitate specific effects on the response inhibition/interference in this group. Previous studies have demonstrated that cognitive performance reflecting Stroop interference as measured by RTs improves significantly following an acute bout of either moderate-intensity aerobic exercise [12,52] or resistance exercise [53]. Quintero et al. [16] also found that acute aerobic HIIE and PRE + HIIE exercise interventions induce behavioral enhancements in cognitive inhibition in overweight inactive male adults when performing the Stroop test. In addition, overweight/obese female adults with type 2 diabetes showed reduced Stroop interference scores following an acute bout of moderate-intensity aerobic exercise [18]. The present results partly concurred with earlier studies investigating the effects of acute exercise on cognitive performance in older adults [54] or in obese groups [17,18]. For example, Vincent et al. [18] indicated that there was no significant effect of moderate-intensity acute aerobic exercise on Stroop performance among young overweight/obese adults or young adults with type II diabetes. Also, Tomporowski et al. [17] found that an acute bout of aerobic exercise did not improve error rates in overweight children when performing a task-switching task. In this study, no relationship was observed between acute exercise and behavioral performance in the obese participants. One plausible reason for the present finding could be that obese individuals with a sedentary lifestyle often exhibit worse VO_{2max} [7,35], and previous studies have suggested that cardiorespiratory fitness, but not acute exercise, could be an important factor modulating cognitive performance [55,56]. This conjecture is somewhat speculative, but provides a basis for future research.

4.2. Cognitive Electrophysiological Performances

An EEG is ideal for capturing the rapid brain neural processes involved in perceptual processing, which requires attention allocation for subsequent inhibitory success (e.g., ERP P2 component) [57–59] and inhibitory control (e.g., ERP N2 and P3 components) [50,51]. In spite of a lack of behavioral improvement in obese women induced by the acute aerobic-and-resistance exercise intervention when performing the Stroop task in the present study, beneficial effects on cognitive electrophysiological signals as measured by brain ERPs were observed in this study. Indeed, increased Stroop interference-related activation in the dorsolateral prefrontal cortices due to an acute bout of a combination of aerobic and resistance exercise was reported in healthy young adults [48]. Although the ERP P2 component is extremely sensitive to arousal levels [60,61], P2 latency and amplitude were not significantly improved after an exercise intervention in the EG in the present study. However, significant effects of acute moderate-intensity exercise on the modulation of the two inhibition-related ERP components (e.g., N2 and P3) were observed. The N2 component, the frontocentral early negative deflection occurring around 200–400 ms post-stimulus, is mainly related to early modality specific inhibition and conflict monitoring processes [49–51]. Drollette et al. [62] found smaller N2 amplitudes induced by acute exercise only for individuals with lower inhibitory capacity but not among those with higher capacity [63,64]. Increased adiposity has been linked with poorer inhibitory control abilities [4,5,7,35]. Although some studies examining the effects of acute exercise on executive function using a neurophysiological approach failed to observe alterations in N2 amplitude after acute aerobic exercise [9,55], the results of the present study showed that the decreased N2 amplitude following acute exercise in the EG was in line with the previous findings [62,65], implying that 30-min of supervised moderate-intensity aerobic dance combined with resistance exercise could enhance response inhibition associated with conflict monitoring [66] in obese women. Concurrently, the EG exhibited shorter N2 latencies after the exercise intervention as compared to the baseline whereas the CG exhibited significantly longer N2 latency in the congruent condition after a 30-min sit-and-rest. The findings suggested that acute exercise may produce more efficient neural processing involving the detection of a response inhibition process/conflict [67] in obese individuals.

The ERP P3 component, a positive component occurring around 300–800 ms post-stimulus, is typically associated with late general inhibition [50,51] and attentional resource allocation [68,69]. Several experimental studies have generally demonstrated increased amplitude and shortened latency of P3 components in relation to cognitive electrophysiological improvements caused by an acute bout of exercise [70–72]. Compatible with many reports of shorter P3 latency and larger P3 amplitude found after acute moderate-intensity aerobic exercise in healthy preadolescent children [62] and young adults [9,70] when performing the Flanker task and the Stroop task, respectively, similar improvements in cognitive electrophysiological signals were also observed following acute aerobic exercise combined with resistance exercise in the obese women in this study. The present findings suggest that faster cognitive processing to detect and process a stimulus in the environment [73] and more attentional resources allocated to process late general inhibition can be induced following acute exercise in obese individuals. Similarly, improvements in inhibition as assessed by the ERP P3 component of the cognitive tasks (e.g., task-switching, visuospatial attention task, and the Flanker task) following acute aerobic and resistance exercise interventions have also been reported in young [14,23,48] and older adults [10] as well as in individuals with developmental coordination disorders [9] and mild cognitive impairment [25], suggesting that acute exercise has a greater influence on cognitive functions involving diverse inhibitory control demands.

In terms of cognitive electrophysiological signals involved in inhibitory control, obese individuals have been demonstrated to show deviant ERP performance when performing the Stroop task [5]. Many empirical studies have reported that an acute bout of moderate-intensity aerobic exercise may elicit improved brain neuroelectric inhibition indices [9,10,23,25,48]. In addition, it has been observed that a single bout of acute resistance exercise effectively enhances cognition [74,75], but not many studies have so far examined the underlying electrophysiological processes, and the available findings are relatively heterogeneous [10,48]. According to the ACSM, moderate-intensity aerobic combined with resistance exercise for weight loss in overweight and obese adults is recommended for a minimum of 150 min each week to improve health [25]. However, among inactive and overweight/obese adults, increased exercise intensity appears to have a negative effect on affective responses [76]. Indeed, it has been reported that moderate-intensity exercise improves cognitive performance and increases prefrontal oxygenation to a greater extent [77]. Furthermore, it has been proposed that the relationship between acute exercise and cognitive performance follows an inverted U-shape [78]. However, it has to be acknowledged that this is not a universal finding since this relationship is influenced by several mediators (e.g., exercise intensity, time between exercise cessation, and cognitive testing) [79,80]. In the present study, we found that a 30-min bout of supervised moderate-intensity aerobic combined with resistance exercise program may have been effective in terms of improving cognitive interference inhibition in the obese female adults when they performed the Stroop task. Accordingly, the exercise prescription adopted in the present study seems to be feasible not only to lose weight but also to remedy the deficits of inhibitory control in such a group.

4.3. Limitations

The effect of exercise on the development of dietary obesity is different in males and females [81], and the adverse effects of obesity on neurocognitive functioning/performance are sex-specific [82]. Gender plays a significant role in pathophysiological changes and clinical manifestations due to a crucial effect of sex hormones on neurohumoral adipose tissue activity [83]. In addition, adiposity-related indices (e.g., body fat % and BMI) and low-grade systemic inflammation are considerably stronger in women than in men [84–86]. Weight reduction as a means to prevent a state of subclinical inflammation may be particularly effective in women [86]. Since inflammatory cytokines (e.g., TNF-α and C-reactive protein) were found to be significantly correlated with cognitive electrophysiological signals (e.g., ERP N2 and P3) in the obese group [7,35], an avenue for future research would be to examine the possibility of interactions among acute exercise, biochemical markers, and neurocognitive performance in both sexes. Additionally, although acute exercise can temporarily improve cognitive performance through arousal, the biochemical indicators that can actually promote the proliferation of brain neurons still cannot be effectively improved in a static state [23,25]. The most important way to improve neurocognitive performance and biochemical indices is to engage in long-term, regular physical exercise [24,26]. Also, a cross-sectional study indicated that, as compared to obese male adults with a sedentary lifestyle, obese individuals engaging in regular exercise can still obtain advantages with regard to neurocognitive performance [35]. Accordingly, further long-term regular exercise interventional studies are needed to understand the neurocognitive benefits for obese sedentary women.

5. Conclusions

This is the first study to investigate the effects of an acute exercise modality combining aerobic and resistance exercise on neurophysiological (i.e., behavioral and cognitive electrophysiological) performance among obese women. We found that brain neural processing related to early and late inhibition (e.g., ERP N2 and P3) were improved by the proposed exercise mode in obese female adults although behavioral benefits were not observed. Given that Stroop task performance may be related to cognitive interference inhibition, the present findings imply that the executive control networks and the efficiency of inhibitory control seem to remediable through an exercise intervention in obese individuals. However, the beneficial effects derived from the present findings through acute exercise and neurocognitive performance are temporary. Regular exercise has been demonstrated to effectively reduce the basal levels of inflammatory cytokines and compromised neural activity in obese individuals [35]. Further research is recommended to determine the long-term effects of a combination of aerobic and resistance exercise on inhibitory control, as well as to advance our present understanding of the real mechanisms and substantial benefits of the exercise–cognition relationships on the neurocognitive problems in individuals with obesity in the clinical setting.

Author Contributions: Conceptualization, H.-J.W. and C.-L.T.; methodology, H.-J.W.; software, H.-J.W.; validation, H.-J.W.; formal analysis, H.-J.W.; investigation, H.-J.W.; resources, H.-J.W.; data curation, H.-J.W.; writing—original draft preparation, review and editing, H.-J.W. and C.-L.T.; visualization, H.-J.W.; supervision H.-J.W.; project administration, H.-J.W.; funding acquisition, H.-J.W. All authors have read and agreed to the published version of the manuscript.

Funding: This research was funded by the Ministry of Science and Technology (MOST 106-2410-H-320-004 and MOST 107-2410-H-320-005), Taiwan.

Acknowledgments: We wish to express our appreciation for the cooperation of all participants and the facility support provided by Tzu Chi University. We also wish to acknowledge graduate student Pei-Qing Lee for assisting with data collection and with the technicians, and the Department of medical imaging at Tzu Chi Hospital for assisting with the DXA measurements.

Conflicts of Interest: The authors declare no conflict of interest.

References

1. Grant, R.W.; Dixit, V.D. Adipose tissue as an immunological organ. *Obesity* **2015**, *23*, 512–518. [CrossRef] [PubMed]
2. Carnell, S.; Gibson, C.; Benson, L.; Ochner, C.N.; Geliebter, A. Neuroimaging and obesity: Current knowledge and future directions. *Obes. Rev.* **2012**, *13*, 43–56. [CrossRef] [PubMed]
3. Hedman, A.M.; van Haren, N.E.M.; Schnack, H.G.; Kahn, R.S.; Hulshoff Pol, H.E. Human brain changes across the life span: A review of 56 longitudinal magnetic resonance imaging studies. *Hum. Brain Mapp.* **2012**, *33*, 1987–2002. [CrossRef] [PubMed]
4. Tsai, C.L.; Chen, F.C.; Pan, C.Y.; Tseng, Y.T. The Neurocognitive Performance of Visuospatial Attention in Children with Obesity. *Front. Psychol.* **2016**, *7*, 1033. [CrossRef]
5. Wen, H.J.; Tsai, C.L. Neurocognitive Inhibitory Control Ability Performance and Correlations with Biochemical Markers in Obese Women. *Int. J. Public Health* **2020**, *17*, 2726. [CrossRef]
6. Syan, S.K.; Owens, M.M.; Goodman, B.; Epstein, L.H.; Meyre, D.; Sweet, L.H.; MacKillop, J. Deficits in executive function and suppression of default mode network in obesity. *Neuroimage Clin.* **2019**, *24*, 102015. [CrossRef]
7. Tsai, C.L.; Huang, T.H.; Tsai, M.C. Neurocognitive performances of visuospatial attention and the correlations with metabolic and inflammatory biomarkers in adults with obesity. *Exp. Physiol.* **2017**, *102*, 1683–1699. [CrossRef] [PubMed]

8. Dietrich, A.; Audiffren, M. The reticular-activating hypofrontality (RAH) model of acute exercise. *Neurosci. Biobehav. Rev.* **2011**, *35*, 1305–1325. [CrossRef] [PubMed]
9. Chang, Y.K.; Alderman, B.L.; Chu, C.H.; Wang, C.C.; Song, T.F.; Chen, F.T. Acute exercise has a general facilitative effect on cognitive function: A combined ERP temporal dynamics and BDNF study. *Psychophysiology* **2017**, *54*, 289–300. [CrossRef] [PubMed]
10. Tsai, C.L.; Wang, C.H.; Pan, C.Y.; Chen, F.C.; Huang, T.H.; Chou, F.Y. Executive function and endocrinological responses to acute resistance exercise. *Front. Behav. Neurosci.* **2014**, *8*, 262. [CrossRef]
11. Pontifex, M.B.; Parks, A.C.; Henning, D.A.; Kamijo, K. Single bouts of exercise selectively sustain attentional processes. *Psychophysiology* **2015**, *52*, 618–625. [CrossRef] [PubMed]
12. Yanagisawa, H.; Dan, I.; Tsuzuki, D.; Kato, M.; Okamoto, M.; Kyutoku, Y.; Soya, H. Acute moderate exercise elicits increased dorsolateral prefrontal activation and improves cognitive performance with Stroop test. *NeuroImage* **2010**, *50*, 1702–1710. [CrossRef] [PubMed]
13. Ludyga, S.; Gerber, M.; Brand, S.; Holsboer-Trachsler, E.; Pühse, U. Acute effects of moderate aerobic exercise on specific aspects of executive function in different age and fitness groups: A meta-analysis. *Psychophysiology* **2016**, *53*, 1611–1626. [CrossRef] [PubMed]
14. Tsai, C.L.; Chen, F.C.; Pan, C.Y.; Wang, C.H.; Huang, T.H.; Chen, T.C. Impact of acute aerobic exercise and cardiorespiratory fitness on visuospatial attention performance and serum BDNF levels. *Psychoneuroendocrinology* **2014**, *41*, 121–131. [CrossRef]
15. Fearnbach, S.N.; Silvert, L.; Keller, K.L.; Genin, P.M.; Morio, B.; Pereira, B.; Duclos, M.; Boirie, Y.; Thivel, D. Reduced neural response to food cues following exercise is accompanied by decreased energy intake in obese adolescents. *Int. J. Obes.* **2016**, *40*, 77–83. [CrossRef]
16. Quintero, A.P.; Bonilla-Vargas, K.J.; Correa-Bautista, J.E.; Domínguez-Sanchéz, M.A.; Triana-Reina, H.R.; Velasco-Orjuela, G.P.; García-Hermoso, A.; Villa-González, E.; Esteban-Cornejo, I.; Correa-Rodríguez, M.; et al. Acute effect of three different exercise training modalities on executive function in overweight inactive men: A secondary analysis of the BrainFit study. *Physiol. Behav.* **2018**, *197*, 22–28. [CrossRef]
17. Tomporowski, P.D.; Davis, C.L.; Lambourne, K.; Gregoski, M.; Tkacz, J. Task switching in overweight children: Effects of acute exercise and age. *J. Sport Exerc. Psychol.* **2008**, *30*, 497–511. [CrossRef]
18. Vincent, C.M.; Hall, P.A. Cognitive effects of a 30-min aerobic exercise bout on adults with overweight/obesity and type 2 diabetes. *Obes. Sci. Pract.* **2017**, *3*, 289–297. [CrossRef]
19. Parris, B.A.; Wadsley, M.G.; Hasshim, N.; Benattayallah, A.; Augustinova, M.; Ferrand, L. An fMRI study of response and semantic conflict in the Stroop task. *Front. Psychol.* **2019**, *10*, 2426. [CrossRef]
20. Paszkiel, S. *Analysis and Classification of EEG Signals for Brain–Computer Interfaces*; Springer Nature: Cham, Switzerland, 2020.
21. Donnelly, J.E.; Blair, S.N.; Jakicic, J.M.; Manore, M.M.; Rankin, J.W.; Smith, B.K. American College of Sports Medicine Position Stand. Appropriate physical activity intervention strategies for weight loss and prevention of weight regain for adults. *Med. Sci. Sports Exerc.* **2009**, *41*, 459–471. [CrossRef]
22. Berthoud, H.R. Metabolic and hedonic drives in the neural control of appetite: Who is the boss? *Curr. Opin. Neurobiol.* **2011**, *21*, 888–896. [CrossRef] [PubMed]
23. Tsai, C.L.; Pan, C.Y.; Chen, F.C.; Wang, C.H.; Chou, F.Y. Effects of acute aerobic exercise on a task-switching protocol and brain-derived neurotrophic factor concentrations in young adults with different levels of cardiorespiratory fitness. *Exp. Physiol.* **2016**, *101*, 836–850. [CrossRef] [PubMed]
24. Herold, F.; Schega, L.; Müller, N.G. Functional and/or structural brain changes in response to resistance exercises and resistance training lead to cognitive improvements—A systematic review. *Eur. Rev. Aging Phys. Act.* **2019**, *16*, 10. [CrossRef] [PubMed]
25. Tsai, C.L.; Ukropec, J.; Ukropcová, B.; Pai, M.C. An acute bout of aerobic or strength exercise specifically modifies circulating exerkine levels and neurocognitive functions in elderly individuals with mild cognitive impairment. *Neuroimage Clin.* **2018**, *17*, 272–284. [CrossRef]
26. Tsai, C.L.; Wang, C.H.; Pan, C.Y.; Chen, F.C. The effects of long-term resistance exercise on the relationship between neurocognitive performance and GH, IGF-1, and homocysteine levels in the elderly. *Front. Behav. Neurosci.* **2015**, *9*, 23. [CrossRef]
27. Marzolini, S.; Oh, P.; McIlroy, W.; Brooks, D. The effects of an aerobic and resistance exercise training program on cognition following stroke. *Neurorehabil. Neural. Repair* **2013**, *27*, 392–402. [CrossRef]

28. Bossers, W.J.; Scherder, E.J.; Boersma, F.; Hortobágyi, T.; van der Woude, L.H.; van Heuvelen, M.J. Feasibility of a combined aerobic and strength training program and its effects on cognitive and physical function in institutionalized dementia patients. A pilot study. *PLoS ONE* **2014**, *9*, e97577. [CrossRef]
29. Costigan, S.A.; Eather, N.; Plotnikoff, R.C.; Hillman, C.H.; Lubans, D.R. High-Intensity Interval Training for Cognitive and Mental Health in Adolescents. *Med. Sci. Sports Exerc.* **2016**, *48*, 1985–1993. [CrossRef]
30. Colcombe, S.; Kramer, A.F. Fitness effects on the cognitive function of older adults: A meta-analytic study. *Psychol. Sci.* **2003**, *14*, 125–130. [CrossRef]
31. Liu-Ambrose, T.; Donaldson, M.G. Exercise and cognition in older adults: Is there a role for resistance training programmes? *Br. J. Sports Med.* **2009**, *43*, 25–27. [CrossRef]
32. Tsai, C.L.; Pai, M.C.; Ukropec, J.; Ukropcova, B. Distinctive Effects of Aerobic and Resistance Exercise Modes on Neurocognitive and Biochemical Changes in Individuals with Mild Cognitive Impairment. *Curr. Alzheimer Res.* **2019**, *16*, 316–332. [CrossRef] [PubMed]
33. Diamond, A. Executive functions. *Annu. Rev. Psychol.* **2013**, *64*, 135–168. [CrossRef] [PubMed]
34. Dai, C.T.; Chang, Y.K.; Huang, C.J.; Hung, T.M. Exercise mode and executive function in older adults: An ERP study of task-switching. *Brain Cogn.* **2013**, *83*, 153–162. [CrossRef] [PubMed]
35. Tsai, C.L.; Pan, C.Y.; Chen, F.C.; Huang, T.H.; Tsai, M.C.; Chuang, C.Y. Differences in neurocognitive performance and metabolic and inflammatory indices in male adults with obesity as a function of regular exercise. *Exp. Physiol.* **2019**, 1–11. [CrossRef]
36. Wen, C.P.; Cheng, T.Y.; Tsai, S.P.; Chan, H.T.; Hsu, H.L.; Hsu, C.C.; Eriksen, M.P. Are Asians at greater mortality risks for being overweight than Caucasians? Redefining obesity for Asians. *Public Health Nutr.* **2009**, *12*, 497–506. [CrossRef]
37. World Health Organization. *The Asia-Pacific Perspective: Redefining Obesity and Its Treatment*; Health Communications Australia: Sydney, Australia, 2000.
38. Oldfield, R.C. The assessment and analysis of handedness: The Edinburgh inventory. *Neuropsychologia* **1971**, *9*, 97–113. [CrossRef]
39. Dragovic, M. Categorization and validation of handedness using latent class analysis. *Acta Neuropsychiatrica* **2004**, *16*, 212–218. [CrossRef]
40. Beck, A.T.; Steer, R.A.; Brown, G.K. *BDI-II: 2nd Edition Manual*; The Psychological Corporation: San Antonio, TX, USA, 1996.
41. Folstein, M.F.; Folstein, S.E.; McHugh, P.R. Mini-mental state. A practical method for grading the cognitive state of patients for the clinician. *J. Psychiatr. Res.* **1975**, *12*, 189–198. [CrossRef]
42. Cohen, J.E. *Statistical Power Analysis for the Behavioral Sciences*; Lawrence Erlbaum Associates: Hillsdale, NJ, USA, 1988.
43. Garber, C.E.; Blissmer, B.; Deschenes, M.R.; Franklin, B.A.; Lamonte, M.J.; Lee, I.M.; Nieman, D.C.; Swain, D.P. American College of Sports Medicine position stand. Quantity and quality of exercise for developing and maintaining cardiorespiratory, musculoskeletal, and neuromotor fitness in apparently healthy adults: Guidance for prescribing exercise. *Med. Sci. Sports Exerc.* **2011**, *43*, 1334–1359. [CrossRef]
44. Rey-Mermet, A.; Gade, M. Inhibition in aging: What is preserved? What declines? A meta-analysis. *Psychon. Bull. Rev.* **2018**, *25*, 1695–1716. [CrossRef]
45. Gajewski, P.D.; Falkenstein, M. Long-term habitual physical activity is associated with lower distractibility in a Stroop interference task in aging: Behavioral and ERP evidence. *Brain Cogn.* **2015**, *98*, 87–101. [CrossRef] [PubMed]
46. MacLeod, C.M. Half a century of research on the Stroop effect: An integrative review. *Psychol. Bull.* **1991**, *109*, 163–203. [CrossRef]
47. Stroop, J.R. Studies of interference in serial verbal reactions. *J. Exp. Psychol.* **1935**, *18*, 643–662. [CrossRef]
48. Wu, C.H.; Karageorghis, C.I.; Wang, C.C.; Chu, C.H.; Kao, S.C.; Hung, T.M.; Chang, Y.K. Effects of acute aerobic and resistance exercise on executive function: An ERP study. *J. Sci. Med. Sport* **2019**, *22*, 1367–1372. [CrossRef] [PubMed]
49. Puglisi, G.; Howells, H.; Sciortino, T.; Leonetti, A.; Rossi, M.; Conti Nibali, M.; Gabriel Gay, L.; Fornia, L.; Bellacicca, A.; Viganò, L.; et al. Frontal pathways in cognitive control: Direct evidence from intraoperative stimulation and diffusion tractography. *Brain* **2019**, *142*, 2451–2465. [PubMed]

50. Tsai, C.L.; Pan, C.Y.; Chang, Y.K.; Wang, C.H.; Tseng, K.D. Deficits of visuospatial attention with reflexive orienting induced by eye-gazed cues in children with developmental coordination disorder in the lower extremities: An event-related potential study. *Res. Dev. Disabil.* **2010**, *31*, 642–655. [CrossRef]
51. Tsai, C.L.; Wang, C.H.; Tseng, Y.T. Effects of exercise intervention on event-related potential and task performance indices of attention networks in children with developmental coordination disorder. *Brain Cogn.* **2012**, *79*, 12–22. [CrossRef]
52. Piepmeier, A.T.; Shih, C.H.; Whedon, M.; Williams, L.M.; Davis, M.E.; Henning, D.A.; Park, S.Y.; Calkins, S.D.; Etnier, J.L. The effect of acute exercise on cognitive performance in children with and without ADHD. *J. Sport Health Sci.* **2015**, *4*, 97–104. [CrossRef]
53. Chang, Y.K.; Etnier, J.L. Exploring the dose-response relationship between resistance exercise intensity and cognitive function. *J. Sport Exerc. Psychol.* **2009**, *31*, 640–656. [CrossRef]
54. Johnson, L.; Addamo, P.K.; Selva Raj, I.; Borkoles, E.; Wyckelsma, V.; Cyarto, E.; Polman, R.C. An Acute Bout of Exercise Improves the Cognitive Performance of Older Adults. *J. Aging Phys. Act.* **2016**, *24*, 591–598. [CrossRef]
55. Fernandes, M.; de Sousa, A.; Medeiros, A.R.; Del Rosso, S.; Stults-Kolehmainen, M.; Boullosa, D.A. The influence of exercise and physical fitness status on attention: A systematic review. *Int. Rev. Sport Exerc. Psychol.* **2019**, *12*, 202–234. [CrossRef]
56. Huang, T.; Tarp, J.; Domazet, S.L.; Thorsen, A.K.; Froberg, K.; Andersen, L.B.; Bugge, A. Associations of Adiposity and Aerobic Fitness with Executive Function and Math Performance in Danish Adolescents. *J. Pediatr.* **2015**, *167*, 810–815. [CrossRef] [PubMed]
57. Benikos, N.; Johnstone, S.J.; Roodenrys, S.J. Varying task difficulty in the Go/Nogo task: The effects of inhibitory control, arousal, and perceived effort on ERP components. *Int. J. Psychophysiol.* **2013**, *87*, 262–272. [CrossRef] [PubMed]
58. Yuan, J.; Zhang, J.; Zhou, X.; Yang, J.; Meng, X.; Zhang, Q.; Li, H. Neural mechanisms underlying the higher levels of subjective well-being in extraverts: Pleasant bias and unpleasant resistance. *Cogn. Affect. Behav. Neurosci.* **2012**, *12*, 175–192. [CrossRef]
59. Zahedi, A.; Stuermer, B.; Hatami, J.; Rostami, R.; Sommer, W. Eliminating stroop effects with post-hypnotic instructions: Brain mechanisms inferred from EEG. *Neuropsychologia* **2017**, *96*, 70–77. [CrossRef] [PubMed]
60. Feng, C.; Li, W.; Tian, T.; Luo, Y.; Gu, R.; Zhou, C.; Luo, Y.J. Arousal modulates valence effects on both early and late stages of affective picture processing in a passive viewing task. *Soc. Neurosci.* **2014**, *9*, 364–377. [CrossRef]
61. Imbir, K.; Spustek, T.; Bernatowicz, G.; Duda, J.; Żygierewicz, J. Two Aspects of Activation: Arousal and Subjective Significance—Behavioral and Event-Related Potential Correlates Investigated by Means of a Modified Emotional Stroop Task. *Front. Hum. Neurosci.* **2017**, *11*, 608. [CrossRef]
62. Drollette, E.S.; Scudder, M.R.; Raine, L.B.; Moore, R.D.; Saliba, B.J.; Pontifex, M.B.; Hillman, C.H. Acute exercise facilitates brain function and cognition in children who need it most: An ERP study of individual differences in inhibitory control capacity. *Dev. Cogn. Neurosci.* **2014**, *7*, 53–64. [CrossRef]
63. Maayan, L.; Hoogendoorn, C.; Sweat, V.; Convit, A. Disinhibited eating in obese adolescents is associated with orbitofrontal volume reductions and executive dysfunction. *Obesity* **2011**, *19*, 1382–1387. [CrossRef]
64. Horstmann, A.; Busse, F.P.; Mathar, D.; Müller, K.; Lepsien, J.; Schlögl, H.; Kabisch, S.; Kratzsch, J.; Neumann, J.; Stumvoll, M.; et al. Obesity-Related Differences between Women and Men in Brain Structure and Goal-Directed Behavior. *Front. Hum. Neurosci.* **2011**, *5*, 58. [CrossRef]
65. Schroder, H.S.; Moser, J.S. Improving the study of error monitoring with consideration of behavioral performance measures. *Front. Hum. Neurosci.* **2014**, *8*, 178. [CrossRef] [PubMed]
66. Peruyero, F.; Zapata, J.; Pastor, D.; Cervelló, E. The Acute Effects of Exercise Intensity on Inhibitory Cognitive Control in Adolescents. *Front. Psychol.* **2017**, *8*, 921. [CrossRef] [PubMed]
67. Harjunen, V.J.; Ahmed, I.; Jacucci, G.; Ravaja, N.; Spapé, M.M. Manipulating Bodily Presence Affects Cross-Modal Spatial Attention: A Virtual-Reality-Based ERP Study. *Front. Hum. Neurosci.* **2017**, *11*, 79. [CrossRef]
68. Gabbard, C.; Cacola, P. Children with developmental coordination disorder have difficulty with action representation. *Rev. Neurol.* **2010**, *50*, 33–38.

69. Anokhin, A.P.; Golosheykin, S.; Grant, J.D.; Heath, A.C. Heritability of brain activity related to response inhibition: A longitudinal genetic study in adolescent twins. *Int. J. Psychophysiol.* **2017**, *115*, 112–124. [CrossRef]
70. Hsieh, S.S.; Huang, C.J.; Wu, C.T.; Chang, Y.K.; Hung, T.M. Acute Exercise Facilitates the N450 Inhibition Marker and P3 Attention Marker during Stroop Test in Young and Older Adults. *J. Clin. Med.* **2018**, *7*. [CrossRef]
71. Brush, C.J.; Olson, R.L.; Ehmann, P.J.; Osovsky, S.; Alderman, B.L. Dose-Response and Time Course Effects of Acute Resistance Exercise on Executive Function. *J. Sport Exerc. Psychol.* **2016**, *38*, 396–408. [CrossRef]
72. Moriarty, T.; Bourbeau, K.; Bellovary, B.; Zuhl, M.N. Exercise Intensity Influences Prefrontal Cortex Oxygenation during Cognitive Testing. *Behav. Sci.* **2019**, *9*, 83. [CrossRef]
73. Kutas, M.; McCarthy, G.; Donchin, E. Augmenting mental chronometry: The P300 as a measure of stimulus evaluation time. *Science* **1977**, *197*, 792–795. [CrossRef] [PubMed]
74. Chang, Y.K.; Ku, P.W.; Tomporowski, P.D.; Chen, F.T.; Huang, C.C. Effects of acute resistance exercise on late-middle-age adults' goal planning. *Med. Sci. Sports Exerc.* **2012**, *44*, 1773–1779. [CrossRef]
75. Chang, Y.K.; Tsai, C.L.; Huang, C.C.; Wang, C.C.; Chu, I.H. Effects of acute resistance exercise on cognition in late middle-aged adults: General or specific cognitive improvement? *J. Sci. Med. Sport* **2014**, *17*, 51–55. [CrossRef] [PubMed]
76. Wen, H.J.; Ang, B.S. Does interval duration or intensity during high-intensity interval training affect adherence and enjoyment in overweight and obese adults? *Q. Chin. Phys. Educ.* **2019**, *33*, 73–89. [CrossRef]
77. Chang, H.; Kim, K.; Jung, Y.J.; Kato, M. Effects of acute high-Intensity resistance exercise on cognitive function and oxygenation in prefrontal cortex. *J. Exerc. Nutr. Biochem.* **2017**, *21*, 1–8. [CrossRef] [PubMed]
78. McMorris, T.; Hale, B.J.; Corbett, J.; Robertson, K.; Hodgson, C.I. Does acute exercise affect the performance of whole-body, psychomotor skills in an inverted-U fashion? A meta-analytic investigation. *Physiol. Behav.* **2015**, *141*, 180–189. [CrossRef]
79. Aguirre-Loaiza, H.; Arenas, J.; Arias, I.; Franco-Jímenez, A.; Barbosa-Granados, S.; Ramos-Bermúdez, S.; Ayala-Zuluaga, F.; Núñez, C.; García-Mas, A. Effect of Acute Physical Exercise on Executive Functions and Emotional Recognition: Analysis of Moderate to High Intensity in Young Adults. *Front. Psychol.* **2019**, *10*, 2774. [CrossRef]
80. Harveson, A.T.; Hannon, J.C.; Brusseau, T.A.; Podlog, L.; Papadopoulos, C.; Durrant, L.H.; Hall, M.S.; Kang, K.D. Acute Effects of 30 Minutes Resistance and Aerobic Exercise on Cognition in a High School Sample. *Res. Q. Exerc. Sport* **2016**, *87*, 214–220. [CrossRef]
81. Foright, R.M.; Johnson, G.C.; Kahn, D.; Charleston, C.A.; Presby, D.M.; Bouchet, C.A.; Wellberg, E.A.; Sherk, V.D.; Jackman, M.R.; Greenwood, B.N.; et al. Compensatory eating behaviors in male and female rats in response to exercise training. *Am. J. Physiol. Regul. Integr. Comp. Physiol.* **2020**, *319*, R171–R183. [CrossRef]
82. Chaku, N.; Hoyt, L.T. Developmental Trajectories of Executive Functioning and Puberty in Boys and Girls. *J. Youth Adolesc.* **2019**, *48*, 1365–1378. [CrossRef]
83. Selthofer-Relatić, K.; Radić, R.; Stupin, A.; Šišljagić, V.; Bošnjak, I.; Bulj, N.; Selthofer, R.; Delić Brkljačić, D. Leptin/adiponectin ratio in overweight patients—Gender differences. *Diab. Vasc. Dis. Res.* **2018**, *15*, 260–262.
84. Crush, E.A.; Loprinzi, P.D. Dose-Response Effects of Exercise Duration and Recovery on Cognitive Functioning. *Percept. Mot. Skills* **2017**, *124*, 1164–1193. [CrossRef]
85. Hunma, S.; Ramuth, H.; Miles-Chan, J.L.; Schutz, Y.; Montani, J.P.; Joonas, N.; Dulloo, A.G. Do gender and ethnic differences in fasting leptin in Indians and Creoles of Mauritius persist beyond differences in adiposity? *Int. J. Obes.* **2018**, *42*, 280–283. [CrossRef]
86. Pruijm, M.; Vollenweider, P.; Mooser, V.; Paccaud, F.; Preisig, M.; Waeber, G.; Marques-Vidal, P.; Burnier, M.; Bochud, M. Inflammatory markers and blood pressure: Sex differences and the effect of fat mass in the CoLaus Study. *J. Hum. Hypertens.* **2013**, *27*, 169–175. [CrossRef] [PubMed]

Publisher's Note: MDPI stays neutral with regard to jurisdictional claims in published maps and institutional affiliations.

© 2020 by the authors. Licensee MDPI, Basel, Switzerland. This article is an open access article distributed under the terms and conditions of the Creative Commons Attribution (CC BY) license (http://creativecommons.org/licenses/by/4.0/).

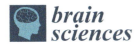

Article

Effects of Mini-Basketball Training Program on Executive Functions and Core Symptoms among Preschool Children with Autism Spectrum Disorders

Jin-Gui Wang [1], Ke-Long Cai [1], Zhi-Mei Liu [1], Fabian Herold [2,3], Liye Zou [4], Li-Na Zhu [5], Xuan Xiong [1] and Ai-Guo Chen [1,*]

- [1] College of Physical Education, Yangzhou University, Yangzhou 225127, China; jinguiwang5715@163.com (J.-G.W.); kelongcai@163.com (K.-L.C.); 15161885591@sohu.com (Z.-M.L.); movmu7@sina.com (X.X.)
- [2] Research Group Neuroprotection, German Center for Neurodegenerative Diseases (DZNE), Leipziger Str. 44, 39120 Magdeburg, Germany; Fabian.herold@dzne.de
- [3] Department of Neurology, Medical Faculty, Otto von Guericke University, Leipziger Str. 44, 39120 Magdeburg, Germany
- [4] Exercise and Mental Health Laboratory, School of Psychology, Shenzhen University, Shenzhen 518060, China; liyezou123@gmail.com
- [5] School of Physical Education and Sports Science, Beijing Normal University, Beijing 100000, China; zhulina827@163.com
- * Correspondence: agchen@yzu.edu.cn; Tel.: +86-514-8797-8013

Received: 6 April 2020; Accepted: 28 April 2020; Published: 30 April 2020

Abstract: This study examined the effects of a 12-week mini-basketball training program (MBTP) on executive functions and core symptoms among preschoolers with autism spectrum disorder (ASD). In this quasi-experimental pilot study, 33 ASD preschoolers who received their conventional rehabilitation program were assigned to either a MBTP group ($n = 18$) or control group ($n = 15$). Specifically, the experimental group was required to take an additional 12-week MBTP (five days per week, one session per day, and forty minutes per session), while the control group was instructed to maintain their daily activities. Executive functions and core symptoms (social communication impairment and repetitive behavior) were evaluated by the Childhood Executive Functioning Inventory (CHEXI), the Social Responsiveness Scale-Second Edition (SRS-2), and the Repetitive Behavior Scale-Revised (RBS-R), respectively. After the 12-week intervention period, the MBTP group exhibited significantly better performances in working memory ($F = 7.51$, $p < 0.01$, partial $\eta^2 = 0.195$) and regulation ($F = 4.23$, $p < 0.05$, partial $\eta^2 = 0.12$) as compared to the control group. Moreover, the MBTP significantly improved core symptoms of ASD preschoolers, including the social communication impairment ($F = 6.02$, $p < 0.05$, partial $\eta^2 = 0.020$) and repetitive behavior ($F = 5.79$, $p < 0.05$, partial $\eta^2 = 0.016$). Based on our findings, we concluded that the 12-week MBTP may improve executive functions and core symptoms in preschoolers with ASD, and we provide new evidence that regular physical exercise in the form of a MBTP is a promising alternative to treat ASD.

Keywords: exercise; executive functions; core symptoms; children; autism spectrum disorders

1. Introduction

Autism spectrum disorder (ASD) is a neurodevelopmental disorder with several core symptoms (social skill deficits, communication problems, stereotyped and repetitive behavior) [1]. Empirical evidence suggests that these problem behaviors do not merely involve the typical clinical manifestations, but also limit opportunities for achieving health benefits, academic achievement, and social integration [2]. Recently, accumulating evidence has indicated that children with ASD have also presented with executive dysfunction [3].

Executive functions are brain-based skills required to successfully carry out goal-directed behaviors, with three primary domains that are generally categorized: (1) inhibition is the ability to voluntarily inhibit impulsive responses, (2) regulation involves the mental ability to selectively shift attention between two tasks, and (3) working memory is the ability to hold the meaningful information for decision making, planning, and organization [4]. In the context of ASD, executive functions are proposed to significantly associate with specific impairments (e.g., theory of mind, social cognition, social impairment, restricted and repetitive behaviors, and quality of life) [5–8]. It is also worth mentioning that the prefrontal cortex as a key structure is extensively investigated to explore neural mechanisms related to executive functions [9]. In line with this, Hill's executive dysfunction theory has proposed that in individuals with ASD, difficulties in initiating new non-routine actions and stereotypical behaviors are linked to frontal lobe dysfunction [10]. According to the above-mentioned evidence concerning social and behavioral deficits as well as executive dysfunction, it is very likely that cognitive deficits in ASD children may persist into adulthood.

Currently, there is no available pharmacological therapy for treating ASD children [11,12]. Hence, ASD children are usually treated by behavioral therapies, but it is difficult for many families to access the time-consuming counseling sessions or to implement long-term and high-quality behavioral interventions in their daily routines. Moreover, those behavioral treatments are relatively expensive and challenging, which may not be affordable for all ASD families. More unfortunately, the conduction of behavioral therapies does not produce significant positive changes in the underlying deficits that promote the behavioral manifestations of ASD in children. To overcome the limitations of these existing behavioral interventions, it is urgently needed to search for effective and alternative therapeutic strategies (like exercise training) for treatment of ASD children [13].

Accumulating evidence has shown that physical exercise interventions could be a valuable alternative to the existing behavioral therapies, as it was observed that acute physical exercises can improve cognitive functions, at least transiently, in ASD children [14–19]. Likewise, previous studies also showed that long-term physical exercise interventions had positive effects on executive functions among school-aged children who were diagnosed with ASD [13,20–23]. Moreover, it is reported that in children with ASD, the rehabilitative effects of physical exercise interventions (e.g., exergaming and Karate techniques training) on social communication, repetitive behaviors, and cognitive performance can be maintained, at least, up to one month after the cessation of the intervention [22].

Notably, previous studies on physical exercise intervention focused on school-aged children with ASD, rather than preschoolers. As it is well-known that preschool age is a critical period for dramatic growth and the development of executive functions [24], thus it would also be appropriate to start intervention programs during this developmental stage. This assumption is supported by the growing evidence suggesting that early intensive interventions would ameliorate symptoms of ASD children, which was associated with an increased likelihood of moving into socialized environments in later life periods [25,26]. Collectively, physical exercise interventions that start at a preschool age stage seem to also be beneficial for this special population. Hence, to fill this knowledge, we aimed to investigate the effects of an exercise intervention program on executive function and core symptoms of ASD in a sample of 3–6-year-old preschoolers with ASD. As it has been speculated [27–29] and demonstrated [30] that cognitively and/or coordinatively demanding physical exercises are more efficient to improve executive functioning in children than purely aerobic exercises, we implemented a mini-basketball training program (MBTP) in this intervention study. Mini-basketball is a cognitively challenging and coordination training program which trains speed and strength, as well as social and cognitive skills [31,32]. Based on the promising evidence which suggests that physical exercise can improve social skills and cognitive performance, we hypothesized that the 12-week MBTP would result in improvements of executive functioning and core symptoms in preschoolers with ASD as compared to the control group.

2. Materials and Methods

2.1. Study Design

The study was a quasi-experimental design in which "between-subject factor" was "group/condition" and "within-subject factor" is "time". This study was conducted between October and December 2018 in Yangzhou, China, with ethics approval from the Ethics and Human Protection Committee of the Affiliated Hospital of Yangzhou University. Study protocol was registered with the Chinese Clinical Trial Registry (ChiCTR1900024973) before initiating our experiments and all study procedures are in accordance with the latest version of the Declaration of Helsinki. Written informed consent were obtained from parents of ASD children.

2.2. Participants

Children aged 3–6 years, meeting the Diagnostic and Statistical Manual of Mental Disorders, 5th edition, criteria for ASD [1], were recruited from Yangzhou Chuying Child Development Center and Starssailor Education Institute (Yangzhou, P. R. China). Children were not eligible if they met one of the following exclusion criteria: (1) received basketball training or regular participation in physical exercise in the past 6 months, (2) one or more co-morbid psychiatric disorders, (3) a neurological disorder (e.g., epilepsy, phenylketonuria, fragile X syndrome, tuberous sclerosis), (4) visual and auditory disorders, (5) a medical history of head trauma, and (6) any medical condition that does not allow exercise participation (e.g., heart disease, operations or fractures within the last six months).

Ninety-four children who met the diagnosis for ASD were initially screened in the two institutes. Of the initially diagnosed ASD preschoolers, 35 children who did not meet study criteria or declined to participate in this study were excluded so that 59 participants were finally eligible. Given that this is a pilot study, a quasi-experimental design was adopted in which eligible participants were geographically arranged into two groups: (1) participants from the Chuying Child Development Center were considered as the control group ($n = 29$), and (2) participants from the Starssailor Education Institution were chosen as the MBTP group ($n = 30$). Notably, only 33 participants (28 boys and 5 girls; 4.924 ± 0.697 years) were finally included for data analysis (Figure 1) after removal of 26 participants due to (1) injury that was not related to basketball ($n = 1$); (2) sickness ($n = 4$); (3) schedule conflict of parents ($n = 6$); (4) and unwillingness to participate in the functional magnetic resonance imaging (fMRI) task ($n = 15$).

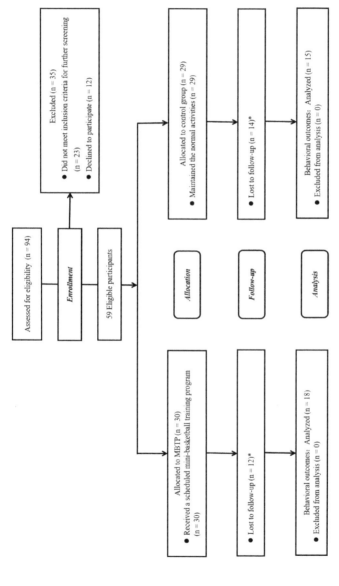

Figure 1. Participant flow chart. * Twenty-six children's parents did not finish the assessment in the post-test.

2.3. Power Calculation

Prior sample size was calculated using G*Power [33] while we selected key parameters: (1) a medium effect size (Cohen's f = 0.25), (2) power of 0.80, (3) alpha of 0.05, and (4) repeated measures analysis of variance (ANOVA) with the two groups (MBTP and control). This indicated that a sample of twenty-four (twelve participants in each of the two groups) can generate a statistical significance. Given that ASD children might drop out over a 12-week intervention period, we increased this by 37.5%, which has yielded the final sample of thirty-three that should be included in this study.

2.4. Mini-Basketball Training Program

In this present study, the mini-basketball training program (MBTP) was adopted from previous studies [31,32,34]. This exercise program has been shown to be a safe, enjoyable, readily accessible, and easy-to-administer program, which is popular among preschool children and their parents. This program with various levels of difficulty is appropriately designed for this special group and ASD children were taught in a progressive manner (three stages are detailed in Appendix A). As they progressed, cognitively demanding game play was arranged to train the executive functions of ASD children. Each training session was carried out in collective classes, which could facilitate social interaction and communication among the participating children with ASD [35]. Parents of the participating children were encouraged to join each training session, which could create a more enjoyable and positive climate, leading to more effective social interactions among all participants. On the other hand, if their parents were present, it potentially makes ASD children feel more comfortable so that they are more likely to succeed in motor skill learning. As recommended by the American College of Sports Medicine, moderate exercise intensity was set, with 60–69% of maximum heart rate (MHR; MHR was determined by the formula: MHR = 220 − age of the participant) [36]. Exercise intensity was monitored using heart rate monitors (POLAR M430) throughout all sessions of the experiment.

In this pilot study, the 12-week MBTP was arranged for ASD children in the experimental group. Weekly five sessions (60 sessions = 12 weeks × 5 sessions) were carried out, with each session lasting 40 min. Specifically, each session included four stages of (a) 5-min warm-up, (b) 20-min basic basketball skill learning, (c) 10-min basketball games, and (d) 5-min cool-down. Parts (b) and (c) involved 30 min of moderate-intensity physical activity, indicated by 129–149 heart beats per minute on average.

2.5. Measurements

Demographic information (age, gender, weight and height) were obtained at baseline and are presented in Table 1. Severity of participant was assessed using the Childhood Autism Rating Scale (CARS) [37] and clinical assessment report. Additionally, previous studies have indicated that core symptoms were associated with sleep disorders and eating behaviors in children with ASD [38,39]. To control for these potential confounding variables, sleep problems and eating behavior were collected at baseline assessment. First, sleep problems were assessed using the Children's Sleep Habits Questionnaire (CSHQ) [40], administered by their parents. Second, eating style was assessed by a parent-report Child Eating Behavior Questionnaire (CEBQ) [41]. Executive functions as primary outcomes and core symptoms as secondary outcomes were also measured in this pilot study. Their assessment tools are discussed below.

2.5.1. Assessment of Executive Functions

In this pilot study, the validated Childhood Executive Functioning Inventory (CHEXI) in Chinese was used to measure severity of executive functions [42]. The revised version consisted of 24 items (1 = completely inconsistent to 5 = completely consistent) within three dimensions (regulation, inhibition, and working memory). A sum score of 120 can be obtained, with higher scores indicating worse executive function [43].

2.5.2. Assessment of Core Symptoms

Social Communication Impairment was measured using the Social Responsiveness Scale Second Edition (SRS-2) [44]. It consisted of 65 items, with each item rated on a 4-point scale ranging from 1 (not true) to 4 (almost always true). It can generate a total score of 75, with higher scores indicating more severe impairment in social communication. Likewise, parent-reported behavioral outcomes were also collected with the validated assessment tool [44].

Repetitive behaviors were measured using the Repetitive Behavior Scale-Revised (RBS-R) [45]. This informant-based questionnaire was designed to provide a quantitative, continuous measure of the full spectrum of various repetitive behaviors among individuals with ASD. In the RSB-R, 43 items are grouped conceptually. Each item is rated on a 4-point Likert scale for severity (0 = behavior does not occur, 1 = behavior occurs and is a mild problem, 2 = behavior occurs and is a moderate problem, 3 = behavior occurs and is a severe problem). Higher scores indicate more severe behaviors.

2.6. Procedure

All potential participants were screened by physicians in the Yangzhou Maternal and Child Care and Service Centre. Meanwhile, written informed consent was obtained from mothers of all participating children after the experimental procedures had been fully explained. Eligible ASD children were assigned to either a MBTP group or control group. During the first visit, their legal guardians completed all paperwork, including the CHEXI, SRS-2, RBS-R, CSHQ, and CEBQ. Both MBTP and control groups had received the similar conventional rehabilitation program. Notably, only ASD preschoolers in the experimental group were arranged to attend the MBTP, whereas the control group maintained their unaltered lifestyle. The intervention duration of the MBTP was 12 weeks in total. Each session was conducted by two certified physical educators. For the safety consideration and teaching effectiveness, at least one parent of the participating children was required to join the class and play with their child throughout the entire training session. The training program was implemented as described previously (see Section 2.4 Mini-Basketball Training Program). ASD children who completed this intervention and all assessments received a basketball as fair remuneration

2.7. Statistical Analysis

A two-way repeated design was employed with group and time as independent variables. To ensure homogeneity, significant group differences on potential confounding variables (age, gender, eating behaviors, and sleep behaviors) were tested using a t-test or a χ^2-test. Then, a mixed ANOVA was employed to determine significant group differences on primary and secondary outcomes between baseline and post-intervention. If significant interaction effects existed, simple effects were performed. Effect sizes (Cohen's d) that reflect the magnitude of the intervention effect were calculated and partial eta-squared (η^2) values were reported for significant main effects and interactions. Data was presented as descriptive statistics: mean ± standard deviation (M ± SD). An α of 0.05 was used as the level of statistical significance for all statistical analyses, which were conducted using jamovi 1.0.7 (Retrieved from https://www.jamovi.org).

3. Results

3.1. Participant Characteristics

There was no significant group difference on gender (chi-square = 0.07, $p > 0.05$), age ($t(1,31) = 1.74$, $p > 0.05$), height ($t(1,31) = 1.96$, $p > 0.05$), weight ($t(1,31) = 1.64$, $p > 0.05$), severity (CARS) ($t(1,31) = 1.08$, $p > 0.05$), physical fitness ($t(1,31) = 1.59$, $p > 0.05$), sleep problems (CSHQ) ($t(1,31) = -0.92$, $p > 0.05$), and eating behavior (CEBQ) ($t(1,31) = -0.03$, $p > 0.05$). Results indicated homogeneity between the two groups. The demographic characteristics of participants in both groups are summarized in Table 1.

Table 1. Baseline characteristics of participants (M ± standard deviation (SD)).

Measure	MBTP Group	Control Group	p
N	18	15	-
Gender (boys/girls)	15/3	13/2	0.790
Age(years)	5.11 ± 0.65	4.70 ± 0.70	0.092
Body height (cm)	113.94 ± 8.49	108.93 ± 5.57	0.059
Body mass (kg)	20.63 ± 3.32	18.89 ± 2.90	0.112
CARS	45.94 ± 21.37	39.80 ± 5.24	0.287
Physical Fitness	20.39 ± 2.87	18.73 ± 3.15	0.125
CSHQ	55.72 ± 4.73	58.60 ± 12.29	0.366
CEBQ	54.22 ± 8.88	54.40 ± 20.05	0.973

MBTP: mini-basketball training program; CARS: Childhood Autism Rating Scale; CSHQ: The Children's Sleep Habits Questionnaire; CEBQ: Children's Eating Behavior Questionnaire. p-Values are calculated using independent samples t-tests for continuous variables and chi-square tests for categorical variables between groups.

3.2. Executive Functions

A significant group × time interaction ($F(1,31) = 7.51$, $p < 0.05$, partial $\eta^2 = 0.195$) was found on working memory (Table 2). Results from the follow-up analysis have shown no significant group differences on baseline scores between the MBTP and control groups. Notably, significantly lower scores in the MBTP were observed at the post-intervention as compared to the baseline ($t(1,32) = 1.57$, $p < 0.05$, $d = 0.274$), but not in the control group.

Table 2. Analysis of MBTP and Control groups for executive functions and core symptoms variables (M ± SD).

Variable	MBTP Group (n = 18) Baseline	MBTP Group (n = 18) Posttest	Control Group (n = 15) Baseline	Control Group (n = 15) Posttest
Executive Functions				
Working memory	47.67 ± 7.71	43.44 ± 8.42	43.60 ± 7.47	46.40 ± 5.36
Inhibition	21.94 ± 4.29	20.33 ± 3.25	20.27 ± 2.66	22.40 ± 2.67
Regulation	19.67 ± 3.11	17.67 ± 2.99	18.53 ± 3.42	21.13 ± 8.25
Core Symptoms				
SRS-2	93.28 ± 28.75	82.22 ± 27.55	93.72 ± 12.92	95.93 ± 19.47
RBS-R	15.50 ± 9.34	11.22 ± 9.31	21.47 ± 11.45	23.13 ± 14.19

SRS-2: Social Responsiveness Scale Second Edition; RBS-R: Repetitive Behavior Scale-Revised.

A significant group × time interaction ($F(1,31) = 5.66$, $p < 0.05$, partial $\eta^2 = 0.08$) was found on inhibition (Table 2). Results from the follow-up analysis have shown no significant group differences at the baseline assessment. Notably, significantly higher scores in the control group were observed at the post-intervention as compared to the baseline ($t(1,32) = -1.84$, $p < 0.05$, $d = 0.320$), but not in the MBTP group.

A significant group × time interaction ($F(1,31) = 4.23$, $p < 0.05$, partial $\eta^2 = 0.12$) was found on regulation (Table 2). Results from the follow-up analysis have shown no significant group differences at the baseline. Notably, significantly lower scores in the MBTP were observed at the post-intervention as compared to the baseline ($t(1,32) = -2.06$, $p < 0.05$, $d = 0.359$), but not in the control group (Figure 2).

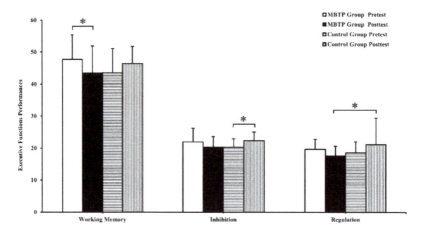

Figure 2. Performances for executive functions (mean and standard deviation) of time point (baseline versus post-test) and group (MBTP versus Control), * $p < 0.05$.

3.3. Core Symptoms

For social communication, a statistically significant group × time interaction was present ($F(1,31) = 6.02$, $p < 0.05$, partial $\eta^2 = 0.020$) (Table 2). Results from the follow-up analysis have shown no significant group differences at the baseline. Notably, significantly lower scores in the MBTP were observed at the post-intervention, as compared to the baseline ($t(1,32) = 3.04$, $p < 0.05$, $d = 0.528$), but not in the control group.

For repetitive behavior, a significant statistical difference between the groups ($F(1,31) = 5.93$, $p < 0.05$, partial $\eta^2 = 0.144$) was found. A statistically significant group × time interaction was present ($F(1,31) = 5.79$, $p < 0.05$, partial $\eta^2 = 0.016$) (Table 2). Results from the follow-up analysis have shown no significant group differences at the baseline. Notably, significantly lower scores in the MBTP were observed at the post-intervention as compared to the baseline ($t(1,32) = 2.57$, $p < 0.05$, $d = 0.447$), but not in the control group.

For the primary and secondary outcomes, means and standard deviations at the baseline and post-intervention are presented in Table 2. The follow-up contrasts are show in Figures 2 and 3.

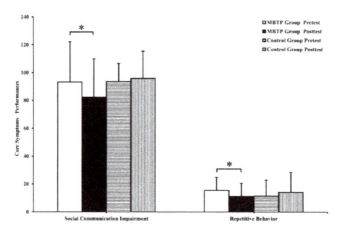

Figure 3. Performances for core symptoms (mean and standard deviation) of time point (baseline versus post-test) and group (MBTP versus control), * $p < 0.05$.

4. Discussion

The present study investigated the effects of a 12-week MBTP on executive functions and core symptoms among preschoolers with ASD. With the continual employment of fundamental movement skill training and basketball games in MBTP, the main findings revealed that MBTP improved executive function, social communication, and repetitive behavior. Potential explanations for our results are discussed below.

4.1. Executive Functions

All aspects of executive functions improved following the 12-week intervention, including working memory, inhibition, and regulation. Recent studies in children with and without disabilities showed that fundamental motor training (e.g., speed-agility, strength training, and coordinating upper- and lower-extremity movements) and complex motor skills training could benefit cognitive performance, which is consistent with our findings [20,21,35,46–49]. Furthermore, our results are in line with previous studies investigating the beneficial effects of cognitive-motor exercise training for executive function [27–30,50]. The superior effects of cognitively engaging exercise training might be related to the neurocognitive demands which are posed to the brain in order to execute the motor-cognitive tasks [51]. In the literature, this effect has also been referred to as the "guidance effect" [52–54]. In particular, MBTP includes the learning of new and complex motor skills (inter-limb coordination), which demands various cognitive domains during the game playing part of the exercise sessions. The cognitive demands posed by the MBTP might train more or less indirectly specific aspects of executive functions (e.g., inhibition or working memory). For instance, the basketball game play requires working memory to update and store the new and old information alternately (position of the players on the field). However, further investigations are needed to provide empirical support for our assumptions.

Another possible explanation for cognitive benefits is the "facilitation effect". It has emphasized the pronounced release of neurochemicals such as brain-derived neurotrophic factor (BDNF) in response to physical exercise and physical training [52–54]. In this regard, it was observed that after 12 weeks of endurance training, the resting concentration of the serum level of BDNF and the working memory performance increased in a sample of healthy adolescent subjects [55]. Whether such changes in serum or plasma levels of BDNF occur after the MBTP in preschoolers with ASD and how these changes might positively influence cognitive performance would be an interesting topic for further studies in this field. In addition, neural correlates (e.g., changes in functional brain activity patterns) of the observed cognitive improvements need to be further investigated. Speculatively, MBTP might positively influence functional brain activation since previous studies reported that in overweight children, significant functional brain changes had occurred after an eight-month aerobic training intervention [56,57].

4.2. Core Symptoms

The findings of the current study support our hypothesis that a 12-week MBTP improved social communication and repetitive behavior among preschoolers with ASD. These findings were similar to previous studies suggesting that social behavior improved after prolonged training in horse riding [58], aquatic group exercise [59], or movement skills [22]. In addition, martial arts training (e.g., techniques training) for children with ASD effectively reduced their repetitive behavior [60]. Such observed improvements in social communication may be attributed to that ASD children who were repeatedly exposed to a rich environment had the opportunity to improve imitation skills, potentially leading to better social skills. This assumption is buttressed by one study which reported that imitation treatment was an effective approach to improve social communication in ASD children [61]. An alternative exploratory approach is that MBTP was implemented in a positive and collaborative environment (individual games, collaborative games, and competitive games) which, in turn, may promote their social and emotional health. Besides, MBTP contains many repeated body movements that are similar to repetitive behavior, which may contribute to physical exhaustion so that frequency of stereotypic behaviors were reduced in this study.

Leung et al. had found that executive dysfunction is often predictive for the core symptoms of children with ASD. In other words, children with superior executive functions were more likely to have lower core symptoms of ASD [6]. Given that the time from birth to 8 years is a critical period in the brain development, starting interventions in early age stages (preschool age in the current study) is probably more beneficial for the development of executive functioning in children with ASD. Likewise, our results suggest that preschoolers with ASD who participated in a 12-week MBTP have shown improved executive functions and reduced core symptoms of ASD. Hence, our promising findings support the idea that physical exercise interventions such as MBTP can be considered as a therapeutic tool for treating ASD preschoolers.

In summary, the findings of the present study suggest that the 12-week MBTP effectively improved executive function and core symptoms in preschoolers with ASD. Thus, this study provides initial evidence that MBTP serves as an effective, inexpensive, easily accessible intervention that can be applied in various settings across different cultures and countries. MBTP is a promising alternative intervention program that meets the need for a globally applicable intervention model for ASD preschoolers.

4.3. Strengths and Limitations

A clear strength of our study is the application of an alternative approach to treat ASD preschoolers. Specifically, we implemented a multidimensional physical exercise program, namely a mini-basketball training program that did not simply include the training of basic movement skills, but were also designed to promote behavior reinforcement. Hence, MBTP is different from previous training programs that were applied to treat preschool children with ASD. A further strength of this study is the rigorous control for several potential confounders, which could strengthen the assumption that the observed training-related gains in executive function and social communication can be attributed to the conduction of the MBTP. Nevertheless, it is important to emphasize that there are still several limitations in the current study which need further discussion. Firstly, we used a quasi-experimental design and thus the participants were not randomly assigned. On the other hand, since baseline scores were not significantly different between the two groups, this non-random assignment may not affect our findings. Secondly, although CHEXI, SRS-2, and RBS-R were validated scales to specifically assess executive functions and core symptoms, they are subjective measures, administered by parents of the participating children. It must be admitted that there is currently no other tool available which would allow for a more objective assessment of social communication impairments of individuals with ASD. Thus, positive effects on social communication in this study should be interpreted cautiously. Finally, except for age and gender, other demographic information including IQ, language level, and severity of symptoms were not collected in this pilot study. Future studies on this topic should include these variables.

5. Conclusions

The present study provides initial evidence that 12 weeks of MBTP may positively influence executive functions and core symptoms in preschoolers with ASD. These promising findings suggest that a mini-basketball training program can be used as a complementary intervention to alleviate core symptoms of ASD and to enhance executive functioning in preschoolers with ASD. Further research is needed to investigate the underlying neurobiological processes of the observed behavioral improvements.

Author Contributions: A.-G.C. and Z.-M.L. designed the study and oversaw the data collection; J.-G.W. and K.-L.C. analyzed the data and wrote the initial manuscript; A.-G.C., L.-N.Z., X.X., F.H., and L.Z. revised the manuscript for intellectual content. All authors have read and agreed to the published version of the manuscript.

Funding: This research was supported by grants from the National Natural Science Foundation of China (31771243) and the Fok Ying Tong Education Foundation (141113) to Ai-Guo Chen.

Acknowledgments: The authors would like to thank A.-G.C. and L.-N.Z. for their help with different aspects of this study. We would like to express our sincerest appreciation to the children and parents who generously gave their time and courage to participate in this study.

Conflicts of Interest: The authors declare no conflict of interest.

Appendix A

Stage I (2 Weeks)

To arouse children's interest in mini-basketball, and to standardize classroom routines in children and their parents, the main content was interesting and simple basketball training. Children in this stage were supposed to learn standard behavior and classroom routines such as taking turns, waiting and obeying.

Stage II (8 Weeks)

To improve children's motor skills, executive ability and flexibility, and to alleviate their core symptoms, the main content was basic basketball skill (dribbling, passing, shooting, etc.) and peer coordination training (e.g., passing and catching ball, relay racing).

Stage III (2 Weeks)

To improve children's cooperation and collectivization, the main content was basketball games such as basketball-dribbling relay, basketball-passing relays, basket-moving shooting, and basketball games.

References

1. American Psychiatric Association. *Diagnostic and Statistical Manual of Mental Disorders (DSM-5®)*; American Psychiatric Association: Washington, DC, USA, 2013.
2. Prelock, P.; Paul, R.; Allen, E.M. Evidence-Based Treatments in Communication for Children with Autism Spectrum Disorders. *Evid.-Based Pract. Treat. Child. Autism* **2010**, 93–169. [CrossRef]
3. Kenny, L.; Cribb, S.J.; Pellicano, E. Childhood Executive Function Predicts Later Autistic Features and Adaptive Behavior in Young Autistic People: A 12-Year Prospective Study. *J. Abnorm. Child Psychol.* **2018**, *47*, 1089–1099. [CrossRef] [PubMed]
4. Kaushanskaya, M.; Park, J.S.; Gangopadhyay, I.; Davidson, M.; Weismer, S.E. The Relationship between Executive Functions and Language Abilities in Children: A Latent Variables Approach. *J. Speech Lang. Hear. Res.* **2017**, *60*, 912–923. [CrossRef] [PubMed]
5. Pellicano, E. Links between theory of mind and executive function in young children with autism: Clues to developmental primacy. *Dev. Psychol.* **2007**, *43*, 974–990. [CrossRef]
6. Leung, R.C.; Vogan, V.M.; Powell, T.L.; Anagnostou, E.; Taylor, M.J. The role of executive functions in social impairment in Autism Spectrum Disorder. *Child. Neuropsychol.* **2015**, *22*, 336–344. [CrossRef]
7. Mostert-Kerckhoffs, M.A.L.; Staal, W.G.; Houben, R.H.; De Jonge, M.V. Stop and change: Inhibition and flexibility skills are related to repetitive behavior in children and young adults with autism spectrum disorders. *J. Autism Dev. Disord.* **2015**, *45*, 3148–3158. [CrossRef]
8. De Vries, M.; Geurts, H. Influence of Autism Traits and Executive Functioning on Quality of Life in Children with an Autism Spectrum Disorder. *J. Autism Dev. Disord.* **2015**, *45*, 2734–2743. [CrossRef]
9. Funahashi, S.; Andreau, J.M. Prefrontal cortex and neural mechanisms of executive function. *J. Physiol.* **2013**, *107*, 471–482. [CrossRef]
10. Hill, E. Evaluating the theory of executive dysfunction in autism. *Dev. Rev.* **2004**, *24*, 189–233. [CrossRef]
11. Hsia, Y.; Wong, A.Y.S.; Murphy, D.G.; Simonoff, E.; Buitelaar, J.K.; Wong, I.C. Psychopharmacological prescriptions for people with autism spectrum disorder (ASD): A multinational study. *Psychopharmacol.* **2013**, *231*, 999–1009. [CrossRef]
12. Lamy, M.; Erickson, C.A. Pharmacological management of behavioral disturbances in children and adolescents with autism spectrum disorders. *Curr. Probl. Pediatr. Adolesc. Health Care* **2018**, *48*, 250–264. [CrossRef]

13. Tan, B.W.Z.; Pooley, J.A.; Speelman, C. A Meta-Analytic Review of the Efficacy of Physical Exercise Interventions on Cognition in Individuals with Autism Spectrum Disorder and ADHD. *J. Autism Dev. Disord.* **2016**, *46*, 3126–3143. [CrossRef]
14. Ludyga, S.; Koutsandréou, F.; Reuter, E.-M.; Voelcker-Rehage, C.; Budde, H. A Randomized Controlled Trial on the Effects of Aerobic and Coordinative Training on Neural Correlates of Inhibitory Control in Children. *J. Clin. Med.* **2019**, *8*, 184. [CrossRef] [PubMed]
15. Benzing, V.; Chang, Y.-K.; Schmidt, M. Acute Physical Activity Enhances Executive Functions in Children with ADHD. *Sci. Rep.* **2018**, *8*, 12382. [CrossRef]
16. Chen, A.-G.; Zhu, L.-N.; Yan, J.; Yin, H.-C. Neural Basis of Working Memory Enhancement after Acute Aerobic Exercise: fMRI Study of Preadolescent Children. *Front. Psychol.* **2016**, *7*, 39. [CrossRef] [PubMed]
17. Chen, A.-G.; Zhu, L.-N.; Xiong, X.; Li, Y. Acute aerobic exercise alters executive control network in preadolescent children. *J. Sport Psychol.* **2017**, *26*, 132–137.
18. Koutsandréou, F.; Wegner, M.; Niemann, C.; Budde, H. Effects of Motor versus Cardiovascular Exercise Training on Children's Working Memory. *Med. Sci. Sports Exerc.* **2016**, *48*, 1144–1152. [CrossRef]
19. Zou, L.Y.; Xiao, Z.J.; Wang, H.R.; Wang, C.Y.; Hu, X.J.; Shu, Y.K. Martial arts for health benefits in children and youth with autism spectrum disorder: A systematic review. *Sport Sci.* **2017**, *13*, 79–92.
20. Hilton, C.; Cumpata, K.; Klohr, C.; Gaetke, S.; Artner, A.; Johnson, H.; Dobbs, S. Effects of Exergaming on Executive Function and Motor Skills in Children With Autism Spectrum Disorder: A Pilot Study. *Am. J. Occup. Ther.* **2013**, *68*, 57–65. [CrossRef]
21. Phung, J.N.; Goldberg, W.A. Promoting Executive Functioning in Children with Autism Spectrum Disorder Through Mixed Martial Arts Training. *J. Autism Dev. Disord.* **2019**, *49*, 3669–3684. [CrossRef]
22. Bahrami, F.; Movahedi, A.; Marandi, M.; Sorensen, C. The Effect of Karate Techniques Training on Communication Deficit of Children with Autism Spectrum Disorders. *J. Autism Dev. Disord.* **2015**, *46*, 978–986. [CrossRef] [PubMed]
23. Anderson-Hanley, C.; Tureck, K.; Schneiderman, R.L. Autism and exergaming: Effects on repetitive behaviors and cognition. *Psychol. Res. Behav. Manag.* **2011**, *4*, 129–137. [CrossRef]
24. Smithson, P.E.; Kenworthy, L.; Wills, M.C.; Jarrett, M.; Atmore, K.; Yerys, B.E. Real world executive control impairments in preschoolers with autism spectrum disorders. *J. Autism Dev. Disord.* **2013**, *43*, 1967–1975. [CrossRef] [PubMed]
25. Charman, T.; Baird, G. Practitioner Review: Diagnosis of autism spectrum disorder in 2- and 3-year-old children. *J. Child Psychol. Psychiatry* **2002**, *43*, 289–305. [CrossRef]
26. High, P.C. The Effectiveness of Early Intervention. *J. Dev. Behav. Pediatr.* **1999**, *20*, 294–295. [CrossRef]
27. Diamond, A. Effects of Physical Exercise on Executive Functions: Going beyond Simply Moving to Moving with Thought. *Ann. Sports Med. Res.* **2015**, *2*, 1011.
28. Diamond, A.; Ling, D.S. Aerobic-Exercise and resistance-training interventions have been among the least effective ways to improve executive functions of any method tried thus far. *Dev. Cogn. Neurosci.* **2018**, *37*, 100572. [CrossRef]
29. Pesce, C. Shifting the Focus from Quantitative to Qualitative Exercise Characteristics in Exercise and Cognition Research. *J. Sport Exerc. Psychol.* **2012**, *34*, 766–786. [CrossRef]
30. Ms, J.W.D.G.; Bosker, R.J.; Oosterlaan, J.; Visscher, C.; Hartman, E. Effects of physical activity on executive functions, attention and academic performance in preadolescent children: A meta-analysis. *J. Sci. Med. Sport* **2018**, *21*, 501–507. [CrossRef]
31. Fotrousi, F.; Bagherly, J.; Ghasemi, A. The Compensatory Impact of Mini-Basketball Skills on the Progress of Fundamental Movements in Children. *Procedia-Soc. Behav. Sci.* **2012**, *46*, 5206–5210. [CrossRef]
32. Zhu, Y.; Xu, C.; Wan, Q.; Guo, L.Y. Effects of adapted physical exercise intervention on visual working memory in children with autism spectrum disorder. *China Sport Sci. Technol.* **2017**, *53*, 55–62. [CrossRef]
33. Faul, F.; Erdfelder, E.; Buchner, A.; Lang, A.-G. Statistical power analyses using G*Power 3.1: Tests for correlation and regression analyses. *Behav. Res. Methods* **2009**, *41*, 1149–1160. [CrossRef]
34. Lambert, J.M.; Copeland, B.A.; Karp, E.L.; Finley, C.I.; Houchins-Juarez, N.J.; Ledford, J.R. Chaining Functional Basketball Sequences (with Embedded Conditional Discriminations) in an Adolescent with Autism. *Behav. Anal. Pract.* **2016**, *9*, 199–210. [CrossRef]
35. Chen, A.-G.; Yan, J.; Yin, H.-C.; Pan, C.-Y.; Chang, Y.-K. Effects of acute aerobic exercise on multiple aspects of executive function in preadolescent children. *Psychol. Sport Exerc.* **2014**, *15*, 627–636. [CrossRef]

36. Whaley, M.H.; Brubaker, P.H.; Otto, R.M.; Armstrong, L.E. *ACSM's Guidelines for Exercise Testing and Prescription*, 7th ed.; Lippincott Williams & Wilkins: Philadelphia, PA, USA, 2006.
37. Schopler, E.; Reichler, R.J.; DeVellis, R.F.; Daly, K. Toward objective classification of childhood autism: Childhood Autism Rating Scale (CARS). *J. Autism Dev. Disord.* **1980**, *10*, 91–103. [CrossRef]
38. Angriman, M.; Caravale, B.; Novelli, L.; Ferri, R.; Bruni, O. Sleep in Children with Neurodevelopmental Disabilities. *Neuropediatrics* **2015**, *46*, 199–210. [CrossRef]
39. Kral, T.V.; Eriksen, W.T.; Souders, M.C.; Pinto-Martin, J.A. Eating Behaviors, Diet Quality, and Gastrointestinal Symptoms in Children With Autism Spectrum Disorders: A Brief Review. *J. Pediatr. Nurs.* **2013**, *28*, 548–556. [CrossRef]
40. Owens, J.A.; Spirito, A.; McGuinn, M. The Children's Sleep Habits Questionnaire (CSHQ): Psychometric properties of a survey instrument for school-aged children. *Sleep* **2000**, *23*, 1043–1051. [CrossRef]
41. Wardle, J.; Guthrie, C.A.; Sanderson, S.; Rapoport, L. Development of the Children's Eating Behaviour Questionnaire. *J. Child Psychol. Psychiatry* **2001**, *42*, 963–970. [CrossRef]
42. Thorell, L.B.; Nyberg, L. The Childhood Executive Functioning Inventory (CHEXI): A New Rating Instrument for Parents and Teachers. *Dev. Neuropsychol.* **2008**, *33*, 536–552. [CrossRef]
43. Wei, W.; Xie, Q.B.; Zhu, J.J.; He, W.; Li, Y. The Psychometric Characteristics of Childhood Executive Functioning Inventory among Chinese Preschoolers. *Chin. J. Clin. Psychol.* **2018**, *26*, 26–29.
44. Constantino, J.; Gruber, C.P. *The Social Responsiveness Scale (SRS) Manual*; Western Psychological Services: Los Angeles, CA, USA, 2005.
45. Bodfish, J.W.; Symons, F.J.; Parker, D.E.; Lewis, M.H. Varieties of repetitive behavior in autism: Comparisons to mental retardation. *J. Autism Dev. Disord.* **2000**, *30*, 237–243. [CrossRef] [PubMed]
46. Pan, C.-Y.; Chu, C.-H.; Tsai, C.-L.; Sung, M.-C.; Huang, C.-Y.; Ma, W.-Y. The impacts of physical activity intervention on physical and cognitive outcomes in children with autism spectrum disorder. *Autism* **2016**, *21*, 190–202. [CrossRef]
47. Pan, C.-Y.; Tsai, C.-L.; Chu, C.-H.; Sung, M.-C.; Huang, C.-Y.; Ma, W.-Y. Effects of Physical Exercise Intervention on Motor Skills and Executive Functions in Children with ADHD: A Pilot Study. *J. Atten. Disord.* **2015**, *23*, 384–397. [CrossRef]
48. Tsai, C.-L.; Wang, C.-H.; Tseng, Y.-T. Effects of exercise intervention on event-related potential and task performance indices of attention networks in children with developmental coordination disorder. *Brain Cogn.* **2012**, *79*, 12–22. [CrossRef]
49. Ziereis, S.; Jansen, P. Effects of physical activity on executive function and motor performance in children with ADHD. *Res. Dev. Disabil.* **2015**, *38*, 181–191. [CrossRef]
50. Alesi, M.; Bianco, A.; Luppina, G.; Palma, A.; Pepi, A. Improving Children's Coordinative Skills and Executive Functions. *Percept. Mot. Ski.* **2016**, *122*, 27–46. [CrossRef]
51. Netz, Y. Is There a Preferred Mode of Exercise for Cognition Enhancement in Older Age?—A Narrative Review. *Front. Med.* **2019**, *6*, 57. [CrossRef]
52. Bamidis, P.; Vivas, A.; Styliadis, C.; Frantzidis, C.A.; Klados, M.; Schlee, W.; Siountas, A.; Papageorgiou, S. A review of physical and cognitive interventions in aging. *Neurosci. Biobehav. Rev.* **2014**, *44*, 206–220. [CrossRef]
53. Fissler, P.; Küster, O.; Schlee, W.; Kolassa, I.-T. Novelty Interventions to Enhance Broad Cognitive Abilities and Prevent Dementia. *Prog. Brain Res.* **2013**, *207*, 403–434. [CrossRef]
54. Herold, F.; Hamacher, D.; Schega, L.; Müller, N.G. Thinking While Moving or Moving While Thinking—Concepts of Motor-Cognitive Training for Cognitive Performance Enhancement. *Front. Aging Neurosci.* **2018**, *10*, 228. [CrossRef]
55. Jeon, Y.K.; Ha, C.H. The effect of exercise intensity on brain derived neurotrophic factor and memory in adolescents. *Environ. Health Prev. Med.* **2017**, *22*, 27. [CrossRef]
56. Krafft, C.E.; Pierce, J.E.; Schwarz, N.F.; Chi, L.; Weinberger, A.L.; Schaeffer, D.J.; Rodrigue, A.L.; Camchong, J.; Allison, J.D.; Yanasak, N.E.; et al. An eight month randomized controlled exercise intervention alters resting state synchrony in overweight children. *Neuroscience* **2013**, *256*, 445–455. [CrossRef]
57. Krafft, C.E.; Schwarz, N.F.; Chi, L.; Weinberger, A.L.; Schaeffer, D.J.; Pierce, J.E.; Rodrigue, A.L.; Yanasak, N.E.; Miller, P.H.; Tomporowski, P.D.; et al. An 8-month randomized controlled exercise trial alters brain activation during cognitive tasks in overweight children. *Obesity* **2013**, *22*, 232–242. [CrossRef]

58. Bass, M.M.; Duchowny, C.A.; Llabre, M.M. The Effect of Therapeutic Horseback Riding on Social Functioning in Children with Autism. *J. Autism Dev. Disord.* **2009**, *39*, 1261–1267. [CrossRef]
59. Pan, C.-Y. Effects of water exercise swimming program on aquatic skills and social behaviors in children with autism spectrum disorders. *Autism* **2010**, *14*, 9–28. [CrossRef]
60. Lang, R.; Koegel, L.K.; Ashbaugh, K.; Regester, A.; Ence, W.; Smith, W. Physical exercise and individuals with autism spectrum disorders: A systematic review. *Res. Autism Spectr. Disord.* **2010**, *4*, 565–576. [CrossRef]
61. Ferraioli, S.J.; Harris, S.L. Treatments to Increase Social Awareness and Social Skills. In *Evidence-Based Practices and Treatments for Children with Autism*; Reichow, B., Ed.; Springer Science + Business Media: New York, NY, USA, 2011; pp. 171–196.

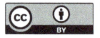

© 2020 by the authors. Licensee MDPI, Basel, Switzerland. This article is an open access article distributed under the terms and conditions of the Creative Commons Attribution (CC BY) license (http://creativecommons.org/licenses/by/4.0/).

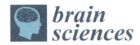

Article

Behavioral and Cognitive Electrophysiological Differences in the Executive Functions of Taiwanese Basketball Players as a Function of Playing Position

Yi-Kang Chiu [1], Chien-Yu Pan [2], Fu-Chen Chen [2], Yu-Ting Tseng [3,4] and Chia-Liang Tsai [1,*]

[1] Institute of Physical Education, Health and Leisure Studies, National Cheng Kung University, Tainan 701, Taiwan; yigang3654@gmail.com
[2] Department of Physical Education, National Kaohsiung Normal University, Kaoshiung 802, Taiwan; chpan@nknucc.nknu.edu.tw (C.-Y.P.); kiddlovejean@gmail.com (F.-C.C.)
[3] Department of Physical Education, National Tsing Hua University, Hsinchu 300, Taiwan; yuting75111@hotmail.com
[4] Research Center for Education and Mind Sciences, National Tsing Hua University, Hsinchu 300, Taiwan
* Correspondence: andytsai@mail.ncku.edu.tw; Tel.: +886-933-306-059 or +886-6275-7575 (ext. 81809); Fax: +886-6276-6427

Received: 14 May 2020; Accepted: 17 June 2020; Published: 19 June 2020

Abstract: The effect of the predominant playing position of elite basketball players on executive functions using both behavioral and electrophysiological measurements was investigated in the present study. Forty-six elite basketball players, including 27 guards and 19 forwards, were recruited. Event-related potential (ERP) signals were simultaneously recorded when the athletes performed the visual Go/NoGo task. Analyses of the results revealed that the guards and forwards groups exhibited comparable behavioral (i.e., reaction time (RTs) and accuracy rates (ARs)) performance. With regards to the electrophysiological indices, the guards relative to the forwards exhibited a shorter N2 latency in the Go condition, a longer N2 latency in the NoGo condition, and a smaller P3 amplitude across the two conditions. These results suggested that although the guards and forwards exhibited similar abilities in terms of behavioral inhibition, different neural processing efficiencies still exist in the basketball playing positions, with guards showing divergent efficiencies in the target evaluation and response selection of the target and non-target stimuli and fewer cognitive resources during premotor preparation and decision-making as compared to the forwards.

Keywords: cognition; inhibition; basketball; playing positions; Go/NoGo; event-related potential

1. Introduction

Sports training can positively influence the brain related to neural functioning and cognitive performance [1–3]. Prolonged engagement within specific sports training processes and deliberate practice contribute to domain-specific expertise, resulting in elaborate cognitive performance [4]. However, the effects of sports training on cognition can vary across various types of sports due to the different amount of cognitive loads required for each sports type [3,5,6].

In general, a large range of sports can be roughly categorized into two types: open-skill and closed-skill sports [2,5–7]. Players in an open-skill sport are required to constantly adapt their actions and switch their strategies and skills according to the fast-changing, unpredictable environment [2,7]. These environments are usually externally paced [6]. On the contrary, closed-skill types of exercise take place in a relatively stable, predictable environment, in which performers behave at their own pace [5–7].

Considering the skills required in these two different domains, engaging in open-skilled sports requires various sets of motor skills (e.g., inhibiting movement from a proponent to an appropriate action in response to cues coming from teammates, opponents, and ball movements) and additional cognitive loads (e.g., planning and cognitive flexibility), while close-skilled athletes should require abilities related to attention maintenance in order to control their pace and concentrate on their own movements [6]. Therefore, open-skilled exercises participants experience greater cognitive loads and open-skilled sports affect cognitive abilities, especially executive functions, more than closed-skilled exercises [7]. Based on these concepts, different levels of executive functions can thus be modulated as a function of the different cognitive load requirements for various types of sports [6].

Executive functions (EF) are higher-order cognitive functions that regulate attention and actions, for which specific processes are especially necessary when individuals have to pay attention and concentrate in atypical situations [8–10]. Evidence has elucidated the effects of different sport types on inhibitory control via event-related potentials (ERPs) performance [5,11]. ERPs are defined as neural electrophysiological signals that reflect the brain's electrical activity occurring during sensory, cognitive, or motoric processing [12,13]. The ERP N2 component is thought to reflect the conflict monitoring in early visual processing, which is a crucial process for early stage inhibitory control [14–17]. Di Russo et al. (2010) found that N2 latencies were significantly shorter for disabled basketball players compared to disabled swimmers [7]. However, basketball players did not significantly differ from healthy non-athletes. In addition, they also found that swimmers' N2 amplitudes were significantly lower than those for basketball players and healthy non-athletes. The reduced N2 amplitudes and the slower N2 latencies shown by swimmers were interpreted as difficulty related to inhibiting intended actions. By contrast, the fact that basketball players' N2 amplitudes and latencies corresponded with healthy non-athletes suggested that open skill sports training increases inhibitory ability by compensating for a disability [7]. Given the superior inhibitory controls of open-skilled athletes, the finding provided evidence that open-skilled training can benefit executive functioning [5,7].

However, playing positions in open-skilled sports features specific tasks, roles, and jobs [18]. For players to exhibit successful performance in a specific position, extended exposure to practices that conform to the demands of specific tasks are necessary. These procedures ultimately contribute to expert performance (i.e., physical skills) associated with a specific playing position [4]—that is, position-specific expertise [19]. In addition, the development of position-specific expertise is due to the neurocognitive adaptation of the cognitive function that characterizes such expert performance [4]. Therefore, it is the cognitive differences that can be differentiated among playing positions, which is in keeping with the differences in positional behavioral patterns.

Studies have confirmed that diverse cognitive styles exist between playing positions in open-skilled sports. For example, Montuori et al. (2019) investigated positional effects on cognitive flexibility in elite volleyball players and reported that mixed players had a longer reaction time (RT) and higher accuracy rates (ARs) compared to strikers and defenders [10]. Another study conducted by Schumacher et al. (2018) investigating the potential effects of general attention, anticipation, and reaction in soccer players with different playing positions found that midfielders only showed a significantly faster reaction time (RT) in an acoustic RT test (ART) as compared to defenders [20]. These findings supported the supposition that the executive profile in open-skill sports is position-specific. In addition, Vestberg et al. (2017) suggested that, in soccer, attackers require stable executive functions, while midfielders require impulsivity and defenders need inhibitory control [21]. Despite the evidence demonstrating that playing positions induce divergent cognitive benefits, these positional effects may vary across different types of open-skilled sports due to the nuances specific to a type of sport [3,11]. Accordingly, more studies that investigate the positional effects of open-skilled sports other than volleyball and soccer are still needed. Most importantly, previous works regarding this issue were primarily focused on behavioral performance, in which instantaneous shifts in attention and the consequences of visual stimulation processes cannot be observed independently [1,5]. Thus far, the neural mechanism that modulates the executive functions as a function of playing position is still unclear. Hence, the further exploration of positional effects on cognition in open-skilled athletes is necessary.

Basketball is a team sport that consists of two teams opposing one another. Teams compete for primary goals by making successful shots with a ball through their opponents' hoop and preventing their opponents scoring through their own. Hence, physical skills or strategies related to scoring and defense, tactical execution, and team cooperation are crucial for basketball players [19]. During basketball matches, players are continuously bombarded with both relevant and distractive information that may potentially imperil their response execution [22]. These contrasting sources of information put substantial loads on the executive abilities of basketball players that require critical focus, carrying out actions, and concurrently controlling attention while being distracted by conflicting information (i.e., inhibitory controls) [22].

In general basketball competitions, basketball players can be precisely categorized into five positions: (1) point guard (PG), (2) shooting guard (SG), (3) small forward (SF), (4) power forward (PF), and (5) center (C). Traditional classifications tend to further classify players into guards (SG and PG), forwards (SF), and centers (PF and C) due to the similarities in their assignments in a match [18,19]. Since physical skills can differentiate playing positions in basketball [19,23], we hypothesized that there would be executive differences in relation to behavioral inhibition exhibited between basketball player positions due to the contrasting physical skill sets that underlie inhibitory controls. For example, penetration requires instant responses to external cues [24], where penetrators have to suppress their ongoing movement (e.g., moving direction, skills, or velocities) in response to defenders and execute more effective movements. In the analysis of the physical skills required for successful performance in a given playing position, penetration movements are executed by players in all positions, while guards penetrate primarily facing the basket and centers penetrate with their back to the basket [19]. It is worth noting that contrasting differences exist between facing or backing penetration. Penetration facing the basket requires instant execution and the suppression of movements, emphasizing both velocity and immediate responses, while penetration with the back to the basket requires powerful force to squeeze into the painted area, stressing physical collision and lower limb stability [18]. Additionally, centers execute more static tasks (e.g., gaining position, blocking, and screening) than guards, for which the movements require a significant amount of physical resistance and contact [19], with relatively fewer uncertain factors as compared to penetration. In addition, the evidence of physical activities can also provide the foundations for positional differences. Basketball exercises generally include substantial changes of direction in response to environmental stimuli; these changes may be related to information processing that involves visual scanning, decision-making, and reactive movements [25]. However, substantial environmental-stimuli from frequent directional changes may positively affect the cognitive abilities of basketball players. Previous studies have reported that guards tend to execute more frequent movement and directional changes than centers [24,26]. Given the greater numbers of changes in directions, accelerations, and decelerations executed by guards when performing at a higher movement speed than centers, the cognitive loads suffered by guards may be therefore greater than those imposed on centers. Taken together, differences in physical skills may potentially modulate the inhibitory control of basketball players based on the different playing positions.

Inhibitory control requires the control of the attentional ability to be unaffected by a strong internal inclination or an external temptation, making it possible to control actions; suppress automatic, dominant, or prepotent responses; and instead act appropriately [8,9,14]. Inhibitory ability is rather critical to athletes due to a positive association with successful performance in open-skilled experts, so successful players can make quick decisions while instantly inhibiting planned movements [8,9,22]. Such a cognitive function is necessary to the successful performances of basketball players in practical competitions and can be differentiated based on basketball playing positions. Accordingly, determining whether inhibitory controls may be modulated by different playing positions owing to several position-specific features of physical skills and motor executions needs to be explored.

The Go/NoGo task is a perceptual discriminative task that is frequently used to investigate inhibitory ability [14,27], especially in elite athletes [7,11,28]. In this paradigm, an individual has to produce a speedy covert response to a target stimulus and must refrain from responding to a non-target stimulus [14,27,29,30]. The procedures in the task mimic the complex visual motor behavior patterns of basketball players, including task preparation, stimulus identification and evaluation, response selection, and response execution or inhibition [7,30].

As mentioned above, ERP signals have been used to detect the dynamic brain activity reflecting instant neural cognitive processing [12,13]. Its excellent temporal resolution allows for determining the time sequences of neural and psychological processes from millisecond to millisecond [12], which behavioral measurement techniques leave blank [27,31]. ERP recordings reflect the timing and organization of several information processes in the brain's networks. These sensitive indices have been widely applied to evaluate cognitive differences across exercise groups [3,6]. Two ERP components (e.g., N2 and P3) are activated when performing the Go/NoGo task coupled with ERP recording. The N2 components are defined as the peak negative voltage evoked after the appearance of the stimuli during a time window of 200–350 ms, whereas the P3 components are the positive deflection that peaks after the appearance of the target in a time window of 350–600 ms [15]. In addition, N2 and P3 can reflect the mental processes involved in conflict monitoring [14–17], as well as premotor evaluations and decision-making [2,3,15,27,29,30,32], respectively.

Notwithstanding the fact that previous studies have revealed divergent executive profiles across playing positions in open-skill sports [10,20], extended investigations are still needed for the following reasons: (1) nuances that are different across various types of open-skilled sports may cause diverse positional effects on cognition [3,11]; and (2) previous findings only emphasized behavioral performance [10,20], leaving the actual neuronal mechanism still unclear. To the best of our knowledge, no research has yet been conducted to demonstrate inhibitory ability as a function of basketball playing position using a Go/NoGo paradigm coupled with neural electrophysiological techniques. Therefore, the aim of the present study was to investigate the effects of predominant playing positions on inhibitory controls using both behavioral (i.e., RT and AR) and electrophysiological (i.e., N2 and P3 latencies and amplitudes) measurements in elite basketball players when performing the visual Go/NoGo task. In the present study, basketball players were classified into two groups: guards (i.e., PG, SG, and SF) and centers (i.e., PF and C), given that this classification is the one that experts and coaches most commonly adopt [18,19]. We hypothesized that significant positional effects would be observed, showing that guards exhibit superior performance in neurocognitive (i.e., behavioral and electrophysiological) measurements as compared to forwards.

2. Materials and Methods

2.1. Participants

Forty-six male elite players (mean age 20.57 ± 1.13 years) participating in the highest level of basketball competitions in Taiwan were recruited from six University Basketball Association (UBA) basketball teams in this study. Since previous research has revealed that differences in neuropsychological and neurophysiological characteristics exist between genders [33] and that differences in training loads also occur between male and female basketball players [34], the experimental design of mixed-gender groups may result in unbalanced neuropsychological changes regarding the cognitive measurements [33]. Only male players were thus recruited in the current study. Twenty-seven guards and nineteen forwards were included. The playing positions of the participants were self-reported and reported by the coaches, and those who played multiple positions (e.g., across both guards and forwards, especially between SF and PF) were excluded from this study. Both of the groups were matched for age, level of education, and hand dominance. All the players were non-smokers, with normal or corrected-to-normal vision. In addition, they were free of cardiovascular, psychiatric, metabolic, or neurological diseases, as well as any history of head injuries. Participants who were taking medications that could influence the function of the central nervous system were excluded. The participants were instructed to avoid caffeine, alcohol consumption, and moderate-to-vigorous workouts on the day before the experiment. None of the players exhibited cognitive impairment, as measured by scoring above 26 on the Mini-Mental-State Examination (MMSE) [35]. Written informed consent, which was approved by the Institutional Ethics Committee of National Cheng Kung University (REC 108-567), was obtained from all of the players after a full explanation of the experimental procedure. All of the players obtained payment for their participation.

2.2. Procedure

The participants were asked to visit the cognitive neurophysiology laboratory twice. On the first visit, a demographic questionnaire; an informed consent form; and the MMSE and Beck Depression Inventory, 2nd edition (BDI-II) [36], assessments were completed, and BMI was calculated (weights/heights^2) to avoid confounding effects on cognition [37,38]. The cognitive task was performed in an acoustical shield laboratory with dimmed light. The participants were seated in front of a color computer monitor (with 47.5 × 27 cm) placed approximately 70 cm from the eyes, and an electrocap and electro-oculographic (EOG) electrodes were attached to their faces and scalps before the Go/NoGo task initiated. On the second visit in the same week, the values of the estimated VO$_2$ max were measured using a Yo-Yo intermittent recovery test (Yo-Yo IR1) [39,40].

2.3. Go/NoGo Paradigm

In the Go/NoGo paradigm, either a blue or yellow dot was presented as the visual stimuli using the E-prime 2.0 neural stimulation system (Psychology Software Tools, Inc., 311 23rd Street Ext. Suite 200 Sharpsburg, PA, USA). The stimulus was presented in the center of the computer monitor at a visual angle of 2.5 degrees. There were four blocks with 60 Go (blue dots) and 20 NoGo (yellow dots) stimuli in each trial. The participants were required to respond to the Go stimuli as quickly as possible by pressing the space button with their dominant hand and to refrain from responding when the NoGo stimuli appeared. The order of presentation was random within blocks and across participants. The entire task procedure is illustrated in Figure 1. Each trial was initiated, and a white cross served as the fixation point. The first trial was initiated with the instructions, followed by a 3 s countdown and a 1000 ms period prior to the commencement of the fixation cross. Following the offset of the fixation, either a Go or NoGo stimulus was presented. The Go stimulus was presented for 500 ms, while the NoGo stimulus lasted for 3000 ms. The next trial was initiated once the space button was pressed (in both the Go and NoGo conditions) or withheld for 3000 ms (in the NoGo condition). Consequently, various intertrial intervals were randomly presented at between 1100 and 1700 ms. Before recording the electrophysiological signals, the participants performed practice blocks to ensure that they were familiar with the task. During the task, the participants had to constantly focus on the center of the monitor to avoid body movements and saccades. A duration of two minutes was given to every participant to rest between blocks.

2.4. Cardiorespiratory Fitness Estimation

The Yo-Yo IR1 test was conducted to estimate cardiorespiratory fitness (i.e., VO$_{2max}$) according to procedures described previously (Krustrup et al., 2003). The test consists of repeated shuttle runs (2 × 20 m) that are performed at a progressively increasing velocity interspersed with active recoveries (2 × 5 m, 10-s) until exhaustion. The test was terminated when the players failed to complete the distance on time twice, or they subjectively felt that they were unable to maintain the speed. The total distances covered during the test was considered the players' scores [39]. After measuring the final score of the test, the estimation of VO$_2$ max was quantified using the following formula: VO$_2$ max (ml kg^{-1} min^{-1}) = players' scores (m) × 0.0084 + 36.4 [40].

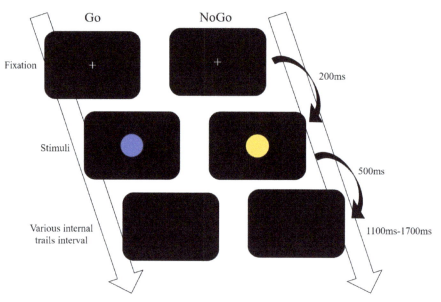

Figure 1. The Go/NoGo paradigm.

2.5. Electrophysiological Recording and Analysis

Electrophysiological data were recorded from participants when they were performing the Go/NoGo task using the Syn-Amps Electroencephalography (EEG) amplifier and the Scan 4.5 package (Neuroscan Inc., El Paso, TX, USA) with 23 electrodes (including Fz, F3, F4, FCz, FC3, FC4, Cz, C3, C4, CPz, CP3, CP4, Pz, P3, P4, PO3, PO4, PO7, PO8, Oz, O1, and O2) according to the International 10-20 System. All the electrodes were referenced to linked bilateral mastoid electrodes. An electrode placed at the mid-frontal scalp served as the ground. The horizontal and vertical electrooculographic (EOG) activities were bipolarly recorded with two pairs of electrodes placed 2 cm from the canthi of both eyes and 2 cm above and below the left eye, respectively. All the electrode impedances were maintained below 5Ω. All the EEG data were digitized with an analog-to-digital (A/D) rate of 500 Hz/channel; amplified with a band-pass filter of 0.1–30 Hz (Zero Phase Shift filtering mode will be adopted), including a notch filter of 60 Hz; and stored for an off-line analysis using the Scan 4.5 analysis software (Neuroscan Inc., El Paso, TX, USA).

Trials with missed Go responses, false NoGo responses, and RTs faster than 150 ms and slower than two standard deviations were excluded from the analysis. The EEG data were segmented into epochs starting from −200 ms prior to and 600 ms after the stimulus onset. Consequently, the epoch trials that were contaminated by ocular artifacts with amplitudes exceeding ± 100 mV were discarded from the analysis. Clean epoch trials were then baseline corrected, averaged to form a grand ERP, and constructed according to various conditions.

Two major stimulus-locked ERP components, N2 and P3, were measured at the Fz, FCz, and Cz electrodes. The mean N2 amplitude and latency were measured within a time window of 200–350 ms, and the mean P3 amplitude and latency were measured within a time window of 350–600 ms [15].

2.6. Statistical Analysis

Between-group comparisons (guards vs. forwards) of the demographic data including age, level of education, height, weight, BMI, estimated VO_2 max, scores on the MMSE and BDI-II, years of playing basketball experience, training frequency per week, and training period were analyzed using an independent t test. Hand dominance was subjected to a Pearson's chi-squared test. A demographic index (e.g., MMSE, BDI-II, BMI, and VO$_{2max}$) served as a confounding variable whenever a significant difference occurred between the two groups [37,38]. RTs were subjected to an independent t test, and the ARs were subjected to a repeated-measured 2 (group: guards and forwards) × 2 (condition: Go and NoGo) ANOVA, with the group as the between-subjects factor and the condition as the within-subjects factor. The electrophysiological indices were subjected to a repeated-measured 2 (group: guards and forwards) × 2 (condition: Go and NoGo) × 3 (electrode: Fz, FCz, and Cz) ANOVA, with group as the between-subjects factor and condition and electrode as the within-subjects factors. A Bonferroni post hoc analysis was performed when a significant difference occurred. A Greenhouse–Geisser correction was adopted to adjust the significance level when the sphericity assumption was violated. The level of significance was set at $p < 0.05$.

3. Results

3.1. Demographic Characteristics

Table 1 provides an overview of the demographic characteristics of the guards and the forwards. The two groups were matched at the group level in terms of age, handedness, BMI, and VO$_2$ max. Basketball experiences, training frequency, and training period were also comparable between the two groups. There were no significant differences in the level of education, mental state, and depression. There were, however, significant between-group differences in height and weight, with forwards being taller ($t_{(1)} = -7.495$, $p < 0.001$) and heavier ($t_{(1)} = -4.561$, $p < 0.001$) than guards.

Table 1. Demographic characteristics (mean ± SD) for the guards and the forward groups.

	Guards (*n* = 27)	Forwards (*n* = 19)	*p*
Age (years)	20.74 ± 1.10	20.26 ± 1.24	0.175
Handiness (R(L))	24 (3)	16 (3)	0.643
Education (years)	14.44 ± 1.37	14.00 ± 0.94	0.199
Height (cm) *	178.59 ± 5.87	190.74 ± 4.65	<0.001
Weight (kg) *	73.54 ± 7.79	86.74 ± 7.33	<0.001
BMI (kg/m^2)	23.04 ± 1.98	23.80 ± 1.61	0.173
MMSE	28.74 ± 1.13	28.33 ± 1.45	0.318
BDI-II	6.89 ± 6.03	9.00 ± 5.95	0.282
BE (years)	7.22 ± 3.27	6.32 ± 2.65	0.324
TF (times/week)	8.48 ± 2.38	7.53 ± 2.72	0.212
TP (hr/time)	2.60 ± 0.46	2.50 ± 0.50	0.480
VO$_2$ max (ml/kg/min)	46.87 ± 3.27	47.79 ± 3.84	0.949

MMSE: Mini Mental State Examination; BDI-II: Beck Depression Inventory, 2nd edition; BE: years of playing basketball experience; TF: Training frequency per week; TP: Training period per session; * $p < 0.05$.

3.2. Behavioral Performance

As illustrated in Figure 2, no significant between-group differences in RT ($t_{(44)} = -0.42$, $p = 0.679$) were observed. A significant main effect of condition on the ARs ($F_{(1,44)} = 8.77$, $p = 0.005$, $\eta_p^2 = 0.17$) was observed, indicating higher ARs in Go conditions (98.08% ± 3.06%) compared to in NoGo conditions (95.94% ± 3.36%) across the two groups. No significant main effects of group or condition × group interactions were observed.

3.3. Electrophysiological Performance

In Figure 3, the grand-average ERP waveforms obtained from the three midline electrodes (e.g., Fz, FCz, and Cz) in the two groups are reillustrated.

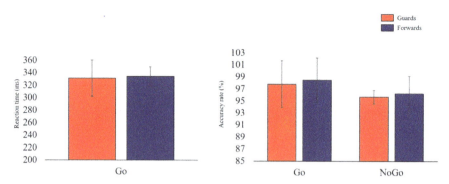

Figure 2. The behavioral performance of the guards and forwards groups.

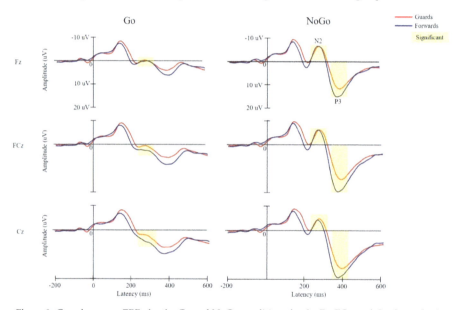

Figure 3. Grand-average ERPs for the Go and NoGo conditions for the Fz, FCz, and Cz electrodes in the guards and forwards groups (red line: guards group; blue line: forwards group).

3.3.1. N2 Latency

There were significant main effects of condition ($F_{(1,44)} = 13.51$, $p = 0.001$, $\eta_p^2 = 0.24$) and electrode ($F_{(1.75, 76.982)} = 18.81$, $p < 0.001$, $\eta_p^2 = 0.47$) on the N2 latencies, indicating that the N2 latencies in the NoGo condition (271.71 ± 2.49 ms) were shorter than those in the Go condition (283.67 ± 3.50 ms) across the two groups. Electrodes on the N2 latency were observed to have the following gradient: Cz (274.67 ± 22.69 ms) < FCz (277.20 ± 21.30 ms) < Fz (280.85 ± 21.47 ms). There was also a significant effect of the group × condition interactions ($F_{(1,44)} = 7.58$, $p = 0.009$, $\eta_p^2 = 0.15$). Post hoc comparisons showed that, in comparison to the forwards, the guards had shorter N2 latencies in the Go condition (guards vs. forwards: 277.64 ± 24.72 vs. 288.82 ± 22.76 ms, $p = 0.007$) and longer N2 latencies in the NoGo condition (guards vs. forwards: 274.54 ± 18.33 vs. 267.89 ± 16.49 ms, $p = 0.030$).

3.3.2. N2 Amplitude

There were significant main effects of electrode ($F_{(1.466, 22.273)} = 22.27$, $p < 0.001$, $\eta_p^2 = 0.34$) and condition ($F_{(1,44)} = 107.68$, $p < 0.001$, $\eta_p^2 = 0.71$) on the N2 amplitudes, indicating that the N2 amplitudes in the NoGo condition (−6.90 ± 6.17 μV) were larger than those in the Go condition (0.44 ± 4.12 μV) across the two group and three electrodes. Electrodes on the N2 amplitudes were observed to have the following gradient: Fz (−4.33 ± 5.36 μV) > FCz (−3.66 ± 6.55 μV) > Cz (−1.70 ± 6.95 μV). There were also significant effects of condition × electrode interactions ($F_{(1.752, 77.096)} = 3.84$, $p = 0.031$, $\eta_p^2 = 0.08$). A post hoc comparison showed that N2 amplitudes in the Fz (−1.08 ± 3.32 μV) were significantly larger than those in the Cz (2.12 ± 4.54 μV) in the Go condition.

3.3.3. P3 Latency

A significant main effect of electrode on the P3 latency ($F_{(1.624, 71.442)} = 11.01$, $p < 0.001$, $\eta_p^2 = 0.20$) was observed, with the following gradient: Fz (381.42 ± 26.17 ms) > FCz (377.97 ± 28.85 ms) > Cz (377.10 ± 27.24 ms). There were also significant effects of group × electrodes interaction on the P3 latencies ($F_{(2,43)} = 6.15$, $p = 0.003$, $\eta_p^2 = 0.12$). A post hoc comparison showed that the P3 latencies in the Fz (380.87 ± 23.16 ms) were slower than those in the FCz (373.82 ± 24.58 ms) and Cz (372.24 ± 23.99 ms) in the forwards group.

3.3.4. P3 Amplitude

There were significant main effects of condition ($F_{(1,44)} = 282.29$, $p < 0.001$, $\eta_p^2 = 0.87$) and electrode ($F_{(1.254, 55.183)} = 50.42$, $p < 0.001$, $\eta = 0.53$), indicating that the P3 amplitudes in the NoGo condition (17.32 ± 6.8 μV) were larger than those in the Go condition (7.8 ± 5.36 μV) across the two group and three electrodes. The electrodes for the N2 amplitudes were observed to have the following gradient: Cz (14.14 ± 7.78 μV) > FCz (13.22 ± 8.1 μV) > Fz (10.31 ± 6.88 μV). A significant main effect of group ($F_{(1,44)} = 5.34$, $p = 0.026$, $\eta_p^2 = 0.11$) was also observed, with the P3 amplitudes being larger in the forwards group (14.64 ± 8.56 μV) than in the guards group (11.10 ± 6.78 μV) across both conditions and electrodes. A significant effect of the conditions × electrodes interaction ($F_{(1.637, 72.02)} = 10.07$, $p < 0.001$, $\eta = 0.19$) was observed. A post hoc comparison showed that the P3 amplitudes at Cz (9.50 ± 5.6 μV) were significantly larger than those at Fz (5.82 ± 4.33 μV) in the Go condition, and the P3 amplitudes at FCz (18.74 ± 6.99 μV) and Cz (18.78 ± 6.86 μV) were significantly larger than those at Fz (14.81 ± 5.91 μV) in the NoGo condition.

4. Discussion

In the present study, we investigated the effects of predominant playing positions on inhibitory controls using both behavioral (i.e., RT and AR) and electrophysiological (i.e., N2 and P3 latencies and amplitudes) measurements in basketball players when the participants were performing the visual Go/NoGo task. The main findings of the present study were as follows: (1) a comparable behavioral performance (i.e., RTs and ARs) was found between the guards and forwards groups, (2) the guards relative to the forwards had a shorter N2 latency in the Go condition and a longer N2 latency in the NoGo condition, (3) the guards group exhibited a smaller P3 amplitudes across the two conditions and three electrodes than the forwards group.

4.1. Behavioral Indices

The present findings, indicating that the guards and forwards groups had comparable RTs and Ars, were inconsistent with the findings of previous works [10,20]. Montuori et al. (2019) suggested that mixed players in volleyball had longer RTs and higher ARs than strikers and defenders when engaged in a sport-specific task-switching task [10]. Schumacher et al. (2018) revealed significant behavioral differences in a visual RT (VRT) task between soccer midfielders and strikers [20]. The lack of differences in behavioral performance was unexpected. We predicted that guards might exhibit a superior behavioral performance compared to the forwards due to the cognitive adaptation resulting from higher levels of cognitive load resulting from their position-specific expertise [19,23] and additional changes in direction while playing basketball [26]. However, this prediction was not consistent with our current findings. Possible interpretations of the comparable behavioral performance may thus be proposed.

Firstly, the way to distinguish the playing positions may be different between basketball and volleyball [10]. In volleyball, players seldom execute tasks that are beyond their positional domain. In other words, attackers seldom play defense, and, conversely, defenders seldom play attackers [10]. Defensive players engage in a judgement that requires continuous reactions to the misdirection and distractions created by the offensive teams [4]. They have to continuously read the intentions of their opponents, process their deceptive actions, and prevent their offensive maneuvers [4,22]. On the other hand, offensive players behave in a selective rather than a passive way due to their possession of the ball. Since they can decide what movements they want to take, offensive players usually play with less uncertainty when executing their decisions because of a lack of illusive schemes from the defensive side [4]. Taken together, given that the tasks required for the playing positions are primarily based on offensive and defensive characteristics, we can tentatively conclude that positional differences in behavioral performance in volleyball are due to the contrasting expertise that is necessitated in offensive vs. defensive schemes. These concepts were supported by investigations of cognitive differences between other offensive and defensive open-skilled players. Wylie et al. (2018) found that defensive football players assume lower interference costs when conducting the Erickson flanker task in comparison to offensive players [22], and Williams et al. (2008) found that defensive soccer players display greater anticipation skills than offensive players in both defensive and offensive situations [4]. Nevertheless, unlike the open-skilled sports mentioned previously, differentiation among basketball positions is based on anthropometrics. In other words, taller, heavier players (as also seen in the present study) are usually placed in the painted area (i.e., forwards), and shorter, lighter players are located in the perimeter area (i.e., guards) [18,19]. It is necessary to mention that task demands based on offensive or defensive plans cannot directly help distinguish between basketball playing positions. Conversely, basketball players all participate in offensive and defensive actions when engaged in the sport. On the offensive side, guards assist, penetrate [23], and perform long-distance shooting [19], and forwards set screens, attack with their back to the basket, and play supportive roles [19]. On the defensive side, guards play one-on-one defenses and prevent their opponents from penetrating their defense [19], and forwards are primarily responsible for blocking, rebounding [23], and cooperative defending [19]. Taken this into consideration, although the division of playing positions on the basis of offensive and defensive schemes served as the primary foundation for interpretation in previous studies, it seems that the effect of different schemes cannot be applied to basketball because of the unique playing position differentiation. As a result, the lack of observation of behavioral differences may be in relation to universal participation in both offensive and defensive tactics for basketball players in all positions, and to a lesser extents, guards and forwards.

The other possible explanation for the inconsistency might be that the positional effect in open-skilled sports on cognitive functions appeared to be selective. In a previous work, Schumacher et al. (2018) found that different playing positions among soccer players could only distinguish RT behavioral performance and could not be used as an indices for sustained attention and anticipation, implying that a selective cognitive advantage can be observed in open-skilled sports [20]. In the present study, only the visual Go/NoGo task was adopted to assess the behavioral differences in executive functions in guards and forwards. Further research is warranted in this area, possibly examining the positional effects on different cognitive domains in basketball.

4.2. Electrophysiological Performance

The present results showed the electrophysiological differences in N2 latency in both the Go and NoGo conditions and the P3 amplitude across the Go and NoGo conditions between guards and forwards, suggesting divergent neural processing efficiency related to player position when performing a cognitive task involving inhibitory control.

We found that the guards had shorter N2 latencies in the Go conditions and longer N2 latencies in the NoGo conditions as compared to the forwards. The N2 components not only reflect conflict monitoring [14,16,17] but also cognitive processes related to stimuli evaluation and response selection [27,41]. To be more specific, the N2 components have been reported have a relationship to the classification of the stimulation [42,43]. Accordingly, the N2 latency reflects the attentional orientation speed in these mental processes [43]. In the present study, we found that, in comparison to forwards, shorter N2 latencies in the Go condition could be observed in the guards, suggesting that they exhibited faster stimuli evaluation and response selection when confronting the target stimuli. Passing is one of the core skills during the offensive stages of games [44]. Appropriate passes facilitate fluent ball movement and allow the ball to move to the other players based on the most optimal offensive opportunity. Passing skills are required in both set plays and transitions. During the set plays, precise timely passes ensure successful tactical enforcement, while during transitions, passes allow quick ball movement down the court, enabling a fast breaker to beat opponents. It should be noted that the execution of passing skills is, at least in part, similar to the mental and response processes to Go and NoGo stimuli. Conditions that passers usually encounter "to pass" (i.e., move the ball to the right man according to tactics) or "not to pass" (i.e., the discovery of the opposites' counter movements) appear to resemble to the decision-making processes between "respond" or "don't respond" when engaging in the Go/NoGo task. Considering that guards are better passers and assisters [19] and that they engage in more passing (especially PG) than forwards [45], performance indicating shorter Go-N2 latencies on the part of guards may reflect their excellent capabilities and efficiencies related to being able to pass whenever an open, appropriate offensive opportunity occurs.

However, the guards had longer N2 latencies than the forwards in the NoGo condition. These findings suggest that the guards require prolonged mental processing when recognizing a need for inhibition. Indeed, the results supported the idea that although there was comparable behavioral inhibition between the guards and forwards, the two groups still showed differences in terms of neural processing efficiency. As mentioned previously, we expected the guards to show superior inhibitory controls compared to forwards owing to their cognitive accommodations to additional environmental interferences (e.g., conflicting situations). Surprisingly, since the NoGo-N2 components reflect conflict detection [14,16,17], it appeared that guards tended to show longer duration for classification and selection of responses when violations of expected actions took place [17,41]. This might point out that, instead of adapting to the extra attentional load, whenever a conflicting situation takes place, these additional interferences might force guards to prolong the time required to evaluate and discriminate between stimuli or situations due to the fact that they are more complex, varied situations [19,26], thus leading to their slower N2 latencies in the NoGo conditions as compared to forwards.

With regards to the P3 components, we found that forwards had larger P3 amplitudes than guards across the Go and NoGo conditions and three electrodes. The P3 components reflect the sequential processes of stimuli evaluation, together with N2 components, as well as the later stages of cognitive processing, including premotor preparation and decision-making [29,30,43]. In these cases, given that the amplitude of the P3 components reflects the amount of attentional resource allocation [30,46], the smaller P3 amplitude pointed out that guards mobilize less attentional resources than forwards during the later stages of premotor cognitive processing. As mentioned above, guards are greater passers and assisters who offensively allocate the ball to the best man in order to create the best offensive opportunities. Notably, offensive strategies in basketball also have an important element, which is time. The team's decision-making will be constrained by the shot clock [47]. Concerning this limitation, teams are often desperate and forced to take a lower quality offensive option that they are previously unwilling to take when the shot clock is going to expire [47]. Accordingly, players who are forced to shoot under the pressure of dwindling time are apt to make rush shot without consideration of whether it is the best choice or not. It is worth noting that players who execute these kinds of risky shots are usually skilled ball handers and shooters [48], or more specifically, guards (especially PG and SG), who can create shooting opportunities even with augmented offensive loadings [47]. That is, when confronted with such circumstances, guards relative to forwards are more likely to make an unreasonable shot rather than to allocate the ball to gain the best offensive opportunity. This might shed light on the tendency of guards to process the perceived stimulus on the basis of rough evaluation and decision-making, allocating less attention during later mental processes. This was supported by Bianco et al. (2017), who found that fencers had greater P3 amplitudes compared to boxers when engaging in the visual Go/NoGo task, since salient incongruencies in exercise strategies differentiate fencing from boxing, with fencers' training emphasizing accuracy to avoid making errors and boxers being trained to make as many attacks as possible that do not require extreme precision [11].

4.3. Limitations

There were some limitations of this study which must be addressed. First, the comparable accuracy rate and scarcity of errors possibly pointed out the simplicity of the task, which could have led to a failure to find between-group behavioral differences [43]. Further work using cognitive tasks with more challenges (e.g., visuospatial attention) is needed to clarify divergent behavioral inhibition [1]. Second, given that the present research was a cross-sectional study, we cannot exclude the superior neurocognitive performance that results from an inherent predisposition toward such performance [22]. Thus, evaluations of the potential contributions of different positions in open-skilled sports to cognitive functioning via longitudinal experiments are needed to clarify this issue [6]. Lastly, the experimental sampling was not completely random due to both the coaches' and players' approvals for collecting data being indispensable, and it could be considered as a non-normal sample set. However, in case the coaches and players agreed, all the qualified players in each team were recruited, which is valid enough to indicate the representation of the data collected.

5. Conclusions

In conclusion, we found that guards relative to forwards had comparable RTs and ARs, a shorter N2 latency in Go conditions, a longer N2 latency in NoGo conditions, and smaller P3 amplitudes across conditions and electrodes. The current findings supported the premise that guards (1) are more efficient in terms of target evaluation and response selection related to non-target stimuli, (2) exhibit prolonged duration in response selection and evaluation when dealing with target stimulation, and (3) use fewer cognitive resources during premotor preparation and decision-making as compared to forwards. The differences in neural processing characteristics between the two positions could provide important information related to elite basketball training, as well as to some degree provide a potential reference value when recruiting players.

Author Contributions: Conceptualization, Y.-K.C. and C.-L.T.; methodology, Y.-K.C. and C.-L.T.; formal analysis, Y.-K.C.; data curation, Y.-K.C.; writing—original draft preparation, Y.-K.C.; writing—review and editing, C.-Y.P., F.-C.C., Y.-T.T., C.-L.T.; supervision, C.-L.T.; project administration, Y.-K.C. and C.-L.T. All authors have read and agreed to the published version of the manuscript.

Funding: This research received no external funding.

Conflicts of Interest: The authors declare no conflict of interest.

References

1. Tsai, C.L.; Chen, F.C.; Pan, C.Y.; Wang, C.H.; Huang, T.H.; Chen, T.C. Impact of acute aerobic exercise and cardiorespiratory fitness on visuospatial attention performance and serum BDNF levels. *Psychoneuroendocrinology* **2014**, *41*, 121–131. [CrossRef]
2. Tsai, C.L.; Wang, W.L. Exercise-mode-related changes in task-switching performance in the elderly. *Front. Behavi. Neurosci.* **2015**, *9*, 56. [CrossRef]

3. Isoglu-Alkac, U.; Ermutlu, M.N.; Eskikutr, G.; Yücesir, L.; Temel, S.D.; Temel, T. Dancers and fastball sports athletes have different spatial visual attention styles. *Cogn. Neurodyn.* **2018**, *12*, 201–209. [CrossRef] [PubMed]
4. Williams, A.M.; Ward, P.; Smeeton, N.; Ward, J. Task specificity, role, and anticipation skill in soccer. *Res. Q. Exerc. Sport.* **2008**, *79*, 428–433. [CrossRef] [PubMed]
5. Tsai, C.L.; Wang, C.H.; Pan, C.Y.; Chen, F.C.; Huang, S.Y.; Tseng, Y.T. The effects of different exercise types on visuospatial attention in the elderly. *Psychol. Sport. Exerc.* **2016**, *26*, 130–138. [CrossRef]
6. Tsai, C.L.; Pan, C.Y.; Chen, F.C.; Tseng, Y.T. Open-and closed-skill exercise interventions produce different neurocognitive effects on executive functions in the elderly: A 6-month randomized, controlled trial. *Front. Aging Neurosci.* **2017**, *9*, 294. [CrossRef] [PubMed]
7. Di Russo, F.; Bultrini, A.; Brunelli, S.; Delussu, A.S.; Polidori, L.; Taddei, F.; Traballesi, M.; Spinelli, D. Benefits of sports participation for executive function in disabled athletes. *J. Neurotrauma* **2010**, *27*, 2309–2319. [CrossRef]
8. Vestberg, T.; Gustafson, R.; Marurex, L.; Ingvar, M.; Petrovic, P. Executive functions predict the success of top-soccer players. *PLoS ONE* **2012**, *7*, e34731. [CrossRef] [PubMed]
9. Diamand, A. Executive function. *Annu. Rev. Psychol.* **2013**, *64*, 135–168. [CrossRef]
10. Montuori, S.; D'Aurizio, G.; Foti, F.; Liparoti, M.; Lardone, A.; Pesoil, M.; Sorrentino, G.; Mandolesi, L.; Curcio, G.; Sorrentino, P. Executive functioning profiles in elite volleyball athletes: Preliminary results by a sport-specific task switching protocol. *Hum. Mov. Sci.* **2019**, *63*, 73–81. [CrossRef]
11. Bianco, V.; Di Russo, F.; Perri, R.L.; Berchicci, M. Different proactive and reactive action control in fencers' and boxers' brain. *Neuroscience* **2017**, *343*, 260–268. [CrossRef] [PubMed]
12. Carrasco, M. Visual attention: The past 25 years. *Vis. Res.* **2011**, *51*, 1484–1525. [CrossRef] [PubMed]
13. Tsai, C.L.; Chang, Y.K.; Hung, T.M.; Tseng, Y.T.; Chen, T.C. The neurophysiological performance of visuospatial working memory in children with developmental coordination disorder. *Dev. Med. Child Neurol.* **2012**, *54*, 1114–1120. [CrossRef] [PubMed]
14. Donkers, F.C.; Van Boxtel, G.J. The N2 in go/no-go tasks reflects conflict monitoring not response inhibition. *Brain Cogn.* **2004**, *56*, 165–176. [CrossRef]
15. Guo, Z.; Chen, R.; Liu, X.; Zhao, G.; Zheng, Y.; Gong, M.; Zhang, J. The impairing effects of mental fatigue on response inhibition: An ERP study. *PLoS ONE* **2018**, *13*, e0198206. [CrossRef]
16. Nieuwenhuis, S.; Yeung, N.; Van Den Wildenberg, W.; Ridderinkhof, K.R. Electrophysiological correlates of anterior cingulate function in a go/no-go task: Effects of response conflict and trial type frequency. *Cogn. Affect. Behav. Neurosci.* **2003**, *3*, 17–26. [CrossRef]
17. Smith, J.L.; Johnstone, S.J.; Barry, R.J. Movement-related potentials in the Go/NoGo task: The P3 reflects both cognitive and motor inhibition. *Clin. Neurophysiol.* **2008**, *119*, 704–714. [CrossRef]
18. Drinkwater, E.J.; Pyne, D.B.; McKenna, M.J. Design and interpretation of anthropometric and fitness testing of basketball players. *Sports Med.* **2008**, *38*, 565–578. [CrossRef]
19. Trninić, S.; Dizdar, D. System of the performance evaluation criteria weighted per positions in the basketball game. *Coll. Antropol.* **2000**, *24*, 217–234.
20. Schumacher, N.; Schmidt, M.; Wellmann, K.; Braumann, K. General perceptual-cognitive abilities: Age and position in soccer. *PLoS ONE* **2018**, *13*, e0202627. [CrossRef]
21. Vestberg, T.; Reinebo, G.; Marurex, L.; Ingvar, M.; Petrovic, P. Core executive functions are associated with success in young elite soccer players. *PLoS ONE* **2017**, *12*, e0170845. [CrossRef] [PubMed]
22. Wylie, S.A.; Bashore, T.R.; Van Wouwe, N.C.; Mason, E.J.; John, K.D.; Neimat, J.S.; Ally, B.A. Exposing an "Intangible" cognitive skill among collegiate football players: Enhanced interference control. *Front. Psychol.* **2018**, *9*, 49. [CrossRef] [PubMed]
23. Köklü, Y.; Alemdaroğlu, U.; Koçak, F.; Erol, A.; Fındıkoğlu, G. Comparison of chosen physical fitness characteristics of Turkish professional basketball players by division and playing position. *J. Hum. Kinet.* **2011**, *30*, 99–106. [CrossRef] [PubMed]
24. Scanlan, A.T.; Tucker, P.S.; Dalbo, V.J. A comparison of linear speed, closed-skill agility, and open-skill agility qualities between backcourt and frontcourt adult semiprofessional male basketball players. *J. Strength Cond. Res.* **2014**, *28*, 1319–1327. [CrossRef]
25. Sheppard, J.M.; Young, W.B. Agility literature review: Classifications, training and testing. *J. Sports Sci.* **2006**, *24*, 919–932. [CrossRef]

26. Puente, C.; Abián-Vicén, J.; Areces, F.; López, R.; Del Coso, J. Physical and physiological demands of experienced male basketball players during a competitive game. *J. Strength Cond. Res.* **2017**, *31*, 956–962. [CrossRef]
27. Cid-Fernández, S.; Lindín, M.; Diaz, F. Effects of amnestic mild cognitive impairment on N2 and P3 Go/NoGo ERP components. *J. Alzheimers Dis.* **2014**, *38*, 295–306. [CrossRef]
28. Di Russo, F.; Taddei, F.; Aprile, T.; Spinelli, D. Neural correlates of fast stimulus discrimination and response selection in top-level fencers. *Neurosci. Lett.* **2006**, *408*, 113–118. [CrossRef]
29. Bruin, K.; Wijers, A.; Van Staveren, A. Response priming in a go/nogo task: Do we have to explain the go/nogo N2 effect in terms of response activation instead of inhibition? *Clin. Neurophysiol.* **2001**, *112*, 1660–1671. [CrossRef]
30. Kok, A. On the utility of P3 amplitude as a measure of processing capacity. *Psychophysiology* **2001**, *38*, 557–577. [CrossRef]
31. Alderman, B.L.; Olson, R.L.; Brush, C.J. Using event-related potentials to study the effects of chronic exercise on cognitive function. *Int. J. Sport Exerc. Psychol.* **2019**, *17*, 106–116. [CrossRef]
32. Dong, G.; Lu, Q.; Zhou, H.; Zhao, X. Impulse inhibition in people with Internet addiction disorder: Electrophysiological evidence from a Go/NoGo study. *Neurosci. Lett.* **2010**, *485*, 138–142. [CrossRef] [PubMed]
33. Rubia, K.; Hyde, Z.; Halari, R.; Giampietro, V.; Smith, A. Effects of age and sex on developmental neural networks of visual–spatial attention allocation. *Neuroimage* **2010**, *51*, 817–827. [CrossRef] [PubMed]
34. Emilija, S.; Nenad, S.; Aaron, T.S.; Vincent, J.D.; Daniel, M.B.; Zoran, M. The activity demands and physiological responses encountered during basketball match-play: A systematic review. *Sports Med.* **2018**, *48*, 111–135.
35. Folstein, M.F.; Folstein, S.E.; McHugh, P.R. "Mini-mental state". A practical method for grading the cognitive state of patients for the clinician. *J. Psychiatr. Res.* **1975**, *12*, 189–198. [CrossRef]
36. Beck, A.T.; Steer, R.A.; Brown, G.K. *BDI-II*, 2nd ed.; The Psychological Corporation: San Antonio, TX, USA, 1996.
37. Tsai, C.L.; Huang, T.H.; Tsai, M.C. Neurocognitive performances of visuospatial attention and the correlations with metabolic and inflammatory biomarkers in adults with obesity. *Exp. Physiol.* **2017**, *102*, 1683–1699. [CrossRef] [PubMed]
38. Tsai, C.L.; Pan, C.Y.; Cen, F.C.; Huang, T.H.; Tsai, M.C.; Chuang, C.Y. Differences in neurocognitive performance and metabolic and inflammatory indices in male adults with obesity as a function of regular exercise. *Exp. Physiol.* **2019**, *104*, 1650–1660. [CrossRef]
39. Krustrup, P.; Mohr, M.; Amstrup, T.; Rysgaard, T.; Johansen, J.; Steensberg, A.; Pedersen, P.K.; Bangsbo, J. The yo-yo intermittent recovery test: Physiological response, reliability, and validity. *Med. Sci. Sports Exerc.* **2003**, *35*, 697–705. [CrossRef]
40. Bangsbo, J.; Iaia, F.M.; Krustrup, P. The Yo-Yo intermittent recovery test. *Sports Med.* **2008**, *38*, 37–51. [CrossRef]
41. Gajewski, P.D.; Stoerig, P.; Falkenstein, M. ERP—Correlates of response selection in a response conflict paradigm. *Brain Res.* **2008**, *1189*, 127–134. [CrossRef]
42. Amenedo, E.; Dıaz, F. Aging-related changes in processing of non-target and target stimuli during an auditory oddball task. *Biol. Psychol.* **1998**, *48*, 235–267. [CrossRef]
43. Piispala, J.; Kallio, M.; Bloigu, R.; Jansson-Verkasalo, E. Delayed N2 response in Go condition in a visual Go/Nogo ERP study in children who stutter. *J. Fluen. Disord.* **2016**, *48*, 16–26. [CrossRef] [PubMed]
44. Maimón, A.Q.; Courel-Ibáñez, J.; Ruíz, F.J.R. The basketball pass: A systematic review. *J. Hum. Kinet.* **2020**, *71*, 275–284. [CrossRef]
45. Ortega, E.; Cárdenas, D.; Saiz de Baranda, P.; Palao, J.M. Analysis of the final actions used in basketball during formative years according to player's. *J. Hum. Mov. Stud.* **2006**, *50*, 427–431.
46. Tsai, C.L.; Pan, C.Y.; Chen, F.C.; Wang, C.H.; Chou, F.Y. Effects of acute aerobic exercise on a task-switching protocol and brain-derived neurotrophic factor concentrations in young adults with different levels of cardiorespiratory fitness. *Exp. Physiol.* **2016**, *101*, 836–850. [CrossRef]

47. Skinner, B.; Goldman, M. Optimal strategy in basketball. In *Handbook of Statistical Methods and Analyses in Sports*; Chapman and Hall/CRC: London, UK, 2017; pp. 245–260.
48. Sindik, J. Performance indicators of the top basketball players: Relations with several variables. *Coll. Antropol.* **2015**, *39*, 617–624.

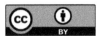

© 2020 by the authors. Licensee MDPI, Basel, Switzerland. This article is an open access article distributed under the terms and conditions of the Creative Commons Attribution (CC BY) license (http://creativecommons.org/licenses/by/4.0/).

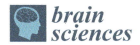

Article

Effects of Various Doses of Caffeine Ingestion on Intermittent Exercise Performance and Cognition

Cuicui Wang, Yuechuan Zhu, Cheng Dong, Zigui Zhou and Xinyan Zheng *

School of Kinesiology, Shanghai University of Sport, Shanghai 200438, China; 1821516026@sus.edu.cn (C.W.); 1821516044@sus.edu.cn (Y.Z.); 1821518006@sus.edu.cn (C.D.); 1921516023@sus.edu.cn (Z.Z.)
* Correspondence: zhengxinyan@sus.edu.cn; Tel.: +86-21-65507360

Received: 2 August 2020; Accepted: 26 August 2020; Published: 28 August 2020

Abstract: To date, no study has examined the effects of caffeine on prolonged intermittent exercise performance that imitates certain team-sports, and the suitable concentration of caffeine for improved intermittent exercise performance remains elusive. The purpose of the present cross-over, double-blind preliminary study was to investigate effects of low, moderate, and high doses of caffeine ingestion on intermittent exercise performance and cognition. Ten males performed a familiarization session and four experimental trials. Participants ingested capsules of placebo or caffeine (3, 6, or 9 mg/kg) at 1 h before exercise, rested quietly, and then performed cycling for 2×30 min. The cycling protocol consisted of maximal power pedaling for 5 s (mass × 0.075 kp) every minute, separated by unloaded pedaling for 25 s and rest for 30 s. At pre-ingestion of capsules, 1 h post-ingestion, and post-exercise, participants completed the Stroop task. The mean power-output (MPO), peak power-output (PPO), and response time (RT) in the Stroop task were measured. Only 3 mg/kg of caffeine had positive effects on the mean PPO and MPO; 3 mg/kg caffeine decreased RTs significantly in the incongruent and congruent conditions. These results indicate that the ingestion of low-dose caffeine had greater positive effects on the participants' physical strength during prolonged intermittent exercise and cognition than moderate- or high-dose caffeine.

Keywords: caffeine; prolonged intermittent exercise; cognition; exercise performance

1. Introduction

As a drug from the methylxanthine family, caffeine ingestion is highly prevalent not only in the general population but also among athletes [1]. In 2004, caffeine was removed from the list of banned substances by the World Anti-Doping Agency and was reaffirmed as a regulatory drug [2]. Since then, many athletes ingest caffeine to improve their exercise performance. Caffeine has shown an ergogenic effect on endurance-based exercise [3–8]. In a study investigating the effects of three different doses of caffeine on prolonged exercise capacity, Graham and Spriet [9] found that the ingestion of a low (3 mg/kg) or a moderate (6 mg/kg) dose of caffeine delayed the time to exhaustion, whereas a high dose (9 mg/kg) did not. These studies indicate that the beneficial effects of caffeine on endurance exercise can be achieved at a low-to-moderate dose, with 6 mg/kg caffeine often suggested. Moreover, lower doses of caffeine do not affect peripheral whole-body responses to exercise and are associated with few, if any, side effects. Spriet [10] suggested low doses of caffeine ingestion for improving exercise performance. Therefore, it is necessary to clarify whether other types of exercise can benefit from a suitable concentration of caffeine.

A successful performance of intermittent exercise is greatly related to an athlete's ability to perform repeated bouts of high-intensity sprint exercises [11]. Therefore, many researchers have studied the effects of caffeine on repetitive high-intensity exercise. For example, Beaven et al. [12] studied 12 trained males who performed 5×6 s sprints interspersed with 24 s of active recovery on a cycle ergometer after the ingestion of caffeine. They found that a 1.2% caffeine solution significantly improved the maximal exercise performance. Another study revealed an increase in the total amount of sprint work and the mean peak power output (PPO) following caffeine supplementation (6 mg/kg), compared with a placebo, during an intermittent sprint test consisting of 2 × 36 min halves, each composed of 18 × 4 s sprints with a 2 min active recovery at 35% of the peak volume of oxygen between each sprint [13]. Using a similar exercise protocol, Crowe et al. [14] demonstrated that the ingestion of 6 mg/kg of caffeine did not improve the results of repeated 60-s maximal cycling tests with a 30 s rest between each exercise. In addition, Salinero et al. [15] reported that caffeine ingestion (3 mg/kg) increased both the PPO and the mean power output (MPO) during the Wingate test in a group of young men and women. Above all, the effects of caffeine on prolonged intermittent exercise performance are inconsistent, and the suitable caffeine concentration for improved intermittent exercise performance remains elusive.

The improvement of exercise performance not only represents the enhancement of physical strength but also includes the development of psychological and cognitive functions necessary in sports [16]. Specially in some team sports, most points are scored in the latter stages of the match; however, the development of fatigue, particularly in the latter half, contributes to decreasing concentration, executive information processing, and decision making [17]. The ergogenic effect of caffeine might not only enhance physical strength but also the development of cognitive functions during exercise. As a stimulant drug, caffeine may have positive effects on cognition [18,19]. Cognition encompasses a great variety of mental processes, including those mediating executive functioning, decision-making, and creativity. Executive functioning is important for athletic performance and can be affected by prolonged physical exertion [20]. Research regarding the effects of caffeine consumption on performance in the Stroop task, a measure of executive function, has been inconsistent. Hogervorst et al. [18] reported that the ingestion of 150 mg of caffeine effectively accelerated response time (RT) in the Stroop task during and after exercise. In addition, Ali et al. [21] observed that a caffeine dose of 6 mg/kg effectively decreased RT in the Stroop task among female football players. However, another study found that caffeine did not have an effect on the Stroop performance after exercise [22]. The differences in these results may be related to the sensitivity of participants to various exercise types, cognitive tests, or caffeine doses. Therefore, it is necessary to compare the effects of different concentrations of caffeine on cognitive function and clarify the optimal concentration of caffeine required to improve cognitive function.

The purpose of the present preliminary study was to investigate the effects of low (3 mg/kg), moderate (6 mg/kg), and high (9 mg/kg) doses of caffeine ingestion on intermittent exercise performance and cognitive performance. We hypothesized that the ingestion of a low dose of caffeine would enhance intermittent exercise performance with a corresponding decrease in RT and the rating of perceived exertion (RPE) compared with the placebo and other doses of caffeine.

2. Materials and Methods

2.1. Participants

Ten healthy, low-caffeine-consuming male soccer players (age: 20.88 ± 2.72 years, height: 176.7 ± 5.1 cm, weight: 72.1 ± 8.7 kg) participated in this study. The sample size used was based on a G*Power 3.1 software calculation (effect size = 0.15) [23,24]. The participants were deemed eligible for this study if their caffeine intake was less than 60 mg/day (did not consume coffee, tea, caffeine-containing energy drinks or supplements, or chocolate; and consumption of cola <330 mL a day), they exercised at least three times/week, they had no injury or surgery in the past six months, they had a normal cognitive function (Mini Mental State Examination score ≥ 26), they were right-handed, and they could perform high-intensity exercise and had normal executive functions. The participants were fully informed of any risks and discomforts associated with the experiment before they provided their informed written consent to participate. The study followed the guidelines of the

Declaration of Helsinki and was approved by the local ethics committee at Shanghai University in Sport, Shanghai, China (No. 2016008).

2.2. Procedures

The participants visited the laboratory five times, including one familiarization trial and four experimental trials. All participants completed all experimental conditions at the same time of the day and at least 2 h after eating to minimize circadian-type variance in body temperature and other biological variables. Meanwhile, in order to better simulate the practical game, the exercise time was in line with the game time at about 3:00 in the afternoon; the exposure to each condition was separated by 1 week to ensure drug washout. The participants abstained from alcohol, food, or drinks containing caffeine (i.e., coffee, tea, cola, energy drinks, caffeine-containing supplements, chocolate), and strenuous exercise for 24 h before the experiment. During the first visit, they were familiarized with the equipment and procedures involved in the study. The participants adjusted the seat and bar heights and positions of their cycle simulator and replicated these positions in the four subsequent experimental exercise trials. After the exercise, the food consumed by each participant during 24 h before the familiarizing experiment was recorded. Participants were asked to replicate this diet prior to subsequent trials.

On the day of the experiment, the participants were asked to go to the toilet and empty their bladder, and then they had their body weight and height measured. The participants were seated in a comfortable chair for the cognitive tasks (Stroop tasks). The Stroop tasks consisted of one practice trial and one baseline (Stroop pre) trial. Following that, the participants ingested capsules containing placebo (calcium carbonate; CON), 3 mg/kg (CAF3), 6 mg/kg (CAF6), or 9 mg/kg (CAF9) of caffeine with 200 mL of water. After a 40-min seated rest, the participants performed the Stroop task, walked to a cycle simulator, and prepared to exercise.

The participants warmed up by cycling for 5 min (body mass × 0.01 kp) and then rested for 5 min. It has been reported that the plasma caffeine concentration is maximal 60 min after ingestion of caffeine [7]. At 1 h after the drug administration, they began to complete a laboratory-based intermittent exercise protocol designed to replicate the demands of an actual sports game [25]. The protocol consisted of two 30-min halves separated by a 15 min half-time break, with each half consisting of two trials separated by a 2 min rest period. One set consisted of maximal pedaling (body mass × 0.075 kp) for 5 s, active recovery (no load, 80 rpm) for 25 s, and resting for 30 s. During the 5 s maximal pedaling, to maintain their effort, verbal encouragement was provided throughout each bout. One trial consisted of 15 sets. The participants performed a total of four trials via a cycling ergometer (Monark 839E, Monark Exercise AB, Vansbro, Sweden). The PPO and MPO were recorded for each 5-s loaded sprint. Finally, the Stroop tasks were repeated. All participants completed all experimental conditions in the normal environment (23 °C, 50% relative humidity, Second Multi air conditioning system, Fuji Medical Science Co. LTD, Tokyo, Japan), and exposures were separated by 1 week to ensure drug washout.

The RPE was recorded at 3 min intervals throughout the cycling process. The Borg 6–20 RPE scale was printed onto a piece of paper, placed on a clipboard, and held in front of each participant when needed during each trial [26]. The heart rate (HR) was monitored via a HR monitor (model RS400; Polar Electro Oy, Kemple, Finland) during the entire process of the experimental trial.

2.3. Drug Treatment

A cross-over, double-blind design was used in the present study. Caffeine hydrate and calcium carbonate were obtained as white powders (034-06782, Wako Pure Chemical Industries, Ltd., Osaka, Japan). The dosages were calculated according to each participant's body weight. The treatments, each of which was delivered in three red capsules, were as follows: CON, 9 mg/kg calcium carbonate; CAF3, a mixture of 3 mg/kg caffeine and 6 mg/kg calcium carbonate; CAF6, a mixture of 6 mg/kg caffeine and 3 mg/kg calcium carbonate; and CAF9, 9 mg/kg caffeine. The researchers and participants could not identify the caffeine dosage by the appearance or taste of the capsules.

2.4. Stroop Task

The Stroop task is widely used to evaluate selective attention, cognitive flexibility, and processing speed [27]. The task was programmed and performed using E-prime 1.0 software (Psychology Software Tools, Pittsburgh, PA, USA). Each trial was displayed as follows: a fixed cross in the center of the screen for 500 ms, followed by a 500-ms stimulus. There were two kinds of stimuli: congruent and incongruent. In the congruent condition, three Chinese color words were shown (绿 for green, 蓝 for blue, and 红 for red), with the font colors matching the colors of each word. In the incongruent condition, the same three words were presented, but the font color did not match the color indicated by the word (e.g., the word "green" was presented in blue or red font). The participants were required to indicate the presentation color of each word on a numeric keypad, wherein the 1, 2, and 3 keys corresponded to the responses of blue, green, and red, respectively. The participants used their index, middle, and ring fingers of their right hand to press the keys, which were situated in the left-to-right order of 1, 2, and 3. The RT and accuracy rate (ACC) were measured.

The participants performed two blocks of 120 trials at pre-ingestion of the capsules, 60 min post-ingestion of the capsules, and post-exercise. Each block included 60 congruent and 60 incongruent trials, which were randomly presented. To prevent the participants from anticipating the stimulus, the interval between the appearance of the fixed cross and the presentation of the stimulus was randomly changed between 300 and 800 ms, with a fixed interstimulus interval duration of 1500 ms. The values for both the RT and ACC were recorded for further analysis.

2.5. Statistical Analyses

All statistical calculations were conducted with SPSS 20.0 software (SPSS Inc., Chicago, IL, USA). The one-sample Kolmogorov–Smirnov test was used to test whether the data were normally distributed. When the data were not normally distributed, statistical analysis was performed on the logarithmic transformation of the data. Alterations in the mean PPO, MPO, RPE, HR, RT, and ACC values were subjected to a two-factor (condition × time) analysis of variance with repeated measures. For cases in which the assumption of sphericity was violated, the Greenhouse–Geisser correction was used to reduce the likelihood of a type I error. If significant main or interaction effects were found, post-hoc analyses were carried out with the Bonferroni correction. For analysis of variance (ANOVA), partial eta^2 (Pη^2) was used as a measure of the effect size. The criteria to interpret the magnitude of the effect size were as follows: small, Pη^2 = 0.01; medium, Pη^2 = 0.06; and large, Pη^2 = 0.14 [28]. Data were summarized as the mean ± standard deviation. Statistical significance was accepted at $P < 0.05$.

3. Results

3.1. Exercise Performance

For the mean PPO, a 4 × 4 mixed ANOVA revealed that there was no significant interaction ($F_{(3, 9)} = 1.12$, $P = 0.36$, Pη^2 = 0.111, Figure 1A), but there was a significant main effect of the condition ($F_{(3)} = 3.83$, $P < 0.05$, Pη^2 = 0.299). For all time points, the mean PPO in the CAF3 group was significantly greater than those in the other groups.

For the mean MPO, a 4 × 4 mixed ANOVA revealed that there was no significant interaction ($F_{(3, 9)} = 0.72$, $p = 0.58$, Pη^2 = 0.074, Figure 1B), but there was a significant main effect of the condition ($F_{(3)} = 7.73$, $p < 0.05$, Pη^2 = 0.518). For all conditions, the mean MPO in the CAF3 group was significantly greater than those in the other groups.

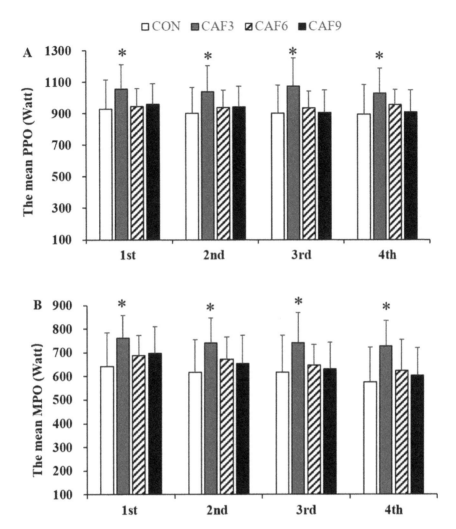

Figure 1. The peak power output (**A**) and mean power output (**B**) per trial. PPO, peak power output; MPO, mean power output; CON, placebo ingestion group; CAF3, 3 mg/kg caffeine ingestion group; CAF6, 6 mg/kg caffeine ingestion group; CAF9, 9 mg/kg caffeine ingestion group. *, vs. CON. Values are mean ± SD, $p < 0.05$.

3.2. HR

For HR, a 4 × 33 mixed ANOVA revealed that there was no significant interaction ($F (3, 96) = 2.038$, $p = 0.156$, $P\eta^2 = 0.337$, Figure 2), but there were significant main effects of condition ($F (3) = 5.57$, $p < 0.05$, $P\eta^2 = 0.582$) and time ($F (32) = 204.25$, $p < 0.001$, $P\eta^2 = 0.981$). The HR changed over time during the exercise protocol. Moreover, all doses of caffeine ingestion induced a significant increase in the HR.

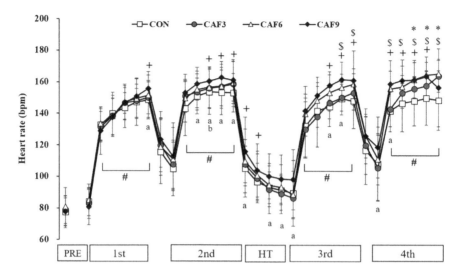

Figure 2. Change in heart rate. CON, placebo ingestion group; CAF3, 3 mg/kg caffeine ingestion group; CAF6, 6 mg/kg caffeine ingestion group; CAF9, 9 mg/kg caffeine ingestion group; PRE, pre ingestion drugs; HT, half time. +, CON vs. CAF9; $, CON vs. CAF6; *, CON vs. CAF3; a, CAF3 vs. CAF9; b, CAF6 vs. CAF9; #, significantly compared with PRE. Values are mean ± SD, $p < 0.05$.

3.3. RPE

Figure 3 summarizes the changes in the mean RPE per trial. For the mean RPE per trial, a 4 × 4 mixed ANOVA revealed that there was no significant interaction (F (3, 9) = 0.33, $p = 0.83$, $P\eta^2 = 0.040$), but there was a significant main effect of time (F (3) = 13.22, $p < 0.001$, $P\eta^2 = 0.623$). The RPE changed over time during the exercise protocol, but none of the caffeine doses affected the RPE.

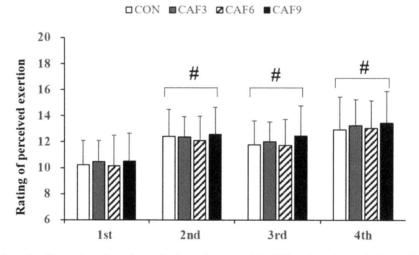

Figure 3. Change in rating of perceived exertion per trial. RPE, rating of perceived exertion; #, compared to 1st. Values are mean ± SD, $p < 0.05$.

3.4. Stroop Task: Incongruent Condition

For the RT in the Stroop task in the incongruent condition, a 4 × 3 mixed ANOVA revealed that there was a significant interaction (F (3, 6) = 3.5, $p < 0.05$, $P\eta^2 = 0.28$, Table 1). The RT at post-ingestion of the capsules in the CAF3 group was significantly faster than those in the other groups, and the RT at post-ingestion in the CAF6 group was significantly faster than those in the CON and CAF9 groups (CON: 603.78 ± 45.15 ms, CAF3: 564.68 ± 41.21 ms, CAF6: 582.75 ± 38.74 ms, CAF9: 609 ± 62 ms, $p < 0.05$). Furthermore, the RT at post-exercise in the CAF3 group was significantly faster than those in the CON and CAF9 groups (CON: 562.2 ± 30.79 ms, CAF3: 529.77 ± 35.94 ms, CAF6: 549.84 ± 37.82 ms, CAF9: 575.6 ± 38.37 ms, $p < 0.05$). For both the CAF3 and CAF6 groups, the RT was significantly faster at post-ingestion and post-exercise than at pre-ingestion. In all of the groups, there was a significantly faster RT at post-exercise compared with post-ingestion. For the ACC, the results from the Stroop task indicated no significant condition × time interaction (F (3, 6) = 0.61, $p = 0.58$, $P\eta^2 = 0.337$, $P\eta^2 = 0.081$, Table 1) or main effects of condition or time in the incongruent condition.

Table 1. Reaction time and accuracy rate of the Stroop task.

Measurements	Condition	Pre-Ingestion	Post-Ingestion	Post-Exercise
RT of incongruent (ms)	CON	604.85 ± 45.39	603.78 ± 45.15 *,#	562.20 ± 30.79 $
	CAF3	614.98 ±50.56	564.68 ± 41.21 !	529.77 ± 35.96 !,$
	CAF6	630.38 ± 61.66	582.75 ± 38.74 *,!	549.84 ± 37.82 !,$
	CAF9	623.96 ± 68.73	609.00 ± 62.00 *,#	575.60 ±38.37 $
RT of congruent (ms)	CON	573.14 ± 32.76	573.08 ± 43.00	547.76 ± 38.09 $
	CAF3	582.61 ± 56.39	537.15 ± 43.01 !	518.58 ± 36.69 !,$
	CAF6	582.31 ± 57.07	566.69 ± 43.99	531.93 ± 56.47 $
	CAF9	577.45 ± 62.58	570.14 ± 45.18	544.71 ± 36.58 $
ACC of incongruent	CON	0.89 ± 0.08	0.91 ± 0.05	0.89 ± 0.07
	CAF3	0.90 ± 0.07	0.90 ± 0.07	0.92 ± 0.06
	CAF6	0.87 ± 0.08	0.90 ± 0.05	0.90 ± 0.06
	CAF9	0.89 ± 0.08	0.91 ± 0.06	0.89 ± 0.11
ACC of congruent	CON	0.93 ± 0.04	0.91 ± 0.06	0.93 ± 0.04
	CAF3	0.93 ± 0.05	0.94 ± 0.04	0.95 ± 0.03
	CAF6	0.91 ± 0.11	0.94 ± 0.03	0.93 ± 0.06
	CAF9	0.92 ± 0.09	0.93 ± 0.04	0.92 ± 0.11

RT, reaction time; ACC, accuracy rate. !, significant vs. Pre-ingestion ($p < 0.05$); $, significant vs. Post-ingestion ($p < 0.05$); *, significant vs. CAF3 ($p < 0.05$); #, significant vs. CAF6 ($p < 0.05$). Values are mean ± SD.

3.5. Stroop Task: Congruent Condition

For the RT in the Stroop task in the congruent condition, a 4 × 3 mixed ANOVA revealed that there was no significant interaction (F (3, 6) = 2.13, $p = 0.11$, $P\eta^2 = 0.192$, Table 1), but there was a significant main effect of time (F (2) = 25.88, $p < 0.001$, $P\eta^2 = 0.742$). For the CAF3 group, the RT was significantly faster at post-ingestion of the capsules and post-exercise compared with that at pre-ingestion (pre-ingestion: 582.61 ± 56.39 ms, post-ingestion: 537.15 ± 43.01 ms, post-exercise: 518.58 ± 36.69 ms, $p < 0.05$). Moreover, the RT was significantly faster at post-exercise compared with post-ingestion in the CON, CAF3, and CAF6 groups. For the ACC, the results from the Stroop task indicated no significant condition × time interaction (F (3, 9) = 0.93, $p = 0.40$, $P\eta^2 = 0.117$, Table 1) or main effects for condition or time in the congruent condition.

4. Discussion

To the best of our knowledge, no study has examined the effects of different doses of caffeine ingestion on prolonged intermittent exercise performance that imitates certain team sports, and the suitable ingestion concentration remains elusive. Data from the current preliminary study showed that only 3 mg/kg of caffeine had positive effects on the mean MPO and PPO, while 6 mg/kg or 9 mg/kg caffeine did not affect these values. These results indicate that the ingestion of a low dose of caffeine had greater positive effects on the participants' physical strength during intermittent exercise than a moderate or high dose of caffeine.

To date, many studies have focused on the effects of caffeine ingestion on intermittent exercise performance [10,13,14,29–35]. In this study, we found that 3 mg/kg of caffeine had positive effects on the mean MPO and PPO. Consistent with our results, Paton et al. [34], Evans et al. [30], and Ranchordas et al. [35] also found that low-dose caffeine ingestion improved an athlete's physical strength during intermittent exercise. Moreover, several groups have reported that 6 mg/kg of caffeine ingestion improves an athlete's physical strength during intermittent exercise [10,13,31], but others have reported no effects of this dose of caffeine ingestion [14,29,32,33]. In this study, ingestion of 6 mg/kg of caffeine failed to affect the participants' physical strength during intermittent exercise, which supports previous studies that this dose has no effects on intermittent exercise performance. The potential ergogenic effects of caffeine may be dependent on the recovery interval, and the ergogenic effects of caffeine may be greater with a long recovery interval [36,37]. If the recovery interval becomes longer than 6 s, a moderate dose of caffeine ingestion may improve exercise performance. Therefore, exercise protocols should be standardized in future studies investigating the effects of a drug on physical strength during intermittent exercise. Unfortunately, a high dose of caffeine failed to affect the participants' physical strength during intermittent exercise and cognitive performance, which could be related, perhaps in part, to the adverse effects of caffeine, such as gastrointestinal upset, nervousness, mental confusion, and an impeded ability to focus [9]. Using the present experimental protocol, we showed that a low dose of caffeine had greater positive effects on the participants' physical strength during intermittent exercise and cognitive performance than a moderate or high dose of caffeine. These results demonstrate that only low-dose caffeine ingestion can improve intermittent exercise performance imitating some team sports. Moreover, the peak plasma caffeine concentrations have been reported to reach maximal levels 60 to 90 min after ingestion [9], indicating that caffeine will exert some biological effects, but their timing might be different between individuals. In order to support our present conclusions, plasma caffeine concentrations should be measured in future studies.

Exercise performance improved by caffeine ingestion is presumed to be due to central nervous system stimulation, not peripheral mechanisms [38]. In the present study, we found that ingestion of 6 mg/kg or 9 mg/kg of caffeine increased the HR but failed to improve the intermittent exercise performance, while 3 mg/kg caffeine did not increase the HR but improved the intermittent exercise performance. These results support the conclusion by Davis and Green [39] that the ergogenic effects of caffeine depend on a mechanism involving the central nervous system, not multiple peripheral mechanisms. Caffeine acts as an antagonist of adenosine receptors, whereby the blockade of adenosine receptors, which have an inhibitory effect on neurons, causes neuronal excitation, enhances brain activation [40], attenuates the RPE [41], and improves cognition and physical ability during exercise. In the present study, we found that 3 mg/kg of caffeine ingestion enhanced the MPO and PPO but failed to affect the RPE. These results are consistent with those reported by Astorino et al. [42]. Their finding that the low dose of caffeine (2mg/kg) enhanced the intermittent exercise performance but did not change the RPE suggests that perceived exertion may be blunted by the low-dose caffeine intake [42]. Moreover, ingestion of 6 mg/kg or 9 mg/kg of caffeine did not affect the RPE or intermittent exercise performance in this study. A possible explanation of this result is that these doses failed to affect brain activation [41].

Previous studies focusing on aerobic exercise have shown that acute moderate aerobic exercise improves executive information processing related to selective attention and inhibitory control [21,43,44].

Different sports may have different effects on cognitive function; thus, recent studies have examined the effects of intermittent exercise on executive function. Consistent with the reports by Kujach et al. [45] and Ichinose et al. [46], the current study found that the RTs under conditions of incongruent or congruent stimuli were significantly shortened after intermittent exercise in all groups. These results indicate that the performance of prolonged intermittent exercise could also improve executive functioning.

By examining participants' cognitive performance at pre-ingestion of the capsules, 60 min post-ingestion, and immediately post-exercise, this study was able to highlight the effects of different doses caffeine ingestion alone and post-exercise. Hogervorst et al. [47] found that participants were significantly faster after a low dose of caffeine ingestion (100 mg) on the computerized complex information processing test (Stroop Color–Word test) and Rapid Visual Information Processing Task, particularly after 140 min and after a time to the exhaustion trial. In the present study, we found that a low-dose caffeine ingestion improved incongruent and congruent conditions. These results are similar to Hogervorst et al. [47] and support that low-dose caffeine may have a direct and specific effect on perceptual-motor speed, efficiency factor, or executive information processing [48]. Moreover, the present finding of 6 mg/kg caffeine decreasing Stroop task RTs in the incongruent condition is consistent with Souissi et al. [49], whose findings showed that 6 mg/kg of caffeine improved RTs. These results suggest that the ingestion of a low or moderate dose of caffeine may reduce interference and thus improve exertive function during exercise. Our finding of no effect of high-dose caffeine on cognitive performance could be related, perhaps in part, to the adverse effects of caffeine. Given that the performance of our participants in both simple and complex task conditions was improved with the 3-mg/kg dose of caffeine, we suggest that low-dose caffeine may have an impact on cognition that is preferable to the effects of a moderate or high dose of caffeine. This hypothesis may be related to the increase in prefrontal cortex activation with lower doses of caffeine [40].

Limitations

Although we used the G-power software to estimate the appropriate sample size, the number of participants only met the minimum sample size requirement. The present results should be replicated in future research with a larger sample size. Furthermore, the peak plasma caffeine concentration has been reported to reach maximal levels 15 to 120 min after ingestion, indicating that caffeine will exert some biological effects, but their timing might be different between individuals. However, in the present study, we did not measure the plasma levels of caffeine. Therefore, analyzing plasma levels of caffeine during intermittent exercise is necessary in future studies.

5. Conclusions

The results of this preliminary study indicate that the ingestion of a low dose of caffeine had greater positive effects on the participants' physical strength during intermittent exercise and cognitive performance than a moderate or high dose of caffeine, suggesting that low-dose caffeine could improve intermittent exercise performance that imitates certain team sports.

Author Contributions: X.Z. conceived and supervised the study. C.W. and X.Z. designed the experiments. C.W., Y.Z., C.D., and Z.Z. carried out the experiments. C.W. and X.Z. analyzed the data. C.W. wrote the manuscript. All authors have read and agreed to the published version of the manuscript.

Funding: This work was supported by the National Natural Science Foundation of China (31701044).

Acknowledgments: We thank the participants for their effort and time.

Conflicts of Interest: The authors declare no conflict of interest.

References

1. Bishop, D. Dietary supplements and team-sport performance. *Sports. Med.* **2010**, *40*, 995–1017. [CrossRef]
2. Chester, N.; Wojek, N. Caffeine consumption amongst british athletes following changes to the 2004 wada prohibited list. *Int. J. Sports. Med.* **2008**, *29*, 524–528. [CrossRef]

3. Pitchford, N.W.; Fell, J.W.; Leveritt, M.D.; Desbrow, B.; Shing, C.M. Effect of caffeine on cycling time-trial performance in the heat. *J. Sci. Med. Sport.* **2014**, *17*, 445–449. [CrossRef]
4. Hodgson, A.B.; Randell, R.K.; Jeukendrup, A.E.; Earnest, C.P. The metabolic and performance effects of caffeine compared to coffee during endurance exercise. *PLoS ONE* **2013**, *38*, e59561. [CrossRef]
5. Hoffmann, R.W.; Haeberlin, E.; Rohde, T. The effect of different dosages of caffeine on endurance performance time. *Int. J Sports Med.* **1995**, *16*, 225–230.
6. Desbrow, B.; Biddulph, C.; Devlin, B.; Grant, G.D.; Anoopkumar-Dukie, S.; Leveritt, M.D. The effects of different doses of caffeine on endurance cycling time trial performance. *J. Sports. Sci.* **2012**, *30*, 115–120. [CrossRef]
7. Graham, T.E. Caffeine and exercise: Metabolism, endurance and performance. *Sports. Med.* **2001**, *31*, 785–807. [CrossRef]
8. Cox, G.R.; Desbrow, B.; Montgomery, P.G.; Anderson, M.E.; Bruce, C.R.; Macrides, T.A.; Burke, L.M. Effect of different protocols of caffeine intake on metabolism and endurance performance. *J. Appl. Physiol.* **2002**, *93*, 990–999. [CrossRef]
9. Graham, T.E.; Spriet, L.L. Metabolic, catecholamine, and exercise performance responses to various doses of caffeine. *J. Appl. Physiol.* **1995**, *78*, 867–874. [CrossRef]
10. Spriet, L.L. Exercise and sport performance with low doses of caffeine. *Sports Med.* **2014**, *2*, 175–184. [CrossRef]
11. Taylor, J.; Macpherson, T.; Spears, I.; Weston, M. The effects of repeated-sprint training on field-based fitness measures: A meta-analysis of controlled and non-controlled trials. *Sports. Med.* **2015**, *45*, 881–891. [CrossRef]
12. Beaven, C.M.; Maulder, P.; Pooley, A.; Kilduff, L.; Cook, C. Effects of caffeine and carbohydrate mouth rinses on repeated sprint performance. *Appl. Physiol. Nutr. Metab.* **2013**, *38*, 633–637. [CrossRef]
13. Schneiker, K.T.; Bishop, D.; Dawson, B.; Hackett, L.P. Effects of caffeine on prolonged intermittent-sprint ability in team-sport athletes. *Med. Sci. Sports Exerc.* **2006**, *38*, 578–585. [CrossRef]
14. Crowe, M.J.; Leicht, A.S.; Spinks, W.L. Physiological and cognitive responses to caffeine during repeated, high-intensity exercise. *Int. J. Sport Nutr. Exerc. Metab.* **2006**, *16*, 528–544. [CrossRef]
15. Salinero, J.; Lara, B.; Ruiz-Vicente, D.; Areces, F.; Puente-Torres, C.; Gallo-Salazar, C.; Coso, J.D. CYP1A2 genotype variations do not modify the benefits and drawbacks of caffeine during exercise: A pilot study. *Nutrients* **2017**, *9*, 269. [CrossRef]
16. Huang, L.; Deng, Y.; Zheng, X.; Liu, Y. Transcranial direct current stimulation with Halo Sport enhances repeated sprint cycling and cognitive performance. *Front. Physiol.* **2019**, *10*, 118. [CrossRef]
17. Bello, M.L.; Walker, A.J.; McFadden, B.A.; Sanders, D.J.; Arent, S.M. Effects of TeaCrine and caffein on endurance and cognitive performance during a simulated match in high-level soccer players. *J. Int. Soc. Sports. Nutr.* **2019**, *16*, 20. [CrossRef]
18. Hogervorst, E.; Riedel, W.J.; Kovacs, E.; Brouns, F.; Jolles, J. Caffeine improves cognitive performance after strenuous physical exercise. *Int. J. Sports. Med.* **1999**, *20*, 354–361. [CrossRef]
19. Smith, A.; Kendrick, A.; Maben, A.; Salmon, J. Effects of breakfast and caffeine on cognitive performance, mood and cardiovascular functioning. *Appetite* **1994**, *22*, 39–55. [CrossRef]
20. Yanagisawa, H.; Dan, I.; Tsuzuki, D.; Kato, M.; Okamoto, M.; Kyutoku, Y.; Soya, H. Acute moderate exercise elicits increased dorsolateral prefrontal activation and improves cognitive performance with stroop test. *Neuroimage* **2010**, *50*, 1702–1710. [CrossRef]
21. Ali, A.; O'Donnell, J.; Hurst, P.V.; Foskett, A.; Rutherfurd-Markwick, K. Caffeine ingestion enhances perceptual responses during intermittent exercise in female team-game players. *J. Sports.* **2016**, *34*, 330–341. [CrossRef]
22. Bottoms, L.; Greenhalgh, A.; Gregory, K. The effect of caffeine ingestion on skill maintenance and fatigue in epee fencers. *J. Sports. Sci.* **2013**, *31*, 1091–1099. [CrossRef]
23. Faul, F.; Erdfelder, E.; Lang, A.G.; Buchner, A. G*Power 3: A flexible statistical power analysis program for the social, behavioral, and biomedical sciences. *Behav. Res. Methods* **2007**, *39*, 175–191. [CrossRef]
24. Faul, F.; Erdfelder, E.; Buchner, A.; Lang, A.G. Statistical power analyses using G*Power 3.1: Tests for correlation and regression analyses. *Behav. Res. Methods* **2009**, *41*, 1149–1160. [CrossRef]
25. Chaen, Y.; Onitsuka, S.; Hasegawa, H. Wearing a cooling vest during half-time improves intermittent exercise in the heat. *Front. Physiol.* **2019**, *10*, 711. [CrossRef]
26. Borg, G.A. Perceived exertion as an indicator of somatic stress. *Scand. J. Rehabil. Med.* **1970**, *2*, 92–98.

27. Pauw, K.D.; Roelands, B.; Knaepen, K.; Polfliet, M.; Stiens, J.; Meeusen, R. Effects of caffeine and maltodextrin mouth rinsing on P300, brain imaging and cognitive performance. *J. Appl. Physiol.* **2015**, *118*, 776–782. [CrossRef]
28. Cohen, J. A power primer. *Psychol. Bull.* **1992**, *112*, 155–159. [CrossRef]
29. Carr, A.; Dawson, B.; Schneiker, K.; Goodman, C.; Lay, B. Effect of caffeine supplementation on repeated sprint running performance. *J. Appl. Physiol.* **2008**, *93*, 990–999.
30. Evans, M.; Tierney, P.; Gray, N.; Hawe, G.; Macken, M.; Egan, B. Acute ingestion of caffeinated chewing gum improves repeated sprint performance of team sports athletes with low habitual caffeine consumption. *Int. J. Sport Nutr. Exerc. Metab.* **2017**, 221–227. [CrossRef]
31. Glaister, M.; Howatson, G.; Abraham, C.S.; Lockey, R.A.; Goodwin, J.E.; Foley, P.; McInnes, G. Caffeine supplementation and multiple sprint running performance. *Med. Sci. Sports Exerc.* **2008**, *20*, 1835–1840. [CrossRef] [PubMed]
32. Kopec, B.J.; Dawson, B.T.; Buck, C.; Wallman, K.E. Effects of sodium phosphate and caffeine ingestion on repeated-sprint ability in male athletes. *J. Sci. Sports* **2016**, *19*, 272–276. [CrossRef]
33. Paton, C.D.; Hopkins, W.G.; Vollebregt, L. Little effect of caffeine ingestion on repeated sprints in team-sport athletes. *Med. Sci. Sports. Exerc.* **2001**, *33*, 822–825. [CrossRef]
34. Paton, C.D.; Lowe, T.; Irvine, A. Caffeinated chewing gum increases repeated sprint performance and augments increases in testosterone in competitive cyclists. *Eur. J. Appl. Physiol.* **2010**, *110*, 1243–1250. [CrossRef]
35. Ranchordas, M.K.; King, G.; Russell, M.; Lynn, A.; Russell, M. Effects of caffeinated gum on a battery of soccer-specific tests in trained university-standard male soccer players. *Int. J. Sport Nutr. Exerc. Metab.* **2018**, *28*, 629–634. [CrossRef]
36. Lee, C.L.; Cheng, C.F.; Lin, L.C.; Huang, H.W. Caffeine's effect on intermittent sprint cycling performance with different rest intervals. *Eur. J. Appl. Physiol.* **2012**, *112*, 2107–2116. [CrossRef]
37. Lee, C.L.; Cheng, C.F.; Astorino, T.A.; Lee, C.J.; Huang, H.W.; Chang, W.D. Effects of carbohydrate combined with caffeine on repeated sprint cycling and agility performance in female athletes. *J. Int. Soc. Sports. Nutr.* **2014**, *11*, 1–7. [CrossRef]
38. Kalmar, J.M.; Cafarelli, E. Caffeine: A valuable tool to study central fatigue in humans? *Exerc. Sport. Sci. Rev.* **2004**, *32*, 143–147. [CrossRef]
39. Davis, J.K.; Green, J.M. Caffeine and anaerobic performance: Ergogenic value and mechanisms of action. *Sports. Med.* **2008**, *39*, 813–832. [CrossRef]
40. Zhang, B.; Liu, Y.; Wang, X.C.; Deng, Y.Q.; Zheng, X. Cognition and brain activation in response to various doses of caffeine: A near-infrared spectroscopy study. *Front. Psychol.* **2020**, *11*, 1393. [CrossRef]
41. Duncan, M.J.; Stanley, M.; Parkhouse, N.; Cook, K.; Smith, M. Acute caffeine ingestion enhances strength performance and reduces perceived exertion and muscle pain perception during resistance exercise. *Eur. J. Appl. Physiol.* **2013**, *13*, 392–399. [CrossRef] [PubMed]
42. Astorino, T.A.; Terzi, M.N.; Roberson, D.W.; Burnett, T.R. Effect of two doses of caffeine on muscular function during isokinetic exercise. *Med. Sci. Sports Exerc.* **2010**, *42*, 2205–2210. [CrossRef] [PubMed]
43. Endo, K.; Matsukawa, K.; Liang, N.; Nakatsuka, C.; Tsuchimochi, H.; Okamura, H.; Hamaoka, T. Dynamic exercise improves cognitive function in association with increased prefrontal oxygenation. *J. Physiol. Sci.* **2013**, *63*, 287–298. [CrossRef]
44. Hogervorst, E.; Riedel, W.; Jeukendrup, A.; Jolles, J. Cognitive performance after strenuous physical exercise. *Percept. Mot. Ski.* **1996**, *83*, 479–488. [CrossRef]
45. Kujach, S.; Byun, K.; Hyodo, K.; Suwabe, K.; Soya, H. A transferable high-intensity intermittent exercise improves executive performance in association with dorsolateral prefrontal activation in young adults. *Neuroimage* **2018**, *169*, 117–125. [CrossRef]
46. Ichinose, Y.; Morishita, S.; Suzuki, R.; Endo, G.; Tsubaki, A. Comparison of the effects of continuous and intermittent exercise on cerebral oxygenation and cognitive function. *Adv. Exp. Med. Biol.* **2020**, *1232*, 209–214.
47. Hogervorst, E.; Bandelow, S.; Schmitt, J.; Jentjens, R.; Oliveira, M.; Allgrove, J.; Carter, T.; Gleeson, M. Caffeine improves physical and cognitive performance during exhaustive exercise. *Med. Sci. Sports Exerc.* **2008**, *40*, 1841–1851. [CrossRef]

48. Nehlig, A. Is caffeine a cognitive enhancer? *J. Alzheimers Dis.* **2010**, *20*, S85–S94. [CrossRef]
49. Souissi, Y.; Souissi, M.; Chtourou, H. Effects of caffeine ingestion on the diurnal variation of cognitive and repeated high-intensity performances. *Biochem. Behav.* **2019**, *177*, 69–74. [CrossRef]

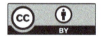 © 2020 by the authors. Licensee MDPI, Basel, Switzerland. This article is an open access article distributed under the terms and conditions of the Creative Commons Attribution (CC BY) license (http://creativecommons.org/licenses/by/4.0/).

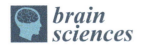

Article

Carbohydrate Mouth Rinse Mitigates Mental Fatigue Effects on Maximal Incremental Test Performance, but Not in Cortical Alterations

Cayque Brietzke [1,2], Paulo Estevão Franco-Alvarenga [1,2], Raul Canestri [1], Márcio Fagundes Goethel [1,3], Ítalo Vínicius [1], Vitor de Salles Painelli [1,4], Tony Meireles Santos [5], Florentina Johanna Hettinga [6] and Flávio Oliveira Pires [1,2,*]

- [1] Exercise Psychophysiology Research Group, School of Arts, Sciences and Humanities, University of São Paulo, São Paulo 05508-060, Brazil; cayquebbarreto@alumni.usp.br (C.B.); francope@gmail.com (P.E.F.-A.); raulcanestri@usp.br (R.C.); gbiomech@usp.br (M.F.G.); italovinicius@usp.br (Í.V.); vitor_pa@hotmail.com (V.d.S.P.)
- [2] Human Movement Science and Rehabilitation Program, Federal University of São Paulo, Avenida Sena Madureira 1500, Brazil
- [3] Porto Biomechanics Laboratory (LABIOMEP), University of Porto, 4000 Porto, Portugal
- [4] Strength Training Study and Research Group, Institute of Health Sciences, Paulista University, Sao Paulo 05347-020, Brazil
- [5] Physical Education Program, Research Center for Performance and Health, Federal University of Pernambuco, Recife 52071-030, Brazil; tonymsantos@gmail.com
- [6] Department of Sport, Exercise and Rehabilitation, Northumbria University, Newcastle NE1 8ST, UK; florentina.hettinga@northumbria.ac.uk
- * Correspondence: piresfo@usp.br; Tel.: +55-11-26480118

Received: 30 June 2020; Accepted: 24 July 2020; Published: 29 July 2020

Abstract: Detrimental mental fatigue effects on exercise performance have been documented in constant workload and time trial exercises, but effects on a maximal incremental test (MIT) remain poorly investigated. Mental fatigue-reduced exercise performance is related to an increased effort sensation, likely due to a reduced prefrontal cortex (PFC) activation and inhibited spontaneous behavior. Interestingly, only a few studies verified if centrally active compounds may mitigate such effects. For example, carbohydrate (CHO) mouth rinse potentiates exercise performance and reduces effort sensation, likely through its effects on PFC activation. However, it is unknown if this centrally mediated effect of CHO mouth rinse may mitigate mental fatigue-reduced exercise performance. After a proof-of-principle study, showing a mental fatigue-reduced MIT performance, we observed that CHO mouth rinse mitigated MIT performance reductions in mentally fatigued cyclists, regardless of PFC alterations. When compared to placebo, mentally fatigued cyclists improved MIT performance by 2.24–2.33% when rinsing their mouth with CHO during MIT. However, PFC and motor cortex activation during MIT in both CHO and placebo mouth rinses were greater than in mental fatigue. Results showed that CHO mouth rinse mitigated the mental fatigue-reduced MIT performance, but challenged the role of CHO mouth rinse on PFC and motor cortex activation.

Keywords: brain regulation; physical performance; cognitive performance; supplementation

1. Introduction

Mental fatigue is a mental state caused by a prolonged, highly demanding cognitive task [1] that induces an increased fatigue sensation and reduced focus on a given task [1–3]. From a physical exercise perspective, mental fatigue has been associated with a reduced exercise capacity [1–3] likely through its effects on cerebral activation [2–4] and effort sensation [2,5]. A recent systematic review has confirmed that detrimental effects of mental fatigue on exercise performance have been well evidenced in endurance exercise modes, such as constant workload and time trial exercises [1,3,5]; however, the effects on maximal incremental test (MIT) performance remain poorly investigated [6,7]. This is a relevant aspect, as MIT is a gold-standard protocol, with intensity gradually increased until exhaustion, to assess cardiopulmonary fitness variables, such as maximal oxygen uptake (VO_{2MAX}) and ventilatory thresholds [8]. Accordingly, potential deleterious mental fatigue effects on MIT performance and cardiopulmonary fitness variables may be important in clinical and sport settings [8,9] and require more investigation.

Despite the number of studies confirming the detrimental effects of mental fatigue on endurance exercise performance [1], only a few have investigated if centrally active compounds may mitigate such effects [2,10]. The suggestion that centrally active compounds may counteract mental fatigue effects is based on the fact that mental fatigue is associated with a reduced prefrontal cortex (PFC) activation [2–4] and inhibits spontaneous behavior [11] due to the increased cerebral ATP hydrolysis and adenosine concentration [12,13]. In a physical exercise scenario, centrally active compounds capable of attenuating the effects of detrimental mental fatigue on cerebral activation may thus be of interest. Recently, Franco-Alvarenga et al. [2] found that caffeine ingestion mitigated the mental fatigue-derived performance reduction in a 20 km cycling time trial. Interestingly, they also found that caffeine-attenuated exercise performance reduction was unrelated to PFC activation, an area involved in perceptual [14], attentional, and inhibitory responses [15]. These results challenged the underlying mechanisms of caffeine effects on exercise performance in mentally fatigued individuals, thus highlighting the need for more investigations on this topic.

Since a seminal study by Carter et al. in 2004 [16], a number of studies have confirmed that carbohydrate (CHO) mouth rinse may potentiate endurance exercise performance [17] likely due to its centrally mediated effects. The underlying mechanisms of the central effects of CHO mouth rinse involve the activation of cerebral areas related to motor planning and emotional responses, such as PFC [18,19]. Therefore, one may suggest that CHO mouth rinse may potentially mitigate the deleterious mental fatigue effects on PFC activation and exercise performance through its beneficial effects on cerebral responses [18,20], endurance exercise performance, and effort sensation [17]. Indeed, a recent study provided insightful results of the CHO mouth rinse effects on cerebral, cognitive, and perceptual responses, as participants improved the accuracy of answers and lowered the mental fatigue sensation when they performed a highly demanding cognitive task while regularly rinsing their mouth with a caffeine-combined CHO solution [20]. Interestingly, the mouth rinses improved some cerebral responses in PFC and other cortex areas, although unchanged responses were observed in other cortex areas. Therefore, despite using a caffeine-combined CHO solution, rather than a CHO solution in isolation, these results may shed light on the potentially beneficial CHO mouth rinse effects on cerebral and perceptual responses in mentally fatigued individuals. However, that study used no exercise performance, so the potential of CHO mouth rinse to mitigate deleterious mental fatigue effects on exercise performance is still unknown.

Two important aspects to consider when designing a straightforward methodology to unravel the CHO mouth rinse effects on exercise performance in mentally fatigued individuals are the use of electroencephalography (EEG) measures and controlled exercise mode. Firstly, it has been observed that an increased EEG theta wave over the PFC is a sensitive method to identify a mental fatigue state at rest [3,4], as this area is involved in inhibitory and sustained attention responses [21]. Moreover, analysis of the entire EEG spectrum may also be insightful in an exercise scenario, as PFC activation has been associated with multiple functions, such as exercise-induced perceptual responses [14], attentional and inhibitory control [15,22], and motor cortex (MC) activation [3,23]. However, given that both CHO mouth rinse and mental fatigue have been suggested to change PFC activation [3,18], it remains to be investigated if rinsing the mouth with CHO may counteract the mental fatigue effects on PFC and MC activation and exercise performance.

Secondly, the use of MIT as exercise mode may be methodologically sound to investigate the mental fatigue-CHO mouth rinse interplay in endurance exercise performance. Different from a ramp test, a graded MIT provides a number of controlled, constant workloads at increasing intensities, thereby allowing studying the CHO mouth rinse effects on physiological variables in a number of controlled intensities. This aspect is relevant, as a study showed that CHO mouth rinse potentiated performance in moderate rather than severe intensities [24], thus indicating the necessity to study the effects of CHO mouth rinse at different exercise intensities. Furthermore, an MIT would allow knowing how the mental fatigue-CHO mouth rinse interplay affects peak power output (W_{PEAK}), peak oxygen comsumption (VO_{2PEAK}), and ventilatory thresholds, a topic poorly investigated, as mentioned earlier.

Therefore, the present study aimed to verify if rinsing the mouth with CHO solution may counteract the deleterious mental fatigue effects on MIT performance and PFC and MC activation. We also aimed to examine if CHO mouth rinse in mentally fatigued individuals may change MIT outcomes, such as W_{PEAK}, VO_{2PEAK}, and ventilatory thresholds, such as the first (VT_1) and second ventilatory threshold (VT_2). We hypothesized that mental fatigue would negatively affect MIT outcomes; however, CHO mouth rinse would mitigate these effects.

2. Materials and Methods

2.1. Participants and Ethics

The sample size was calculated through equation suggested elsewhere as $n = 8e^2/d^2$ [25], where n, e, and d represent sample size, coefficient of variation, and percentage of treatment magnitude, respectively. Participants were invited through social media. After identification of eligible participants, 20 well-trained male cyclists, who attained a W_{PEAK} greater than 325 W in a preliminary MIT, took part in this study. Cyclists were classified within performance levels 2 and 3, according to classification suggested elsewhere [26], and were engaged in regional and national level competitions (7.56 yr ± 5.89 of cycling experience and 310.6 km·week^{-1} ± 128.1 of training volume) at the time the study was conducted. Cyclists should be free from cardiopulmonary, metabolic, and orthopedic diseases and being non-user of prohibited substances. All participants were informed about the risks and benefits before signing the informed written consent. This study was approved by the local Ethics Committee (54910716.4.0000.5390) and conformed the Declaration of Helsinki.

2.2. Study Design

This crossover, counterbalanced, CHO-perceived placebo-controlled study submitted cyclists to 3 experimental sessions after a preliminary and a baseline MIT session (Figure 1). In the first session, cyclists completed an MIT until exhaustion to identify eligible cyclists and habituate them with the MIT procedures. We selected cyclists attaining a $W_{PEAK} \geq 325$ W in this preliminary MIT session, as we intended to reduce the between-subjects performance variability. Additionally, this preliminary MIT served to calculate the percentage of W_{PEAK} (%W_{PEAK}) at which the participants rinsed their mouth with CHO or PLA in the experimental MIT. In the second session, cyclists performed a baseline MIT (BASE), while in sessions 3–5, they performed an MIT with mental fatigue (MF), or combining MF+CHO and MF+placebo (PLA). Importantly, instead of having 1 min steps throughout the MIT protocol, we used extended steps during the MIT in MF, MF+CHO, and MF+PLA sessions, so that steps at 25%, 50%, and 75% of the W_{PEAK} determined in preliminary MIT had 2 min duration. This adaptation was necessary to make possible the CHO mouth rinses every 25% of the trial while recording steady EEG signals during controlled constant workload at different intensities. Sessions 1 and 2 were performed in sequential order, but sessions 3 to 5 were performed in a counterbalanced order. Sessions 2 and 3 provided a proof-of-principle study of the mental fatigue in MIT, as this comparison allowed us to assess deleterious mental fatigue effects on MIT outcomes before studying the combined CHO mouth rinse-mental fatigue effects on this exercise mode.

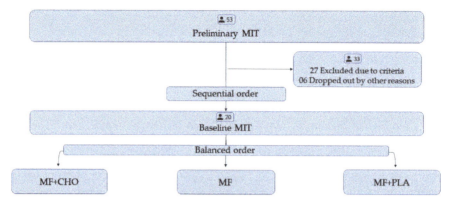

Figure 1. Proof-of-principle and experimental phases of the study. MIT = maximal incremental test. MF = mental fatigue session, MF+CHO = mental fatigue session rinsing carbohydrate, MF+PLA = mental fatigue session rinsing placebo perceived-as-carbohydrate.

Responses, such as gas exchange, as well as PFC and MC EEG, were continuously assessed throughout the MIT, while ratings of perceived exertion (RPE) were obtained at regular intervals. Additionally, EEG, fatigue sensation, and motivation were further obtained before and immediately after the cognitive test-induced mental fatigue. Cyclists were instructed to maintain their regular diet, avoid exhaustive exercise, and refrain from stimulant substances (i.e., energy drink, caffeine, pre-workout beverages) and alcoholic beverages for the 24 h before the sessions. The sessions were performed after a 6–8 h fasting period at the same time of day in a controlled temperature (~22 °C) and relative humidity (~60%) environment. A 3–7 days wash-out interval was observed between sessions.

2.3. Maximal Incremental Test (MIT)

All the MITs were performed on a road bike (Giant®, New York, NY, USA) attached to a cycle simulator (Computrainer, Racer-Mate® 8000, Seattle, WA, USA), calibrated according to manufacturer's instruction before every test. Seat and handlebar positions were individually adjusted before every test, following individual adjustment of the preliminary session. After a 5 min controlled-pace warm-up (100 W at 80 rpm), the workload was increased to 25 W·min^{-1} during the continued MIT until exhaustion, defined as the incapacity to maintain the pedal cadence despite three verbal encouragements (consisted of standardized words). These elongated steps allowed the record of a low-noise, steady time-matched EEG signal just after the mouth rinses. Cyclists were previously familiarized to keep their eyes closed and avoid excessive upper limb movements during exercise at these intensities.

2.4. Mental Fatigue Protocol

In accordance with previous studies [2,3], we used the rapid visual information processing test (RVIP), a high-demanding, sustained attention, and inhibitory control task to induce a mental fatigue state. Cyclists sat down in a comfortable chair in front of a 17-inch monitor, in a quiet and illuminated environment, wearing an earplug to reduce environment noises [2]. The RVIP lasted 40 min and consisted of identifying sequential three odd or even numbers randomly showed in a frequency of one number per 600 ms. Participants used the spacebar of a standard keyboard to indicate the correct answers. Sequences of three odd (i.e., 7, 3, 1; 1, 9, 5) or even (i.e., 8, 6, 2; 2, 8, 4) numbers were shown 8 times per minute. False alarms (a.u), accuracy answers (%), and reaction time (s) were used to assess cognitive performance [2].

2.5. Mouth Rinsing Protocols

Following recommendations from previous studies [18,19,27], we used artificial saliva (0.21 g of $NAHCO_3$ and 1.875 g of KCl per 1 L of ddH_2O) as a base for both CHO and PLA solutions [19,28]. While PLA was formulated as 0.053 g of acesulfame K diluted in 1 L of artificial saliva, the CHO solution was formulated, having 64 g of maltodextrin diluted in 1 L of PLA solution. Before the study, researchers tested these solutions to test the blinding efficacy. The cyclists were asked to rinse their mouth for 10 s with 25 mL CHO or PLA solution at the end of the standard warm-up as well as at 25%, 50%, and 75% of the MIT. The volume was spat into a bowl after each mouth rinse, and then we checked the eventual ingestion of substances by measuring the volume through a 10 mL syringe.

Importantly, we designed this study having a CHO-perceived placebo and a baseline condition as controls, in accordance with a recent placebo intervention consensus [29], suggesting that the expectation of receiving an active compound may be a bias source in sports nutrition studies [30]. Earlier studies had challenged the traditional double-blind, clinical trial design to investigate the ergogenic aid effects on physical performance [31,32], given that the expectancy itself could result in physical performance improvements [33]. In contrast, it has been suggested that the use of an active substance-perceived placebo condition may work as a control for the expectation-induced performance alterations in ergogenic supplement studies [29,30]. Therefore, in the present study, we reinforced the suggestion that CHO mouth rinse is a potential ergogenic aid to improve performance, leading cyclists to believe they would wash their mouths with CHO solution in all experimental sessions (i.e., CHO and PLA trials). We also included a baseline session (BASE) in the design, allowing us to know the effect size of both CHO and PLA mouth rinses relative to a condition totally inert, which had neither expectations nor pharmacological effects.

2.6. Measures and Instruments

2.6.1. Physical Performance

The performance was indicated by W_{PEAK} and time to exhaustion. The W_{PEAK} was defined as the highest power output attained in the last completed stage (60 s), corrected by the time (s) spent in an incomplete stage when necessary. The time to exhaustion was determined when cyclists could no longer maintain the target pedal cadence, despite three strong verbal encouragements provided by a researcher unaware of the substance used in the mouth rinses. Instructions and words used to verbally encourage cyclists were previously standardized.

2.6.2. Gaseous Exchange

The gaseous exchange was recorded breath-by-breath through a mask (Hans Rudolph, Shawnee, KS, USA) coupled to an open circuit gas analyzer (Metalyzer 3B, Cortex, Leipzig, Germany) for minute ventilation (VE), oxygen uptake (VO_2), and carbon dioxide production (VCO_2). The expired air was measured by using a bi-directional flow sensor calibrated before every test. A zirconium sensor analyzed the expired O_2, while the end-tidal CO_2 was analyzed through an infrared sensor. Sensors were calibrated according to the manufacturer's guidelines through a known O_2 (12%) and CO_2 (5%) concentration. Importantly, the mask was briefly removed from the participants' faces at the extended 2 min steps (~15 s), and thus they could rinse their mouth with CHO and placebo solutions. Researchers involved in this part of the study were trained during pilot tests to ensure minimal artifacts during the gaseous exchange and EEG data sampling. Breath-by-breath data were averaged as 10 s intervals so that VO_{2PEAK} and maximal respiratory exchange ratio (RER_{MAX}) were determined as the mean values over the last 30 s of the test during presumed maximal effort [34]. Two experienced researchers visually identified the VT_1 and VT_2 by analyzing the VE/VO_2 and VE/VCO_2 curves, at the first breakpoint in VE/VO_2 and last breakpoint before a systematic raise in VE/VCO_2, respectively. Both RER and VE breakpoints, defined as a systematic raise in these variables, were used to confirm VT_1 and VT_2, respectively. The median between researchers was used in cases of non-agreement between evaluators. Then, thresholds were expressed as absolute power output and VO$_2$ values, as well as relative to W$_{PEAK}$ and VO$_{2PEAK}$.

2.6.3. Electroencephalography

Active electrodes (Ag-AgCl) were placed at Fp1 and Cz positions following the EEG international 10–20 system, oriented by *nasion* and *inion* positions, and referenced to the mastoid process [35]. Electrodes were fixed with medical strips after exfoliation, cleaning, and application of the conductive gel. Resting EEG signal (Emsa®, EEG BNT 36, TiEEG, Rio de Janeiro, Brazil) was recorded during a 180 s time window before and immediately after the RVIP test completion, when cyclists were in absolute rest, with eyes closed, without body or facial movement. Importantly, they maintained their eyes closed during the extended 2 min stages, thus avoiding excessive facial and upper limb movements during EEG capture during MIT. Briefly, a reduced PFC activation, assessed specifically through an increased EEG theta band (3–7 Hz), has been associated with a highly demanding cognitive task-induced mental fatigue [2,3,36]. Hence, we used an increased activity in this particular EEG band over the PFC from pre to post RVIP test to assess mental fatigue. Moreover, PFC activation has been also suggested to play a role in exercise regulation [14,15], as PFC is involved in exercise-induced perceptual responses [11], attentional and inhibitory control [12], and MC activation during exercise [3,13,14]. Earlier studies have suggested that CHO mouth rinse has increased brain activation in PFC [18], so we hypothesized that cortical activation, as measured through the entire EEG power spectrum, would provide a reliable picture of the effects of CHO mouth rinse on cortical activation in mentally fatigued cyclists performing the exercise.

The EEG signal was captured with a Notch filter, before data filtering through a 3–50 Hz band-pass recursive filter. The EEG signal recorded before and after the RVIP test was processed within a 5 s time window (1800 samples) of the most steady signal (lowest local standard deviation) within a −200 and 200 μV amplitude range, after removing the initial and final 30 s time window, a period containing noises related to the individuals' expectancy regarding the start and end of the EEG protocol [37]. The power spectrum within the 3–7 Hz was calculated in PFC through a Fast Fourier Transform so that an increase of the power spectrum within this particular EEG band was interpreted as evidence of mental fatigue [2–4]. In contrast, we further calculated the total power spectrum density (PSD) within the 3–50 Hz band in a 5 s time window in the most steady signal captured immediately after each mouth rinse at the end of the warm-up and at 25%, 50%, and 75% W$_{PEAK}$ during MIT. The use of the entire EEG power spectrum is more meaningful to indicate the exercise-induced alteration in cortical activity. Resting EEG data were expressed as absolute values (dB), while exercise EEG data were expressed as a change (%) from the baseline values recorded before the RVIP test [23,38].

2.6.4. Psychological Responses

Mental fatigue sensation was assessed through a visual analog scale (VAS) before and after the RVIP test. Cyclists were asked to answer "how mentally fatigued you feel now" by using a scale ranging from "0" to "100" mm to rate mental fatigue sensation as "none at all" and "maximal", respectively [2,39]. Moreover, we assessed RPE at the end of extended MIT steps at 25%, 50%, and 75% W$_{PEAK}$ through the 15-point Borg's scale [40], having its anchors as reported elsewhere [41]. The slope of the RPE-exercise relationship (RPE$_{SLOPE}$) was used to indicate how RPE progressed during exercise, while RPE$_{MAX}$ ≥ 18 indicated if the maximal effort was attained.

3. Statistical Analysis

Data were firstly checked for Gaussian distribution; thereafter, they were presented as mean and standard deviation (SD). As a proof-of-principle of the mental fatigue effects on neurophysiological, cognitive, perceptual, and exercise performance variables, we performed a series of comparisons involving BASE and MF exercise sessions before investigating the CHO mouth rinse effects on mentally fatigued individuals. Then, using the MF exercise session, we firstly confirmed the increase of EEG theta band in PFC and mental fatigue sensation from pre to post RVIP test through a paired student *t*-test. Accordingly, we confirmed a likely impairment in cognitive performance over the RVIP test, and thus we compared reaction time, accurate answers, and false alarms through a repeated-measures mixed model design. Secondly, using BASE and MF exercise sessions, we compared MIT outcomes, such as W_{PEAK}, time to exhaustion, VO_{2PEAK}, and RPE_{SLOPE}, through a paired student *t*-test. Given the dependence nature between thresholds, we compared VT_1 and VT_2 between BASE and MF through a repeated-measures mixed model design. In mixed models analysis, we used the restrict Likelihood log criteria to find the covariance matrix that best fitted to the dataset, and cases of significant F-values were corrected by Bonferroni's test. Additionally, we used the BASE MIT session to calculate the mental fatigue-derived smallest worthwhile change on performance, as suggested elsewhere [42].

Using MF, MF+CHO, and MF+PLA exercise sessions, we verified the CHO mouth rinse effects on MIT outcomes, such as W_{PEAK}, time to exhaustion, VO_{2PEAK}, RPE_{SLOPE}, VT_1, and VT_2, in mentally fatigued cyclists through a series of paired student t-tests and repeated-measures mixed models, as detailed above. We also verified the CHO mouth rinse effects on PFC and MC responses to exercise (warm-up, 25%, 50%, 75%, and 100% of the MIT) in mentally fatigued cyclists through repeated-measures mixed model comparisons.

Even performing a prior sample size estimation, we reported the post hoc effect size (ES) to confirm this initial estimation. Regardless of the statistic family test, ES was expressed as Cohens' *d* and interpreted as small ($0 \geq d \leq 0.2$), moderate ($0.3 \geq d \leq 0.6$), large ($0.7 \geq d \leq 1.2$), very large ($1.2 \geq d \leq 1.9$), and extremely large ES ($d \geq 2$), as suggested elsewhere [43]. Statistical significance was set at $p \leq 0.05$, and the analysis was carried out with specific software (v.22 SPSS software, IBM, New York, NY, USA).

4. Results

Twenty-six eligible participants matching the W_{PEAK} criteria were picked out from a broader sample ($n = 53$), after the preliminary MIT. However, six eligible cyclists dropped out from experimental procedures due to personal reasons. Therefore, 20 cyclists (W_{PEAK} of 358.63 W ± 21.96, age of 35 yr ± 7, body mass of 80.5 kg ± 10.4, the height of 176 cm ± 5 and body mass index of 26.04 ± 2.94) completed the experimental procedures.

4.1. Proof-of-Principle of the Mental Fatigue Effects

When compared to pre RVIP test measures, cyclists showed an increased EEG theta band ($p < 0.001$, d = 0.47) and mental fatigue sensation (23.00 ± 24.47 vs. 42.32 ± 26.14, $p = 0.005$) after the cognitive test. Accordingly, the cognitive performance decreased throughout the RVIP test, as the time main effect revealed an impairment in reaction time ($p = 0.04$, d = 2.05) and accurate answers ($p = 0.03$, d = 0.70), although no effect was detected in false alarms ($p = 0.60$).

Comparisons involving BASE and MF sessions revealed that MIT performance was impaired in the MF session (Table 1), either expressed as time to exhaustion ($p = 0.002$, d = 0.24) or W_{PEAK} ($p = 0.002$, d = 0.25). The mean W_{PEAK} difference from BASE to MF trial was 6.99 W, being greater than the smallest worthwhile change estimated as 4.97 W. In contrast, VO_{2PEAK} responses were comparable between BASE and MF trials ($p = 0.80$). Comparisons involving thresholds showed that VT_1 was obviously lower than VT_2 regardless of the condition, and thus the time effects were omitted. Neither VT_1 nor VT_2, expressed either in absolute power output ($p > 0.05$) and VO_2 values ($p > 0.05$) or relative to peak values (i.e., W_{PEAK}, $p > 0.05$; VO_{2PEAK}, $p > 0.05$), were significantly different between BASE and MF sessions. Accordingly, no time by condition interaction effect was observed in VT_1 ($p > 0.05$ for all results) and VT_2 ($p > 0.05$ for all results). The RPE_{SLOPE} was comparable between MF and BASE trials ($p = 0.62$). Table 1 depicts all MIT outcomes between the BASE and MF trials.

Table 1. Proof-of-principle study of the mental fatigue effects on maximal incremental test outcomes.

	Baseline	Mental Fatigue
W_{PEAK}	350.84 ± 24.83	343.85 ± 27.38 *
Time to Exhaustion (seconds)	841.85 ± 59.65	827.75 ± 68.62 *
VO_{2PEAK} (L/min)	4.35 ± 0.37	4.33 ± 0.41
RER_{MAX}	1.16 ± 0.07	1.16 ± 0.06
RPE_{MAX}	19.50 ± 0.63	19.40 ± 0.99
RPE_{SLOPE}	0.89 ± 0.20	0.91 ± 0.21
VT_1 (W)	225.10 ± 27.06	225.21 ± 25.55
VT_2 (W)	283.22 ± 30.03	283.59 ± 29.01
VT_1 (% W_{PEAK})	62.99 ± 7.12	64.62 ± 5.77
VT_2 (% W_{PEAK})	80.11 ± 7.19	82.33 ± 6.79
VT_1 (L/min)	3.04 ± 0.41	3.07 ± 0.39
VT_2 (L/min)	3.57 ± 0.38	3.73 ± 0.39
VT_1 (% VO_{2PEAK})	69.87 ± 7.15	70.87 ± 7.95
VT_2 (% VO_{2PEAK})	82.21 ± 6.37	85.71 ± 4.71

* significantly different in W_{PEAK} (p = 0.002) and time to exhaustion (p = 0.002). W_{PEAK} = peak power output, VO_{2PEAK} = peak oxygen comsumption, RER = respiratory exchange ratio, RPE = ratings of perceived effort, VT = ventilatory threshold.

4.2. Mental Fatigue Responses before the MIT in Mouth Rinse Sessions

In accordance with proof-of-principle results, we also observed an increased EEG theta band in both MF+CHO (p = 0.02, d = 0.56) and MF+PLA sessions (p < 0.001, d = 0.71) from pre to post RVIP test. Likewise, mental fatigue sensation increased from pre to post RVIP test in both MF+CHO (10.82 ± 11.38 vs. 40.58 ± 25.30; p < 0.001, d = 1.44) and MF+PLA sessions (17.18 ± 14.23 vs. 47.65 ± 23.65; p < 0.001, d = 1.49). Together, cognitive performance worsened similarly throughout the RVIP test in both MF+CHO and MF+PLA mouth rinse sessions, as indicated by a time main effect in reaction time (p = 0.003, d = 0.76). In contrast, no time effects were observed in accurate answers (p = 0.12) and false alarms (p = 0.66). Given that no mouth rinses were performed during the cognitive test, no session main effect was observed in reaction time (p = 0.58), accurate answers (p = 0.25), or false alarms (p = 0.06).

4.3. CHO Mouth Rinse Effects on MIT Outcomes in Mentally Fatigued Cyclists

We observed a significant mouth rinse main effect in W_{PEAK} (343.85 ± 27.38 vs. 344.52 ± 24.00 vs. 350.21 ± 21.20 W for MF, PLA+MF, and CHO+MF respectively, p = 0.01, d = 0.72) and time to exhaustion (825.75 ± 65.62 vs. 826.79 ± 57.64 vs. 839.74 ± 50.08 s for MF, PLA+MF, and CHO+MF respectively, p = 0.01, d = 0.70), showing that CHO mouth rinse attenuated the mental fatigue-reduced MIT performance (Figure 2). Thus, as depicted in Figure 3, both the W_{PEAK} and time to exhaustion were greater in MF+CHO than MF+PLA (p = 0.04 and p = 0.04) and MF session (p = 0.02 and p = 0.03), although no difference was observed in VO_{2PEAK} (p = 0.37). Regarding the ventilatory thresholds, VT_1 was obviously lower than VT_2 regardless of the condition, and thus the time effects were omitted. No difference was observed between MF and MF+CHO trial for VT_1 and VT_2, regardless of the variable used to express them. However, VT_1 and VT_2 were greater in MF+PLA than MF trial when expressed as absolute or relative power output values, but not as absolute and relative VO_2. No difference was detected between thresholds identified in MF+CHO and MF+PLA. Comparable RPE_{SLOPE} responses were observed in MF, MF+CHO, and MF+PLA trials (p = 0.79). Table 2 shows the MIT outcomes found in MF, MF+CHO, and MF+PLA trials, except for those outcomes earlier reported as figures.

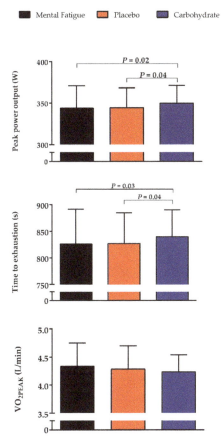

Figure 2. Peak power output (W$_{PEAK}$, **upper panel**), time to exhaustion (**middle panel**), and the peak of O$_2$ uptake (VO$_{2PEAK}$, **bottom panel**) in mental fatigue, and mental fatigue combined with placebo and carbohydrate mouth rinse.

Table 2. Maximal incremental test outcomes during mental fatigue, and mental fatigue combined with carbohydrate and placebo mouth rinses.

	Mental Fatigue	Placebo	Carbohydrate
RER$_{MAX}$	1.16 ± 0.06	1.17 ± 0.07	1.16 ± 0.07
RPE$_{MAX}$	19.40 ± 0.99	19.42 ± 1.50	19.79 ± 0.54
RPE$_{SLOPE}$	0.91 ± 0.21	0.92 ± 0.18	0.88 ± 0.16
VT$_1$ (W)	225.21 ± 25.55	242.43 ± 25.48	237.73 ± 17.52
VT$_2$ (W)	283.59 ± 29.01	297.26 ± 26.63	297.92 ± 19.69
VT$_1$ (% W$_{PEAK}$)	64.62 ± 5.77	70.35 ± 5.49	66.78 ± 7.09
VT$_2$ (% W$_{PEAK}$)	82.33 ± 6.79	86.24 ± 4.32	84.40 ± 3.39
VT$_1$ (L/min)	3.07 ± 0.39	3.30 ± 0.40	3.12 ± 0.40
VT$_2$ (L/min)	3.73 ± 0.39	3.82 ± 0.38	3.85 ± 0.23
VT$_1$ (% VO$_{2PEAK}$)	70.87 ± 7.95	74.78 ± 8.31	71.57 ± 8.70
VT$_2$ (% VO$_{2PEAK}$)	85.71 ± 4.71	87.13 ± 5.12	90.20 ± 4.69

There was a main condition effect (mental fatigue vs. placebo) for VT expressed as %W$_{PEAK}$.

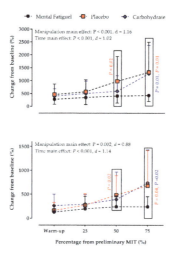

Figure 3. The prefrontal cortex (PFC, **upper panel**) and motor cortex (MC, **bottom panel**) activity throughout the maximal incremental test (MIT) during mental fatigue and mental fatigue combined with carbohydrate and placebo mouth rinse.

Regarding PFC activation during exercise, we found a mouth rinse ($p < 0.001$, d = 1.16) and a time main effect in EEG responses ($p < 0.001$, d = 1.02), as both CHO and PLA mouth rinses changed the PFC activation of mentally fatigued cyclists throughout the MIT. Multiple comparisons showed that PFC activity was higher in MF+CHO ($p = 0.01$) and MF+PLA ($p < 0.001$) than MF, but no difference was detected between MF+CHO and MF+PLA ($p = 0.95$). Time by mouth rinses interaction effects revealed that PFC activity was greater in MF+CHO than MF at 75% of the MIT ($p = 0.01$). Likewise, PFC activity was greater in MF+PLA than MF at 50% ($p = 0.02$) and 75% of the MIT ($p = 0.01$). Figure 3 (upper panel) depicts the results of PFC activation during MIT.

Accordingly, we found a mouth rinse ($p = 0.002$, d = 0.88) and time main effect ($p < 0.001$, d = 1.14) in EEG responses, as both CHO and PLA mouth rinses changed the MC activation of mentally fatigued cyclists throughout the MIT. Additionally, both MF+CHO ($p = 0.01$) and MF+PLA ($p = 0.02$) induced to a greater MC activation when compared to MF trial, as MF+CHO was greater than MF at 75% of the MIT ($p = 0.02$), and MF+PLA was greater than MF at 50% ($p = 0.02$) and 75% of the MIT ($p = 0.04$). No differences were found in MC between MF+CHO and MF+PLA trials ($p > 0.05$). Figure 3 (bottom panel) depicts the results of MC activation during MIT.

Importantly, we checked for eventual solution ingestions during the mouth rinses. Comparisons revealed that spitted volumes were comparable between CHO and PLA mouth rinse sessions ($p = 0.70$), as cyclists ingested 7 mL of solution in both CHO and PLA mouth rinse conditions.

5. Discussion

Given the centrally mediated mental fatigue effects, we hypothesized that CHO mouth rinse could enhance PFC and MC activation and mitigate deleterious mental fatigue effects on exercise performance, as a body of evidence has shown that CHO mouth rinse may potentiate exercise performance through central pathways [17]. We observed that CHO mouth rinse was effective to mitigate the mental fatigue-reduced MIT performance, despite the comparable alterations in PFC and MC activation between CHO and PLA. These results confirmed that CHO mouth rinse might counteract mental fatigue effects on exercise performance, although challenging its role in cortical activation. Additionally, placebo mouth rinse improved the power output corresponding to ventilatory thresholds, even though mental fatigue has not impaired them.

5.1. Proof-of-Principle of the Mental Fatigue Effects on MIT Outcomes

Since an earlier study by Marcora et al. in 2009 [5], mental fatigue effects on endurance exercise performance have been studied in different exercise modes; however, only two included MIT protocols in mental fatigue scenarios [6,7]. Furthermore, only a small number of studies included EEG theta band analysis to verify mental fatigue effects on PFC activation, a cortical area involved in proactive, goal-directed behavior [2,3,36]. It has been suggested that mental fatigue slows down the PFC activity, probably due to the cognitive overload-induced adenosine accumulation, as adenosine accumulation may impair the PFC ability to deal with aversive feelings and attentional control [1,44]. Previous findings showed that the large increase in EEG theta band from pre to post RVIP test was associated with an increased mental fatigue sensation and impaired performance in subsequent endurance exercise [2,3]. Indeed, in the present study, we also observed that the RVIP test induced an increase in EEG theta band over the PFC and led cyclists to report a higher mental fatigue sensation. Accordingly, the mental fatigue impaired exercise performance in MIT.

The results of the effects of mental fatigue on MIT performance are controversial, as some have found that mental fatigue is deleterious to MIT performance [39,45], while others have not [7]. For example, studies have found a decrease in the total distance completed by soccer [39] and cricket players [45] during a Yo-Yo test under mental fatigue. Moreover, Zering et al. [6] observed a reduced W_{PEAK} and VO_{2MAX} in a laboratory cycling MIT, although VT_1 was unchanged. In contrast, Vrijkotte et al. [7] showed no negative effects of mental fatigue on a similar cycling MIT. The reason for such a controversial result involving MIT is unclear [7,39,45], perhaps methodological factors related to the exercise familiarization and experimental conditions might have influenced some results [7]. In the present study, we observed that 40 min RVIP test reduced the time to exhaustion and W_{PEAK} during MIT by around 1.9% and 2.0%, respectively, reinforcing the notion of mental fatigue-impaired performance in MIT [39,45]. Additionally, mental fatigue neither impaired VT_1 and VT_2, regardless of the variable used to express them, nor did change the VO_{2PEAK}. While the VO_2 results agreed with those reported elsewhere [5], thresholds results might suggest that mental fatigue was ineffective in changing these cardiopulmonary fitness variables in well-trained cyclists.

5.2. Effects of CHO Mouth Rinse in Mentally Fatigued Cyclists

Since CHO mouth rinse has been suggested to enhance activation in cortical structures, such as PFC areas [18,19], we hypothesized that CHO mouth rinse could enhance PFC and MC activation and MIT performance in mentally fatigued individuals.

Different from previous studies that have used manipulations to counteract the effects of mental fatigue before or during the cognitive test [2,20], in the present study, cyclists rinsed their mouth with CHO during exercise, when they were already mentally fatigued. As the use of centrally active compounds before or during the RVIP protocol [1,2] could have interfered in cognitive, perceptual, and EEG responses, we designed the CHO mouth rinses only after the RVIP test. Actually, Van Cutsem et al. [20] observed that performing caffeine-CHO mouthwash before and during the high-demanding cognitive task attenuated the mental fatigue sensation and cerebral changes, as measured by EEG, and ameliorated cognitive performance responses. Importantly, in the present study, mental fatigue effects were comparable before the exercise among MF, MF+CHO, and MF+PLA sessions.

To the best of our knowledge, only two studies have investigated the effects of centrally active compounds on exercise performance of mentally fatigued participants [2,10], and no studies have investigated if CHO mouth rinse could attenuate MIT performance reductions in mentally fatigued cyclists, despite evidence for a potential benefit of CHO mouth rinse on exercise performance [17]. Our results showed that mentally fatigued cyclists improved MIT performance by ~2.4% and ~2.3% when compared to MF and MF+PLA trials, respectively, when they rinsed their mouth with CHO. Overall, the beneficial effect of CHO mouth rinse on cycling performance has been reported as ~1.7% [17]. In the present study, the smallest worthwhile change indicated that a change of 1.3% would be needed to detect significant effects on performance.

The underlying pathways of the CHO mouth rinse effects involve the oral receptors-activated brain areas, such as PFC, orbitofrontal cortex, insula, and operculum frontal [14,18,19]. Some of them, such as PFC, composes motor planning [2–4] and exercise regulation areas [14,23], which are similarly affected by mental fatigue, yet in the opposite direction. Interestingly, a recent study by Franco-Alvarenga et al. [2] showed that mentally fatigued cyclists improved their performance when they ingested caffeine, although regardless of alterations in PFC activity. We also observed that CHO mouth rinse improved MIT performance of mentally fatigued cyclists regardless of alterations in PFC and MC activation, as both CHO and PLA mouth rinses similarly improved PFC and MC activation. Somehow, these results challenge the central pathways suggested for CHO mouth rinse [18]. Alternatively, they may be related to the CHO-perceived PLA design used in the present study.

We used a deceptive placebo, as participants were misinformed about the presence of CHO in both mouth rinses sessions. Therefore, they expected a potential benefit when rinsing their mouth with CHO in both sessions. Studies have suggested that participants may improve physical performance when they believe they are receiving the active substance in the placebo session [31,33]. Furthermore, the placebo perceived as the active substance has the potential to induce physiological and brain responses in the same direction of the active substance [31,46]. Thus, these results of cerebral activation may also be related to our placebo design.

It has been traditionally suggested that mental fatigue-reduced performance is associated with a higher than normal RPE, irrespective of alteration in physiological responses, such as VO_2 and heart rate [1,2,5]. Accordingly, our results indicated similar cardiopulmonary responses, given the comparable VO_2, VE, and HR responses among MF, MF+CHO, and MF+PLA trials. Moreover, given that RPE was comparable among these trials, but the performance was reduced with mental fatigue manipulation, one may argue that there was a higher than normal RPE in the MF trial.

Importantly, PLA but not CHO mouth rinse improved the power output at VT_1 and VT_2. The unaltered VT_2 power output combined with an improved W_{PEAK} in the MF+CHO trial might suggest that mentally fatigued cyclists increased the ability to tolerate exercise acidosis-derived aversive sensation after the VT_2 occurrence [47], thus elongating the time spent between VT_2 and W_{PEAK}. Perhaps, mentally fatigued cyclists improved their capacity to resist to intensified body responses, such as hyperventilation, muscle acidosis, cerebral oxygenation, etc., after the VT_2, when they rinsed their mouth with CHO solution [47]. From a practical perspective, these results are relevant and suggest that centrally active compounds may improve MIT outcomes in mentally fatigued individuals, regardless of potential deleterious mental fatigue effects on these outcomes. Interestingly, we also observed that cyclists improved the power output corresponding to VT_1 and VT_2. These results are counterintuitive and require more investigation.

5.3. Methodological Aspects

In the present study, we used a double-controlled experimental design having a baseline and a placebo session as controls. However, instead of using a traditional randomized placebo-controlled clinical trial in which individuals have 50% chances of using CHO vs. 50% changes in using a placebo, we used a CHO-perceived placebo design, as recently suggested elsewhere [29]. Thus, we controlled the active substance-derived expectation effects [29,48]. Although this design has controlled expectations-induced variations in performance responses [31,49], it may have induced particular cerebral responses that may not have been present in a traditional placebo-controlled clinical trial [31], as discussed earlier.

Although we rigorously controlled the internal validity of the study (i.e., characteristic of cyclists, equipment used, environment, etc.) and provided EEG signal with reasonable quality during exercise at increasing controlled intensities, we did not analyze EEG responses from 75% of the W_{PEAK} because artifacts derived from vigorous head and trunk movements could limit the signal quality [50]. Besides, no mouth rinse was performed from this intensity, as the hyperventilation present in the last MIT intensities would have hindered the use of controlled mouth rinses (i.e., no ingestion). Therefore, the present study was unable to unravel the mental fatigue-CHO mouth rinse interplay from intensities above 75% of the W_{PEAK}. However, considering the growing interest in investigating cortical measures during exercise [23,38], the present study provided an example of a rigorous, well-controlled methodology to assess EEG responses at different controlled intensities. In this regard, we used an MIT to investigate the potential effects of CHO mouth rinse on exercise performance in mentally fatigued individuals, as this exercise mode allowed us to know the effects of CHO mouth rinse by exercise intensity interaction on EEG and exercise performance responses [24,51]. Considering that CHO mouth rinse seems to have a timely effect [27] and that most studies have used CHO mouth rinses at regular intervals [16,18], we designed an MIT model to make regular mouth rinses possible (every 25% of the preliminary MIT).

6. Conclusions

In conclusion, the results of the present study showed that CHO mouth rinse is an effective strategy to mitigate deleterious mental fatigue effects on MIT performance, perhaps improving the ability to tolerate aversive sensations above the VT_2. However, our results challenged the role of CHO mouth rinse on PFC and MC activation, highlighting a potential placebo effect on cerebral responses.

Author Contributions: Conceptualization, C.B. and F.O.P.; methodology, C.B., T.M.S., and F.O.P.; software, C.B. and M.F.G.; formal analysis, C.B.; investigation, C.B., P.E.F.-A., R.C., and Í.V.; data curation, C.B. and M.F.G.; writing—original draft preparation, C.B., V.d.S.P., and F.O.P.; writing—review and editing, C.B., F.O.P., and F.J.H.; visualization, C.B.; supervision, F.O.P.; project administration, F.O.P.; funding acquisition, F.O.P. All authors have read and agreed to the published version of the manuscript.

Funding: This research was funded by São Paulo Research Foundation (FAPESP—Brazil), grant number #2016/16496-3, and F.O.P. is grateful to the National Council for Scientific and Technological Development (CNPq—Brazil) for his scholarship. Authors (C.B., P.E.F.-A., R.C., I.V.F.P., and M.F.G.) are grateful for their scholarship from the Coordination of Improvement of Higher Education Personnel (CAPES—Brazil), Finance code 001.

Acknowledgments: We acknowledge Bruno Viana for instructing on initial data processing.

Conflicts of Interest: The authors declare no conflict of interest.

References

1. Van Cutsem, J.; Marcora, S.; De Pauw, K.; Bailey, S.; Meeusen, R.; Roelands, B. The Effects of Mental Fatigue on Physical Performance: A Systematic Review. *Sports Med.* **2017**, *47*, 1569–1588. [CrossRef]
2. Franco-Alvarenga, P.E.; Brietzke, C.; Canestri, R.; Goethel, M.F.; Hettinga, F.; Santos, T.M.; Pires, F.O.; Canestri, R. Caffeine improved cycling trial performance in mentally fatigued cyclists, regardless of alterations in prefrontal cortex activation. *Physiol. Behav.* **2019**, *204*, 41–48. [CrossRef] [PubMed]
3. Pires, F.O.; Silva-Júnior, F.L.; Brietzke, C.; Franco-Alvarenga, P.E.; Pinheiro, F.A.; de França, N.M.; Teixeira, S.; Meireles Santos, T. Mental Fatigue Alters Cortical Activation and Psychological Responses, Impairing Performance in a Distance-Based Cycling Trial. *Front. Physiol.* **2018**, *9*, 227. [CrossRef] [PubMed]
4. Wascher, E.; Rasch, B.; Sänger, J.; Hoffmann, S.; Schneider, D.; Rinkenauer, G.; Heuer, H.; Gutberlet, I. Frontal theta activity reflects distinct aspects of mental fatigue. *Biol. Psychol.* **2014**, *96*, 57–65. [CrossRef] [PubMed]
5. Marcora, S.M.; Staiano, W.; Manning, V. Mental fatigue impairs physical performance in humans. *J. Appl. Physiol.* **2009**, *106*, 857–864. [CrossRef] [PubMed]
6. Zering, J.C.; Brown, D.M.Y.; Graham, J.D.; Bray, S.R. Cognitive control exertion leads to reductions in peak power output and as well as increased perceived exertion on a graded exercise test to exhaustion. *J. Sports Sci.* **2016**, *35*, 1799–1807. [CrossRef] [PubMed]
7. Vrijkotte, S.; Meeusen, R.; Vandervaeren, C.; Buyse, L.; Van Cutsem, J.; Pattyn, N.; Roelands, B. Mental fatigue and physical and cognitive performance during a 2-bout exercise test. *Int. J. Sports Physiol. Perform.* **2018**, *13*, 510–516. [CrossRef]
8. Kunutsor, S.K.; Kurl, S.; Khan, H.; Zaccardi, F.; Laukkanen, J.A. Associations of cardiovascular and all-cause mortality events with oxygen uptake at ventilatory threshold. *Int. J. Cardiol.* **2017**, *236*, 444–450. [CrossRef]
9. Bentley, D.J.; Newell, J.; Bishop, D. Incremental exercise test design and analysis: Implications for performance diagnostics in endurance athletes. *Sport. Med.* **2007**, *37*, 575–586. [CrossRef]

10. Azevedo, R.; Silva-Cavalcante, M.D.; Gualano, B.; Lima-Silva, A.E.; Bertuzzi, R. Effects of caffeine ingestion on endurance performance in mentally fatigued individuals. *Eur. J. Appl. Physiol.* **2016**, *116*, 2293–2303. [CrossRef]
11. Boksem, M.A.; Tops, M. Mental fatigue: Costs and benefits. *Brain Res. Rev.* **2008**, *59*, 125–139. [CrossRef] [PubMed]
12. Dunwiddie, T.V.; Masino, S.A. The role and regulation of adenosine in the central nervous system. *Annu. Rev. Neurosci.* **2001**, *24*, 31–55. [CrossRef] [PubMed]
13. Martin, K.; Meeusen, R.; Thompson, K.G.; Keegan, R.; Rattray, B. Mental Fatigue Impairs Endurance Performance: A Physiological Explanation. *Sports Med.* **2018**, *48*, 2041–2051. [CrossRef] [PubMed]
14. Meeusen, R.; Pires, F.O.; Lutz, K.; Cheung, S.S.; Perrey, S.; Rauch, H.G.L.; Micklewright, D.; Pinheiro, F.A.; Radel, R.; Brisswalter, J.; et al. A role for the prefrontal cortex in exercise tolerance and termination. *J. Appl. Physiol.* **2016**, *120*, 464–466. [CrossRef]
15. Schiphof-Godart, L.; Roelands, B.; Hettinga, F.J. Drive in sports: How mental fatigue affects endurance performance. *Front. Psychol.* **2018**, *9*, 9. [CrossRef]
16. Carter, J.M.; Jeukendrup, A.E.; Jones, D.A. The effect of carbohydrate mouth rinse on 1-h cycle time trial performance. *Med. Sci. Sports Exerc.* **2004**, *36*, 2107–2111. [CrossRef]
17. Brietzke, C.; Franco-Alvarenga, P.E.; Coelho-Júnior, H.J.; Silveira, R.; Asano, R.Y.; Pires, F.O. Effects of Carbohydrate Mouth Rinse on Cycling Time Trial Performance: A Systematic Review and Meta-Analysis. *Sports Med.* **2018**, *49*, 57–66. [CrossRef]
18. Chambers, E.S.; Bridge, M.W.; Jones, D.A. Carbohydrate sensing in the human mouth: Effects on exercise performance and brain activity. *J. Physiol.* **2009**, *587*, 1779–1794. [CrossRef]
19. Turner, C.E.; Byblow, W.D.; Stinear, C.M.; Gant, N. Carbohydrate in the mouth enhances activation of brain circuitry involved in motor performance and sensory perception. *Appetite* **2014**, *80*, 212–219. [CrossRef]
20. Van Cutsem, J.; De Pauw, K.; Marcora, S.; Meeusen, R.; Roelands, B. A caffeine-maltodextrin mouth rinse counters mental fatigue. *Psychopharmacology (Berl)* **2017**, *235*, 947–958. [CrossRef]
21. Carter, C.S.; Braver, T.S.; Barch, D.M.; Botvinick, M.M.; Noll, D.; Cohen, J.D. Anterior cingulate cortex, error detection, and the online monitoring of performance. *Science (80-.)* **1998**, *280*, 747–749. [CrossRef] [PubMed]
22. Brosnan, M.B.; Wiegand, I. The dorsolateral prefrontal cortex, a dynamic cortical area to enhance top-down attentional control. *J. Neurosci.* **2017**, *37*, 3445–3446. [CrossRef]
23. Pires, F.O.; Dos Anjos, C.A.; Covolan, R.J.M.; Pinheiro, F.A.; St Clair Gibson, A.; Noakes, T.D.; Magalhães, F.H.; Ugrinowitsch, C. Cerebral Regulation in Different Maximal Aerobic Exercise Modes. *Front. Physiol.* **2016**, *7*, 253. [CrossRef] [PubMed]
24. Bastos-Silva, V.J.; Melo, A.A.; Lima-Silva, A.E.; Moura, F.A.; Bertuzzi, R.; de Araujo, G.G. Carbohydrate Mouth Rinse Maintains Muscle Electromyographic Activity and Increases Time to Exhaustion during Moderate but not High-Intensity Cycling Exercise. *Nutrients* **2016**, *8*, 49. [CrossRef] [PubMed]
25. Hopkins, W.G. Measures of reliability in sports medicine and science. *Sports Med.* **2000**, *30*, 1–15. [CrossRef]
26. De Pauw, K.; Roelands, B.; Cheung, S.S.; de Geus, B.; Rietjens, G.; Meeusen, R. Guidelines to classify subject groups in sport-science research. *Int. J. Sports Physiol. Perform.* **2013**, *8*, 111–122. [CrossRef]
27. Gant, N.; Stinear, C.M.; Byblow, W.D. Carbohydrate in the mouth immediately facilitates motor output. *Brain Res.* **2010**, *1350*, 151–158. [CrossRef] [PubMed]
28. O'Doherty, J.; Rolls, E.T.; Francis, S.; Bowtell, R.; McGlone, F. Representation of Pleasant and Aversive Taste in the Human Brain. *J. Neurophysiol.* **2001**, *85*, 1315–1321. [CrossRef]
29. Beedie, C.; Benedetti, F.; Barbiani, D.; Camerone, E.; Cohen, E.; Coleman, D.; Davis, A.; Elsworth-Edelsten, C.; Flowers, E.; Foad, A.; et al. Consensus statement on placebo effects in sports and exercise: The need for conceptual clarity, methodological rigour, and the elucidation of neurobiological mechanisms. *Eur. J. Sport Sci.* **2018**, *18*, 1383–1389. [CrossRef]
30. De Painelli, V.S.; Brietzke, C.; Franco-Alvarenga, P.E.; Canestri, R.; Vinícius, Í.; Pires, F.O. Comment on: "Caffeine and Exercise: What next?". *Sports Med.* **2020**, *50*, 1211–1218. [CrossRef]
31. Pires, F.O.; dos Anjos, C.A.S.; Covolan, R.J.M.; Fontes, E.B.; Noakes, T.D.; St Clair Gibson, A.; Magalhães, F.H.; Ugrinowitsch, C. Caffeine and Placebo Improved Maximal Exercise Performance Despite Unchanged Motor Cortex Activation and Greater Prefrontal Cortex Deoxygenation. *Front. Physiol.* **2018**, *9*, 1144. [CrossRef] [PubMed]

32. Saunders, B.; De Oliveira, L.F.; Da Silva, R.P.; De Salles Painelli, V.; Gonçalves, L.S.; Yamaguchi, G.; Mutti, T.; Maciel, E.; Roschel, H.; Artioli, G.G.; et al. Placebo in sports nutrition: A proof-of-principle study involving caffeine supplementation. *Scand. J. Med. Sci. Sports* **2016**, *27*, 1240–1247. [CrossRef] [PubMed]
33. Brietzke, C.; Asano, R.Y.; De Russi de Lima, F.; Pinheiro, F.A.; Franco-Alvarenga; Ugrinowitsch, C.; Pires, F.O. Caffeine effects on VO_{2max} test outcomes investigated by a placebo perceived-as-caffeine design. *Nutr. Health* **2017**, *23*, 231–238. [CrossRef]
34. Mezzani, A. Cardiopulmonary Exercise Testing: Basics of Methodology and Measurements. *Ann. Am. Thorac Soc.* **2017**, *14*, S3–S11. [CrossRef] [PubMed]
35. Pivik, R.T.; Broughton, R.J.; Coppola, R.; Davidson, R.J.; Fox, N.; Nuwer, M.R. Guidelines for the recording and quantitative analysis of electroencephalographic activity in research contexts. *Psychophysiology* **1993**, *30*, 547–558. [CrossRef] [PubMed]
36. Käthner, I.; Wriessnegger, S.C.; Müller-Putz, G.R.; Kübler, A.; Halder, S. Effects of mental workload and fatigue on the P300, alpha and theta band power during operation of an ERP (P300) brain-computer interface. *Biol. Psychol.* **2014**, *102*, 118–129. [CrossRef] [PubMed]
37. Brümmer, V.; Schneider, S.; Strüder, H.K.; Askew, C.D. Primary motor cortex activity is elevated with incremental exercise intensity. *Neuroscience* **2011**, *181*, 150–162. [CrossRef]
38. Robertson, C.V.; Marino, F.E. Prefrontal and motor cortex EEG responses and their relationship to ventilatory thresholds during exhaustive incremental exercise. *Eur. J. Appl. Physiol.* **2015**, *115*, 1939–1948. [CrossRef]
39. Smith, M.R.; Coutts, A.J.; Merlini, M.; Deprez, D.; Lenoir, M.; Marcora, S.M. Mental Fatigue Impairs Soccer-Specific Physical and Technical Performance. *Med. Sci. Sports Exerc.* **2016**, *48*, 267–276. [CrossRef]
40. Borg, G.A. Psychophysical bases of perceived exertion. *Med. Sci. Sports Exerc.* **1982**, *14*, 377–381. [CrossRef]
41. Pageaux, B. Perception of effort in Exercise Science: Definition, measurement and perspectives. *Eur. J. Sport Sci.* **2016**, *16*, 885–894. [CrossRef] [PubMed]
42. Hopkins, W.G. How to Interpret Changes in an Athletic Performance Test. Available online: http://www.sportsci.org/jour/04/wghtests.htm (accessed on 8 November 2019).
43. Hopkins, W.G.; Marshall, S.W.; Batterham, A.M.; Hanin, J. Progressive statistics for studies in sports medicine and exercise science. *Med. Sci. Sports Exerc.* **2009**, *41*, 3–13. [CrossRef]
44. Latini, S.; Pedata, F. Adenosine in the central nervous system: Release mechanisms and extracellular concentrations. *J. Neurochem.* **2008**, *79*, 463–484. [CrossRef] [PubMed]
45. Veness, D.; Patterson, S.D.; Jeffries, O.; Waldron, M. The effects of mental fatigue on cricket-relevant performance among elite players. *J. Sports Sci.* **2017**, *35*, 2461–2467. [CrossRef] [PubMed]
46. Benedetti, F.; Dogue, S. Different Placebos, Different Mechanisms, Different Outcomes: Lessons for Clinical Trials. *PLoS ONE* **2015**, *10*, e0140967. [CrossRef] [PubMed]
47. Vasconcelos, G.; Canestri, R.; Prado, R.C.R.; Brietzke, C.; Franco-Alvarenga, P.; Santos, T.M.; Pires, F.O. A comprehensive integrative perspective of the anaerobic threshold engine. *Physiol. Behav.* **2019**, *210*, 112435. [CrossRef] [PubMed]
48. Foad, A.J.; Beedie, C.J.; Coleman, D.A. Pharmacological and psychological effects of caffeine ingestion in 40-km cycling performance. *Med. Sci. Sports Exerc.* **2008**, *40*, 158–165. [CrossRef]
49. Beedie, C.J.; Stuart, E.M.; Coleman, D.A.; Foad, A.J. Placebo effects of caffeine on cycling performance. *Med. Sci. Sports Exerc.* **2006**, *38*, 2159–2164. [CrossRef]
50. Thompson, T.; Steffert, T.; Ros, T.; Leach, J.; Gruzelier, J. EEG applications for sport and performance. *Methods* **2008**, *45*, 279–288. [CrossRef]
51. Duncan, M.J.; Fowler, N.; George, O.; Joyce, S.; Hankey, J. Mental Fatigue Negatively Influences Manual Dexterity and Anticipation Timing but not Repeated High-intensity Exercise Performance in Trained Adults. *Res. Sports Med.* **2015**, *23*, 1–13. [CrossRef]

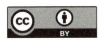

© 2020 by the authors. Licensee MDPI, Basel, Switzerland. This article is an open access article distributed under the terms and conditions of the Creative Commons Attribution (CC BY) license (http://creativecommons.org/licenses/by/4.0/).

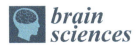

Perspective

New Directions in Exercise Prescription: Is There a Role for Brain-Derived Parameters Obtained by Functional Near-Infrared Spectroscopy?

Fabian Herold [1,2,*], **Thomas Gronwald** [3], **Felix Scholkmann** [4,5], **Hamoon Zohdi** [5], **Dominik Wyser** [4,6], **Notger G. Müller** [1,2,7] and **Dennis Hamacher** [8]

1. Department of Neurology, Medical Faculty, Otto von Guericke University, Leipziger Str. 44, 39120 Magdeburg, Germany; notger.mueller@dzne.de
2. Research Group Neuroprotection, German Center for Neurodegenerative Diseases (DZNE), Leipziger Str. 44, 39120 Magdeburg, Germany
3. Department Performance, Neuroscience, Therapy and Health, MSH Medical School Hamburg, University of Applied Sciences and Medical University, Am Kaiserkai 1, 20457 Hamburg, Germany; Thomas.Gronwald@medicalschool-hamburg.de
4. Department of Neonatology, Biomedical Optics Research Laboratory, University Hospital Zurich, University of Zurich, 8091 Zurich, Switzerland; felix.scholkmann@usz.ch (F.S.); dominik.wyser@hest.ethz.ch (D.W.)
5. Institute for Complementary and Integrative Medicine, University of Bern, 3012 Bern, Switzerland; hamoon.zohdi@ikim.unibe.ch
6. ETH Zurich, Rehabilitation Engineering Laboratory, Department of Health Sciences and Technology, 8092 Zurich, Switzerland
7. Center for Behavioral Brain Sciences (CBBS), Universitätsplatz 2, 39106 Magdeburg, Germany
8. German University for Health and Sports, (DHGS), Vulkanstraße 1, 10367 Berlin, Germany; Dennis.Hamacher@dhgs-hochschule.de
* Correspondence: fabian.herold@st.ovgu.de

Received: 29 April 2020; Accepted: 29 May 2020; Published: 3 June 2020

Abstract: In the literature, it is well established that regular physical exercise is a powerful strategy to promote brain health and to improve cognitive performance. However, exact knowledge about which exercise prescription would be optimal in the setting of exercise–cognition science is lacking. While there is a strong theoretical rationale for using indicators of internal load (e.g., heart rate) in exercise prescription, the most suitable parameters have yet to be determined. In this perspective article, we discuss the role of brain-derived parameters (e.g., brain activity) as valuable indicators of internal load which can be beneficial for individualizing the exercise prescription in exercise–cognition research. Therefore, we focus on the application of functional near-infrared spectroscopy (fNIRS), since this neuroimaging modality provides specific advantages, making it well suited for monitoring cortical hemodynamics as a proxy of brain activity during physical exercise.

Keywords: cognition; personalized training; personalized medicine; exercise prescription

---

1. Introduction

There is a robust body of literature suggesting that regularly conducted physical activity (typically engendered through regular physical exercise) promotes brain health and cognitive performance regardless of age [1–11]. However, the multilevel mechanisms driving exercise-induced neurocognitive changes across different age groups are not well understood [7,12,13] and little is known about which exercise prescription (e.g., intensity, duration, type of exercise) might be optimal to promote neurocognitive changes [1,7,8,14–23]. An adequate exercise prescription is the key to appropriately individualize physical exercise [15,24,25], but there is an ongoing debate about the optimal selection of parameters to do so [26–36]. This debate has now reached the field of exercise–cognition science [37–39] and could be a promising starting point to optimize exercise prescription.

To prescribe physical exercise, both parameters of external load (e.g., workload in Watts) and indicators of internal load (e.g., changes in heart rate) can be used. In this regard, external load is defined as work that an individual performs regardless of internal characteristics, whereas internal load encompasses the individual and acute psychophysiological responses to the external load, as well as influencing factors (environmental factors and lifestyle factors that amplify or diminish the physical exercise stimuli) [15,25,40–47]. In addition, it is important to emphasize that the external load has to be carefully adjusted to achieve a specific internal load. More importantly, specific indicators of internal load can be used as a proxy of the dose [15,25], which influences the effectiveness of an intervention [15,48,49]. However, it is currently not clear which indicator of internal load is the most suitable one to prescribe, for instance, exercise intensity in exercise–cognition science [15]. To extend this debate, we will discuss in this perspective article the role of brain-derived parameters as indicators of internal load and how these parameters serve to prescribe, rather than to solely monitor physical exercises (i.e., exercise intensity). Therefore, (i) we review which portable neuroimaging method would currently be the most suitable to monitor brain activity during physical exercise, (ii) we describe the neurophysiological background of this neuroimaging method and selected application-relevant methodological details, (iii) we explain the advantages of brain-derived parameters compared to conventional indicators of internal load (e.g., heart rate), and (iv) we outline potential opportunities for further investigation.

2. Which Portable Neuroimaging Tools Can Be Used to Assess Brain Activation During Physical Exercises?

Currently, there exist two portable neuroimaging modalities, namely electroencephalography (EEG) and functional near-infrared spectroscopy (fNIRS), to investigate brain activity during physical exercises in relatively unconstrained environments [50–52]. An overview on commercially available systems can be found in the review of Peake et al. [53]. Using EEG, brain activity is directly assessed by measuring electric changes in cortical layers [54]. Using fNIRS, brain activity is indirectly assessed by measuring cortical hemodynamic changes as a proxy of brain activity [50,55]. EEG has been applied in a variety of physical tasks and/or physical exercises (for review see [56]), such as balancing [57–63], walking [64–69], resistance exercises [70–72], or cycling [73–79]. Compared to fNIRS, EEG provides the advantage of a high temporal resolution (e.g., >1000 Hz) [80–85]. On the downside, EEG has the drawbacks of (i) a low spatial resolution (i.e., ~5 to 9 cm; with Laplacian transformation ~3 cm) [80–87], (ii) a time-consuming preparation when gel is used with wet electrodes [84,86], (iii) a high susceptibility to artefacts arising from motion, muscles, or sweat [80,81,87–90], and (iv) a hard interpretability of obtained signals for non-experts [91]. In contrast, fNIRS provides the advantages of a relatively high spatial resolution (i.e., ~1–3 cm) and a relatively high tolerance against motion artefacts [81,83,84,86,92–98], but suffers from a susceptibility to systemic physiological artefacts (e.g., superficial blood flow) [83,94,95,99–101]. Based on the drawbacks of EEG and the advantages of fNIRS, fNIRS is currently better suited for measurements of changes in cortical brain activity during physical exercises in unconstrained environments [50,102,103]. In fact, fNIRS has been applied during a variety of physical exercises such as juggling [104], balancing [105–110], walking (for review see [111,112]), resistance exercises [113–116], dancing [117–119], tai chi [120,121], climbing [122], synchronized swimming routines [123], table tennis [124], running [125–127], and predominantly during cycling [128–165]. Furthermore, fNIRS was used to monitor cerebral oxygenation during stationary cycling even in special cohorts, such as cardiac patients [166–169]. However, in the mentioned studies, fNIRS was only utilized to monitor brain activity during exercising, while, to our knowledge, no study so far has used fNIRS-based parameters to prescribe exercise variables (e.g., exercise intensity).

3. Neurophysiological Mechanisms and Physical Principles of fNIRS

The optical neuroimaging technique fNIRS allows the non-invasive imaging of cerebral hemodynamics from cortical layers in the human brain [83,111]. Neuroimaging based on fNIRS utilizes the physical principles of optical spectroscopy and the physiological processes of neurometabolic and neurovascular coupling [83], which are illustrated in Figure 1a. The execution of a distinct task (e.g., a motor–cognitive exercise such as dancing) causes a higher neural activation in specific brain regions. In order to supply the energy needed to satisfy the energetic demands of the activated neuronal tissue, the oxygen metabolism (neurometabolic coupling) is increased [83,170,171], leading to a higher metabolization rate of oxygen [170–172]. In consequence of the higher rate of oxygen metabolization, the local concentration of oxygenated hemoglobin (oxyHb) decreases and the local concentration of deoxygenated hemoglobin (deoxyHb) increases [170–173]. Furthermore, as shown in Figure 1a, an increase in neural activity also triggers local changes in cerebral hemodynamics and induces an intensified blood flow to the activated brain regions [83,170,174–176]. As a sequel of the locally increased blood flow, the local supply of oxygen is greater than its metabolization and, thus, a higher concentration of oxyHb and a decreased concentration in deoxyHb is to be observed in activated brain regions (see Figure 1a) [83,171,176]. These neural activity-dependent changes in oxyHb and deoxyHb concentrations can be used as indirect indicators of brain activation. To assess the neural activity-dependent changes in oxyHb and deoxyHb with fNIRS, light with distinct wavelengths in the near-infrared spectrum is emitted by a source (e.g., laser or light emitting diodes (LED)) on the scalp into the skull (see Figure 1b) [83,177,178]. Inside the skull, the emitted light travels through different layers (e.g., cerebrospinal fluid) and ideally penetrates the neural tissue [83,177,178]. In all the tissues of the head (intracerebral and extracerebral), the emitted near-infrared light undergoes scattering events and absorption processes, leading to light attenuation at the detectors [92,178,179]. Scattering events increase the length of their traveled photon paths as it forces the photons to deviate from their initial straight trajectories [83,92]. Absorption processes lead to a transformation of the initial energy of the photons into the internal energy of the respective medium (e.g., neural tissue) [83]. Based on the different absorption spectra of the chromophores (e.g., $\lambda > 800$ nm mainly oxyHb, $\lambda < 800$ nm mainly deoxyHb), neural activity-dependent changes in the local concentration of oxyHb and deoxyHb influence the local light absorption rate and, in turn, the regional magnitude of light attenuation [83,93,178]. These neural activity-dependent changes in light attenuation can be assessed by measuring the non-absorbed components of the emitted light using a detector that is placed on the head's surface (see Figure 1b) [177,178]. Changes in light attenuation can be linked to local changes in cortical oxyHb and deoxyHb concentrations by means of the modified Beer–Lambert law, enabling a non-invasive quantification of the "indirect" indicators of brain activity changes [83,177,178].

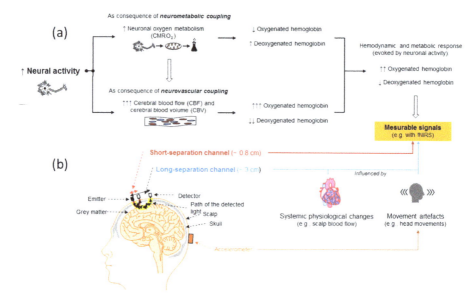

Figure 1. Schematic illustrations of (**a**) changes in cerebral hemodynamics and oxygen, induced by neural activity. (**b**) Depiction of a possible NIRS montage on the human head showing the assumed banana-shaped course of detected light of "short separation channels" and of "long separation channels"; fNIRS, functional near-infrared spectroscopy; $CMRO_2$, cerebral metabolic rate of oxygen; ↑, increase; ↓, decrease.

With regard to the technical implementation of (functional) near-infrared spectroscopy ((f)NIRS), it is important to emphasize that the following four different methods exist. These different methods have unique advantages and disadvantages with respect to the usage in the field of exercise(–cognition) science: (i) continuous-wave NIRS (CW-NIRS), (ii) spatially resolved NIRS (SRS-NIRS), (iii) frequency domain NIRS (FD-NIRS) and (iv) time domain NIRS (TD-NIRS).

(i) In CW-NIRS devices, the changes in light intensity (i.e., attenuation) are used to calculate the relative concentration changes in chromophores (e.g., oxyHb and deoxyHb) [98,171,174,180,181]. Light with a distinct intensity is emitted into the tissue (e.g., brain and scalp tissue) via an emitter (e.g., placed on the scalp) and the non-absorbed light components leaving the tissue at a distinct point are measured via a detector, from which the intensity of outgoing light is obtained. By using CW-NIRS, changes in the attenuation coefficient can be calculated and used to determine the relative concentration changes in the chromophores (e.g., relative to baseline) [171,182].

(ii) SRS-NIRS is a special type of CW-NIRS. In SRS-NIRS, at least two detectors (e.g., placed on the head surface) are used to measure the light which leaves the examined tissue after traveling through it (e.g., brain and scalp tissue) [183]. The information of the two detectors is used to determine the local gradients of light attenuation which, in turn, can be used to calculate the absolute concentration changes in chromophores (e.g., oxyHb and deoxyHb) and the tissue oxygenation index (TOI) [184,185]. TOI is the ratio of oxyHb to total hemoglobin (sum of oxy- and deoxyHb) and is also known as the tissue saturation index (TSI) and regional tissue oxygen saturation (StO_2, and rSO_2).

(iii) In FD-NIRS, the source(s) (e.g., placed on the scalp) continuously emit(s) light with a distinct intensity into the tissue, whose amplitude is modulated at a specific frequency in the MHz range. A detector (e.g., placed on the head's surface) measures the phase shift (delay) and light attenuation of the measured and non-absorbed light components, which, in turn, are used to determine the absorption and scattering properties of the specific tissue (e.g., brain tissue).

Using the individual-specific information about the scattering and absorption properties of the distinct tissue allows the quantification of absolute concentration changes in the chromophores (e.g., oxyHb and deoxyHb) [98,171,174,180,181,186,187].

(iv) In TD-NIRS, multiple sources emit extremely short light impulses into the tissue (e.g., brain and scalp tissue) and detectors, placed at a certain distance from the light emitting source, quantify the time of flight, the temporal distribution, and the shape of the temporal distribution of the non-absorbed photons, which leave the examined tissue (e.g., brain and scalp tissue). The information about the time of flight, temporal distribution, and shape of the temporal distribution of the non-absorbed photons are used to determine the scattering and absorption properties of the distinct tissue (e.g., brain tissue). In general, photons that travelled through the cerebral tissue are more delayed than photons that are only traveling through the scalp. The obtained information about scattering and absorption enables the calculation of absolute concentrations changes in chromophores (e.g., oxyHb and deoxyHb) [98,171,174,180,181,186,187].

With regard to the application of fNIRS in the field of exercise science (in particular to prescribe exercise), SRS-NIRS is the most promising of the four NIRS methods. SRS-NIRS allows, compared to CW-NIRS, the quantification of absolute changes in the concentration of chromophores [184,185], and, compared to FD-NIRS and TD-NIRS, SRS-NIRS devices are less expensive, have a higher acquisition rate, and are less bulky [98,180,188]. Furthermore, TD-NIRS suffers from the drawback that it is not able to detect small functional activation changes due to its working principle, which is based on time of flight photon detection. The latter returns a noisier parameter compared to SRS-NIRS, which is based on light attenuation measurement [171,180,188]. Moreover, multi-distance configurations of NIRS channels, as used in SRS-NIRS, allow measurements that are more robust against motion artefacts, resulting in a more stable acquisition of the signals [184]. In addition, in the field of exercise science, NIRS systems with LED sources (e.g., SRS-NIRS) are more suitable because they allow smaller and portable instrumentation and are safer in their application, as compared to NIRS systems with laser sources (e.g., FD-NIRS and TD-NIRS) [171,189]. More detailed information about the differences between CW-NIRS, SRS-NIRS, FD-NIRS, and TD-NIRS can be found in the referenced literature [98,171,174,180,181,183,185,186,190–196].

4. Advantages of Brain-Derived Indicators of Internal Load

In this section, we discuss the advantages of brain-derived indicators of internal load to prescribe physical exercise in exercise–cognition research. Therefore, we focus on the exercise variable *exercise intensity* because a full discussion of all exercise variables is beyond the scope of this perspective article. It is undoubted that the established approach prescribing the exercise intensity using specific indicators of internal load, such as percentages of maximal heart rate (HR_{max}) or maximal oxygen uptake ($VO_{2\,max}$), which were obtained during a preceding graded exercise test, has its merits. However, this established approach for the prescription of exercise intensity can cause a considerable amount of interindividual heterogeneity in neurocognitive outcomes [15]. Hence, we recommend alternative approaches to exercise prescription, which make use of specific indicators of internal load, and which are known to be causally related to the intended outcome [15]. In this respect, fNIRS-derived brain parameters (e.g., oxyHb, deoxyHb, totHb, or StO_2) can be a promising option for prescribing exercise intensity because they are more closely related to the organic system which is intended to be modulated (i.e., brain). This assumption is supported by the evidence outlined in the following:

(a) cortical hemodynamics are sensitive to the level of physical load (e.g., exercise intensity) [125,126,128,139] and a decline in prefrontal oxygenation (i.e., oxyHb and StO_2/TOI) at very high exercise intensities was observed [126,158,164,197,198]. The latter corroborates the notion of a "central governor" limiting maximal exercise performance [198–205],

(b) cortical hemodynamics are sensitive to the influence of psychophysiological parameters (e.g., exercise tolerance) [129,206],

(c) cortical hemodynamics during physical exercise are indicators of responsiveness, as levels of oxyHb in the right ventrolateral prefrontal cortex (PFC) during exercise are higher in individuals who show superior performance in a spatial memory task (e.g., being responders) after an acute bout of physical exercise [207],

(d) the level of cortical hemodynamics during physical exercise might act as an indicator of the optimal brain state since lower levels of oxygenated hemoglobin in the PFC during physical exercise were associated with slower reaction times in an executive function task (i.e., Stroop task [208].

Regarding (c) and (d), comparable findings have, to the best of our knowledge, not been reported for conventional parameters of exercise prescription (e.g., heart rate (HR)) when neurocognitive outcomes were considered. Hence, (c) and (d) of the above-mentioned points especially support the idea that brain-derived parameters may be superior when prescribing physical exercise (e.g., exercise intensity) in the setting of exercise–cognition research. Moreover, commonly used conventional parameters of exercise prescription, such as HR, also suffer from the drawback that they are not able to sufficiently reflect psychophysiological responses to non-cardiorespiratory demands (e.g., cognitive load), which are posed by non-endurance exercises, such as simultaneous motor–cognitive exercise (e.g., dancing [14]). However, these demands are mirrored in brain-derived measures. Regarding fNIRS-derived brain parameters, it was reported that they are sensitive to:

(e) the level of cognitive load [209–212],
(f) the level of cognitive fatigue [213–215],
(g) the influence of stress [216–220],
(h) the influence of expertise level [104,122,212,221] or skill level [106,222],
(i) training-related changes in motor–cognitive performance [105,117].

Accordingly, the provided evidence further buttresses the idea to use brain-derived parameters in exercise prescription. Brain-derived parameters, as compared to conventional parameters, have, at least theoretically, an added value in exercise prescription. Both the monitoring of brain parameters (e.g., during the course of a physical intervention) and the use of brain parameters to prescribe physical exercises (i.e., exercise intensity) are valuable options to gain more knowledge about the exercise–cognition interaction. The first approach (i.e., solely monitoring cerebral hemodynamics) can help us to answer specific research questions related to the effects of exercise on the brain which, in turn, can later be used to inform exercise prescription (e.g., *To what extent does an exercise prescription based on conventional parameters cause interindividual heterogeneity concerning cerebral hemodynamics?*). The second approach (i.e., brain-derived parameters to prescribe exercise) opens a new perspective, as it allows the study of the effects of an alternative exercise prescription on specific outcome measures (e.g., *To what extent does an exercise prescription based on brain-derived parameters influence interindividual heterogeneity in cognitive performance changes in response to an acute bout of physical exercise?*). Hence, both approaches should be seen as complementary options, which enable us to study the subject of exercise–cognition from two different perspectives.

5. Practical Implementation of Brain-Derived Parameters to Prescribe Physical Exercise

In the previous section, we have outlined that there is a strong theoretical rationale to use brain-derived parameters to prescribe exercise variables (e.g., exercise intensity), but this approach is currently underutilized. As this approach will open a new perspective on exercise–cognition interaction, we highlight potential areas of application by answering the following questions, which seem relevant for the practical implementation: *(i) How Can We Prescribe Exercise Intensity by Using fNIRS-Derived Brain Parameters?*, *(ii) Which Cortical Brain Area Should Be Targeted?*, *(iii) How Can We Minimize Confounders in Order to Successfully Apply fNIRS During Physical Exercise?* and *(iv) Which Additional Internal Load Indicators Should Be Recorded Alongside fNIRS?*

5.1. How Can We Prescribe Exercise Intensity by Using fNIRS-Derived Brain Parameters?

In our opinion, a prescription of exercise intensity using fNIRS-derived brain parameters can be implemented in a manner comparable to routinely used conventional indicators of internal load (HR). To test the practicability of the novel approach to prescribe exercise intensity by using fNIRS-derived brain parameters, continuous endurance exercises (e.g., cycling) could be a good starting point. Similar to the conventional approach of exercise prescription, the individual firstly performs a graded exercise test in which brain-derived indicators of internal load (e.g., StO_2) can be measured alongside conventional ones (e.g., HR or VO_2). Based on this graded exercise test, the external load (e.g., workload) can be identified, which corresponds, for instance, to the highest StO_2 or to a specific percentage of a maximal StO_2 (see Figure 2). This external load (i.e., workload) can then, in turn, be used to set the initial exercise intensity in an exercise session. Importantly, as fNIRS allows a non-invasive online monitoring of brain parameters, such as StO_2 while exercising, the external load can be individually adjusted during the course of the exercise session, in order to ensure that the target StO_2 is achieved (e.g., comparable to HR monitoring). Hence, using brain parameters, such as StO_2, allows one to account for daily variations in performance capacity in the same manner as the established conventional approaches (e.g., heart rate monitoring). However, before the application of fNIRS can be recommended unreservedly, further research is necessary. Such research should aim, for instance, at investigating the reproducibility of fNIRS-derived brain parameters in the exercise setting, at studying the relationship between fNIRS-derived brain parameters and conventional parameters of exercise prescription (e.g., HR, level of peripheral blood lactate, and relative perceived exertion (RPE)), and at examining whether this novel approach of exercise prescription may be superior in inducing neurocognitive changes (e.g., acute influence on cognitive performance or blood-based markers), as compared to conventional approaches of exercise prescription.

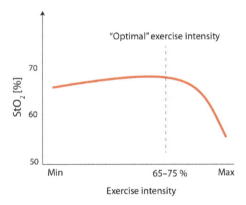

Figure 2. Schematic illustration of the time course of StO_2 during a graded exercise test to exhaustion. The optimum is tentatively defined as the lowest exercise intensity leading to the highest cerebral oxygenation (marked by the dashed line).

5.2. Which Cortical Brain Area Should Be Targeted?

The exact placement of fNIRS optodes is crucial to obtaining cerebral hemodynamic signals from a specific brain area. To test the practicability of an exercise prescription which is based on brain-derived measures, we propose that the PFC could be a promising initial target area. The PFC is a key structure for the performance of cognitive control/executive functions [223,224], which is the most investigated cognitive domain in acute exercise–cognition studies [225]. More specifically, and based on evidence that is outlined in more detail below, the ventrolateral PFC, dorsolateral PFC, and the frontopolar area (FPA) are promising brain areas for investigations:

(a) Regarding the ventrolateral PFC; it was observed that young adults with superior performance in a spatial memory tasks in response to an acute bout of endurance exercise (i.e., responders) exhibited higher levels of oxyHb in the right ventrolateral PFC during the exercise [207].
(b) Regarding the dorsolateral PFC; it was noticed that in young adults, higher levels of oxyHb in the left dorsolateral PFC (measured during a cognitive test after exercising) [226–228] were associated with exercise-induced behavioral changes in the performance of the Stroop test.
(c) Regarding the FPA; it was observed that in young adults, higher levels of oxyHb in the left FPA (measured during a cognitive test after exercising) [227] were associated with exercise-induced behavioral changes in the performance of the Stroop test. Similar findings have been observed for older adults regarding the right FPA [229].

In addition, more detailed information regarding an accurate and standardized placement of fNIRS optodes can be found in the referenced literature [176].

5.3. How Can We Minimize Confounders in Order to Successfully Apply fNIRS during Physical Exercise?

With respect to the practical application of fNIRS during physical exercising, it is mandatory to emphasize that movement artefacts or systemic physiological artefacts, which occur during physical exercising, influence the accuracy of the brain signal measurement of fNIRS significantly [99,101,149,151, 230–235]. To minimize the influence of such signal confounders, appropriate data processing techniques should be applied (e.g., short-separation channel regression (SSR) to account for superficial blood flow [99,111,176,235,236] or SSR in conjunction with accelerometer signals to account for superficial blood flow and motion artefacts in CW-NIRS [237]). Furthermore, the application of other NIRS methods, namely SRS-NIRS, should be considered in the context of physical exercise, since they are less influenced by systemic physiological interference [238] and motion-related artefacts [184].

In addition, it is strongly recommended to record multiple physiological signals along with fNIRS signals (e.g., HR and heart rate variability (HRV), electrodermal activity (skin conductance), mean arterial blood pressure, systolic and diastolic blood pressure, respiration rate, and partial pressure of exhaled CO_2 ($P_{ET}CO_2$)) to make valid assumptions about the physiological origin of the observed changes in fNIRS signals and, in turn, to improve the interpretation of fNIRS signals [99]. This approach has been recently termed systematic physiological augmented functional near-infrared spectroscopy (SPA-fNIRS) [239,240]. However, the study of Tempest et al. [108] supports the application of fNIRS, for instance, during motor–cognitive exercises, as robust cognitive task-evoked changes in cortical cerebral hemodynamics during cycling were measured by fNIRS, which are comparable to cortical hemodynamic changes observed without exercise [131]. Notwithstanding, it is important to emphasize that further efforts are necessary to improve the signal quality of fNIRS-based brain monitoring devices, which would allow for the more reliable conclusion of the origin of observed signal changes [99].

5.4. Which Additional Internal Load Indicators Should Be Recorded Alongside fNIRS?

In order to quantify the state of organic systems more comprehensively, it seems useful to complement the measures of the central nervous system (e.g., StO_2 in the PFC) with (easily quantifiable) measures of the autonomous nervous system. A promising indicator of the state of the autonomous nervous system is the HRV, which is operationalized by the beat-to-beat variations of the heart rate over a specific time period (e.g., during a resting state or during physical exercises) [45,241–245]. HRV is considered to be a proxy of the actual health state [246–249] and stress level [247,250] of an individual. HRV also reflects, at least partly, the fitness level and daily readiness [243,244,251–255] of an individual, as well as the organismic demands [256–260]. There are numerous non-linear analysis approaches to appraise HRV, which reflect the systemic character of the organism [245,248,249,261–263]. Moreover, HRV is linked to cognitive performance in specific cognitive domains (e.g., during a resting state) [245,264–273] and it is, as outlined in the neurovisceral integration model, associated with the integrity of specific subareas of the PFC (e.g., medial PFC) [247,273–280]. In summary, this evidence suggests that HRV is a valuable parameter which should be recorded along with fNIRS in order to assess changes in the autonomic system more precisely. However, there is, to the best of our knowledge, no study available using HRV as an indicator of internal load to directly prescribe exercise intensity. Existing studies used resting-state HRV to guide the exercise prescription, but exercise intensity was prescribed with other parameters than HRV (e.g., HR or running velocity) [252,281–283].

Another parameter of interest is the pulse–respiration quotient, which provides a unique measure of the physiological state and traits [284,285] and which, therefore, should be more often assessed in physical exercise studies.

6. Summary and Conclusion

The optimal exercise prescription in the field of exercise–cognition is a topic of emerging interest, and a lively discussion on the matter has started. However, the question about which indicators of internal load may be the most appropriate ones remains open [15]. In this perspective article, we discuss and advocate for the use of brain-derived parameters in the exercise prescription of exercise–cognition studies (e.g., to prescribe exercise intensity). Brain-derived parameters provide the advantages that they are more closely related to the organic system that is aimed to be influenced and that they are sensitive to demands (e.g., cognitive load), which are not sufficiently reflected in conventional measures (e.g., HR). In particular, we discuss the promising potential of fNIRS-derived brain parameters (e.g., oxyHB, deoxyHb, totHb, and StO_2) to prescribe physical exercise (e.g., exercise intensity) and we encourage the research community to test the practicability and effectiveness of this novel approach of exercise prescription.

Author Contributions: F.H. and D.H. developed the idea of the manuscript. F.H. wrote and edited the manuscript. F.H., F.S., H.Z., and D.W. created the figures. T.G., F.S., H.Z., D.W., N.G.M., and D.H. reviewed and edited the drafted versions. All authors have read and agreed to the published version of the manuscript.

Funding: This article was partially supported by the joint project "Autonomy in Old Age" (AiA) funded by the European Regional Development Fund (grant number: ZS/2019/07/99755; to N.G.M.). The authors are solely responsible for the work and the funders had no role in the preparation of the manuscript, the analysis of the studies, and the decision to publish.

Acknowledgments: The authors have nothing to acknowledge.

Conflicts of Interest: The authors have no conflict of interest to disclose.

References

1. Hillman, C.H.; Erickson, K.I.; Kramer, A.F. Be smart, exercise your heart: Exercise effects on brain and cognition. *Nat. Rev. Neurosci.* **2008**, *9*, 58–65. [CrossRef] [PubMed]
2. Liu-Ambrose, T.; Barha, C.; Best, J.R. Physical activity for brain health in older adults. *Appl. Physiol. Nutr. Metab.* **2018**, *43*, 1105–1112. [CrossRef] [PubMed]
3. Erickson, K.I.; Hillman, C.; Stillman, C.M.; Ballard, R.M.; Bloodgood, B.; Conroy, D.E.; Macko, R.; Marquez, D.X.; Petruzzello, S.J.; Powell, K.E.; et al. Physical Activity, Cognition, and Brain Outcomes. *Med. Sci. Sports Exerc.* **2019**, *51*, 1242–1251. [CrossRef] [PubMed]
4. Jackson, P.; Pialoux, V.; Corbett, D.; Drogos, L.; Erickson, K.I.; Eskes, G.A.; Poulin, M.J. Promoting brain health through exercise and diet in older adults: A physiological perspective. *J. Physiol.* **2016**, *594*, 4485–4498. [CrossRef]
5. Tyndall, A.V.; Clark, C.M.; Anderson, T.J.; Hogan, D.B.; Hill, M.D.; Longman, R.S.; Poulin, M.J. Protective Effects of Exercise on Cognition and Brain Health in Older Adults. *Exerc. Sport Sci. Rev.* **2018**, *46*, 215–223. [CrossRef]
6. Liu-Ambrose, T.; Best, J.R. Exercise is Medicine for the Aging Brain. *Kinesiol. Rev.* **2017**, *6*, 22–29. [CrossRef]
7. Stillman, C.M.; Esteban-Cornejo, I.; Brown, B.; Bender, C.M.; Erickson, K.I. Effects of Exercise on Brain and Cognition Across Age Groups and Health States. *Trends Neurosci.* **2020**. [CrossRef] [PubMed]
8. Esteban-Cornejo, I.; Tejero-González, C.M.; Sallis, J.F.; Veiga, O.L. Physical activity and cognition in adolescents: A systematic review. *J. Sci. Med. Sport* **2015**, *18*, 534–539. [CrossRef]

9. Greeff, J.W.D.; Bosker, R.J.; Oosterlaan, J.; Visscher, C.; Hartman, E. Effects of physical activity on executive functions, attention and academic performance in preadolescent children: A meta-analysis. *J. Sci. Med. Sport* **2018**, *21*, 501–507. [CrossRef]
10. Hillman, C.H.; Logan, N.E.; Shigeta, T.T. A Review of Acute Physical Activity Effects on Brain and Cognition in Children. *Transl. J. Acsm* **2019**, *17*, 132–136. [CrossRef]
11. Ludyga, S.; Gerber, M.; Pühse, U.; Looser, V.N.; Kamijo, K. Systematic review and meta-analysis investigating moderators of long-term effects of exercise on cognition in healthy individuals. *Nat. Hum. Behav.* **2020**, 1–10. [CrossRef] [PubMed]
12. Stillman, C.M.; Cohen, J.; Lehman, M.E.; Erickson, K.I. Mediators of Physical Activity on Neurocognitive Function: A Review at Multiple Levels of Analysis. *Front. Hum. Neurosci.* **2016**, *10*, 626. [CrossRef]
13. Stimpson, N.J.; Davison, G.; Javadi, A.-H. Joggin' the Noggin: Towards a Physiological Understanding of Exercise-Induced Cognitive Benefits. *Neurosci. Biobehav. Rev.* **2018**, *88*, 177–186. [CrossRef] [PubMed]
14. Herold, F.; Hamacher, D.; Schega, L.; Müller, N.G. Thinking While Moving or Moving While Thinking—Concepts of Motor-Cognitive Training for Cognitive Performance Enhancement. *Front. Aging Neurosci.* **2018**, *10*, 228. [CrossRef]
15. Herold, F.; Müller, P.; Gronwald, T.; Müller, N.G. Dose-Response Matters!—A Perspective on the Exercise Prescription in Exercise-Cognition Research. *Front. Psychol.* **2019**, *10*, 2338. [CrossRef]
16. Rolland, Y.; Van Kan, G.A.; Vellas, B. Healthy Brain Aging: Role of Exercise and Physical Activity. *Clin. Geriatr. Med.* **2010**, *26*, 75–87. [CrossRef]
17. Bherer, L.; Erickson, K.I.; Liu-Ambrose, T. A Review of the Effects of Physical Activity and Exercise on Cognitive and Brain Functions in Older Adults. *J. Aging Res.* **2013**, *2013*, 1–8. [CrossRef]
18. Voelcker-Rehage, C.; Niemann, C. Structural and functional brain changes related to different types of physical activity across the life span. *Neurosci. Biobehav. Rev.* **2013**, *37*, 2268–2295. [CrossRef]
19. Lauenroth, A.; Ioannidis, A.E.; Teichmann, B. Influence of combined physical and cognitive training on cognition: A systematic review. *BMC Geriatr.* **2016**, *16*, 141. [CrossRef]
20. Cai, Y.; Abrahamson, K. Does Exercise Impact Cognitive Performance Research Article Op in Community-dwelling Older Adults with Mild Cognitive Impairment? A Systematic Review. *Qual. Prim. Care* **2015**, *23*, 214–222.
21. Tait, J.; Duckham, R.L.; Milte, C.M.; Main, L.C.; Daly, R.M. Influence of Sequential vs. Simultaneous Dual-Task Exercise Training on Cognitive Function in Older Adults. *Front. Aging Neurosci.* **2017**, *9*, 368. [CrossRef]
22. Herold, F.; Törpel, A.; Schega, L.; Müller, N.G. Functional and/or structural brain changes in response to resistance exercises and resistance training lead to cognitive improvements—Asystematic review. *Eur. Rev. Aging Phys. Act.* **2019**, *16*, 10. [CrossRef]
23. Soga, K.; Masaki, H.; Gerber, M.; Ludyga, S. Acute and Long-term Effects of Resistance Training on Executive Function. *J. Cogn. Enhanc.* **2018**, *2*, 200–207. [CrossRef]
24. Wollesen, B.; Voelcker-Rehage, C. Training effects on motor–cognitive dual-task performance in older adults. *Eur. Rev. Aging Phys. Act.* **2013**, *11*, 5–24. [CrossRef]
25. Gronwald, T.; Budde, H. Commentary: Physical Exercise as Personalized Medicine for Dementia Prevention? *Front. Physiol.* **2019**, *10*, 1358. [CrossRef] [PubMed]
26. Hofmann, P.; Tschakert, G. Special Needs to Prescribe Exercise Intensity for Scientific Studies. *Cardiol. Res. Pract.* **2010**, *2011*, 1–10. [CrossRef] [PubMed]
27. Mann, T.N.; Lamberts, R.P.; Lambert, M. Methods of Prescribing Relative Exercise Intensity: Physiological and Practical Considerations. *Sports Med.* **2013**, *43*, 613–625. [CrossRef] [PubMed]
28. Gass, G.C.; McLellan, T.M.; Gass, E.M. Effects of prolonged exercise at a similar percentage of maximal oxygen consumption in trained and untrained subjects. *Eur. J. Appl. Physiol. Occup. Physiol.* **1991**, *63*, 430–435. [CrossRef]
29. Katch, V.; Weltman, A.; Sady, S.; Freedson, P. Validity of the relative percent concept for equating training intensity. *Eur. J. Appl. Physiol. Occup. Physiol.* **1978**, *39*, 219–227. [CrossRef]
30. Meyer, T.; Gabriel, H.H.; Kindermann, W. Is determination of exercise intensities as percentages of VO2max or HRmax adequate? *Med. Sci. Sports Exerc.* **1999**, *31*, 1342–1345. [CrossRef]
31. Scharhag-Rosenberger, F.; Meyer, T.; Gäßler, N.; Faude, O.; Kindermann, W. Exercise at given percentages of VO2max: Heterogeneous metabolic responses between individuals. *J. Sci. Med. Sport* **2010**, *13*, 74–79. [CrossRef]

32. Weltman, A.; Weltman, J.; Rutt, R.; Seip, R.; Levine, S.; Snead, D.; Kaiser, D.; Rogol, A. Percentages of Maximal Heart Rate, Heart Rate Reserve, and VO2peak for Determining Endurance Training Intensity in Sedentary Women*. *Int. J. Sports Med.* **1989**, *10*, 212–216. [CrossRef] [PubMed]

33. Weltman, A.; Snead, D.; Seip, R.; Schurrer, R.; Weltman, J.; Rutt, R.; Rogol, A. Percentages of Maximal Heart Rate, Heart Rate Reserve and VO 2 max for Determining Endurance Training Intensity in Male Runners. *Int. J. Sports Med.* **1990**, *11*, 218–222. [CrossRef]

34. Weatherwax, R.; Harris, N.; Kilding, A.E.; Dalleck, L. The incidence of training responsiveness to cardiorespiratory fitness and cardiometabolic measurements following individualized and standardized exercise prescription: Study protocol for a randomized controlled trial. *Trials* **2016**, *17*, 601. [CrossRef]

35. Tschakert, G.; Hofmann, P. High-Intensity Intermittent Exercise: Methodological and Physiological Aspects. *Int. J. Sports Physiol. Perform.* **2013**, *8*, 600–610. [CrossRef] [PubMed]

36. Schneider, J.; Schlüter, K.; Sprave, T.; Wiskemann, J.; Rosenberger, F. Exercise intensity prescription in cancer survivors: Ventilatory and lactate thresholds are useful submaximal alternatives to VO2peak. *Support. Care Cancer* **2020**, 1–8. [CrossRef]

37. Gronwald, T.; Velasques, B.; Ribeiro, P.; Machado, S.; Murillo-Rodríguez, E.; Ludyga, S.; Yamamoto, T.; Budde, H. Increasing exercise's effect on mental health: Exercise intensity does matter. *Proc. Natl. Acad. Sci. USA* **2018**, *115*, E11890–E11891. [CrossRef]

38. Suwabe, K.; Byun, K.; Hyodo, K.; Reagh, Z.M.; Roberts, J.M.; Matsushita, A.; Saotome, K.; Ochi, G.; Fukuie, T.; Suzuki, K.; et al. Reply to Gronwald et al.: Exercise intensity does indeed matter; maximal oxygen uptake is the gold-standard indicator. *Proc. Natl. Acad. Sci. USA* **2018**, *115*, E11892–E11893. [CrossRef]

39. Gronwald, T.; Alves, A.C.D.B.; Murillo-Rodríguez, E.; Latini, A.; Schuette, J.; Budde, H. Standardization of exercise intensity and consideration of a dose-response is essential. Commentary on "Exercise-linked FNDC5/irisin rescues synaptic plasticity and memory defects in Alzheimer's models", by Lourenco et al., published 2019 in Nature Medicine. *J. Sport Health Sci.* **2019**, *8*, 353–354. [CrossRef]

40. Burgess, D.J. The Research Doesn't Always Apply: Practical Solutions to Evidence-Based Training-Load Monitoring in Elite Team Sports. *Int. J. Sports Physiol. Perform.* **2017**, *12*, S2136–S2141. [CrossRef]

41. Bourdon, P.C.; Cardinale, M.; Murray, A.; Gastin, P.; Kellmann, M.; Varley, M.; Gabbett, T.J.; Coutts, A.J.; Burgess, D.J.; Gregson, W.; et al. Monitoring Athlete Training Loads: Consensus Statement. *Int. J. Sports Physiol. Perform.* **2017**, *12*, S2161–S2170. [CrossRef] [PubMed]

42. McLaren, S.J.; MacPherson, T.; Coutts, A.J.; Hurst, C.; Spears, I.R.; Weston, M. The Relationships Between Internal and External Measures of Training Load and Intensity in Team Sports: A Meta-Analysis. *Sports Med.* **2017**, *48*, 641–658. [CrossRef]

43. Vanrenterghem, J.; Nedergaard, N.J.; Robinson, M.A.; Drust, B. Training Load Monitoring in Team Sports: A Novel Framework Separating Physiological and Biomechanical Load-Adaptation Pathways. *Sports Med.* **2017**, *47*, 2135–2142. [CrossRef] [PubMed]

44. Wallace, L.K.; Slattery, K.; Coutts, A.J. The Ecological Validity and Application of the Session-RPE Method for Quantifying Training Loads in Swimming. *J. Strength Cond. Res.* **2009**, *23*, 33–38. [CrossRef] [PubMed]

45. Halson, S. Monitoring training load to understand fatigue in athletes. *Sports Med.* **2014**, *44*, S139–S147. [CrossRef]

46. Impellizzeri, F.M.; Marcora, S.M.; Coutts, A.J. Internal and External Training Load: 15 Years On. *Int. J. Sports Physiol. Perform.* **2019**, *14*, 270–273. [CrossRef]

47. Soligard, T.; Schwellnus, M.; Alonso, J.-M.; Bahr, R.; Clarsen, B.; Dijkstra, H.P.; Gabbett, T.; Gleeson, M.; Hägglund, M.; Hutchinson, M.R.; et al. How much is too much? (Part 1) International Olympic Committee consensus statement on load in sport and risk of injury. *Br. J. Sports Med.* **2016**, *50*, 1030–1041. [CrossRef]

48. Maslov, P.Z.; Schulman, A.; Lavie, C.J.; Narula, J. Personalized exercise dose prescription. *Eur. Heart J.* **2017**, *39*, 2346–2355. [CrossRef]

49. Pickering, C.; Kiely, J. Do Non-Responders to Exercise Exist—And If So, What Should We Do About Them? *Sports Med.* **2018**, *49*, 1–7. [CrossRef]

50. Perrey, S.; Besson, P. Studying brain activity in sports performance: Contributions and issues. *Prog. Brain Res.* **2018**, *240*, 247–267. [CrossRef]

51. Tan, S.J.; Kerr, G.; Sullivan, J.P.; Peake, J.M. A Brief Review of the Application of Neuroergonomics in Skilled Cognition During Expert Sports Performance. *Front. Hum. Neurosci.* **2019**, *13*, 278. [CrossRef] [PubMed]

52. Wang, C.-H.; Moreau, D.; Kao, S.-C. From the Lab to the Field: Potential Applications of Dry EEG Systems to Understand the Brain-Behavior Relationship in Sports. *Front. Mol. Neurosci.* **2019**, *13*, 893. [CrossRef] [PubMed]
53. Peake, J.M.; Kerr, G.; Sullivan, J.P. A Critical Review of Consumer Wearables, Mobile Applications, and Equipment for Providing Biofeedback, Monitoring Stress, and Sleep in Physically Active Populations. *Front. Physiol.* **2018**, *9*, 743. [CrossRef] [PubMed]
54. Cohen, M.X. Where Does EEG Come From and What Does It Mean? *Trends Neurosci.* **2017**, *40*, 208–218. [CrossRef]
55. Yucel, M.; Selb, J.J.; Huppert, T.J.; Franceschini, M.A.; Boas, D. Functional Near Infrared Spectroscopy: Enabling routine functional brain imaging. *Curr. Opin. Biomed. Eng.* **2017**, *4*, 78–86. [CrossRef]
56. Rahman, M.; Karwowski, W.; Fafrowicz, M.; Hancock, P.A. Neuroergonomics Applications of Electroencephalography in Physical Activities: A Systematic Review. *Front. Hum. Neurosci.* **2019**, *13*, 182. [CrossRef]
57. Hülsdünker, T.; Mierau, A.; Neeb, C.; Kleinöder, H.; Strüder, H. Cortical processes associated with continuous balance control as revealed by EEG spectral power. *Neurosci. Lett.* **2015**, *592*, 1–5. [CrossRef]
58. Collado-Mateo, D.; Adsuar, J.C.; Olivares, P.R.; Cano-Plasencia, R.; Gusi, N. Using a dry electrode EEG device during balance tasks in healthy young-adult males: Test-retest reliability analysis. *Somat. Mot. Res.* **2015**, *32*, 219–226. [CrossRef]
59. Slobounov, S.; Sebastianelli, W.; Hallett, M. Residual brain dysfunction observed one year post-mild traumatic brain injury: Combined EEG and balance study. *Clin. Neurophysiol.* **2012**, *123*, 1755–1761. [CrossRef]
60. Choi, W.; Lee, S.; Park, J. EEG-biofeedback Intervention Improves balance in Stroke Survivor. *Indian J. Sci. Technol.* **2015**, *8*, 8. [CrossRef]
61. Hülsdünker, T.; Mierau, A.; Strüder, H.K. Higher Balance Task Demands are Associated with an Increase in Individual Alpha Peak Frequency. *Front. Hum. Neurosci.* **2016**, *9*, 85. [CrossRef] [PubMed]
62. Mierau, A.; Hülsdünker, T.; Strüder, H.K. Changes in cortical activity associated with adaptive behavior during repeated balance perturbation of unpredictable timing. *Front. Behav. Neurosci.* **2015**, *9*, 233. [CrossRef] [PubMed]
63. Mierau, A.; Pester, B.; Hülsdünker, T.; Schiecke, K.; Strüder, H.K.; Witte, H. Cortical Correlates of Human Balance Control. *Brain Topogr.* **2017**, *30*, 434–446. [CrossRef] [PubMed]
64. Beurskens, R.; Steinberg, F.; Antoniewicz, F.; Wolff, W.; Granacher, U. Neural Correlates of Dual-Task Walking: Effects of Cognitive versus Motor Interference in Young Adults. *Neural Plast.* **2016**, *2016*, 1–9. [CrossRef] [PubMed]
65. Bruijn, S.; Van Dieën, J.; Daffertshofer, A. Beta activity in the premotor cortex is increased during stabilized as compared to normal walking. *Front. Hum. Neurosci.* **2015**, *9*, 321. [CrossRef] [PubMed]
66. Castermans, T.; Duvinage, M.; Cheron, G.; Dutoit, T. About the cortical origin of the low-delta and high-gamma rhythms observed in EEG signals during treadmill walking. *Neurosci. Lett.* **2014**, *561*, 166–170. [CrossRef]
67. Nordin, A.D.; Hairston, W.D.; Ferris, D.P. Human electrocortical dynamics while stepping over obstacles. *Sci. Rep.* **2019**, *9*, 4693. [CrossRef]
68. Oliveira, A.S.; Schlink, B.R.; Hairston, W.D.; Konig, P.; Ferris, D.P. Restricted vision increases sensorimotor cortex involvement in human walking. *J. Neurophysiol.* **2017**, *118*, 1943–1951. [CrossRef]
69. Peterson, S.M.; Ferris, D.P. Differentiation in Theta and Beta Electrocortical Activity between Visual and Physical Perturbations to Walking and Standing Balance. *eNeuro* **2018**, *5*, 207–218. [CrossRef]
70. Flanagan, S.D.; Dunn-Lewis, C.; Comstock, B.A.; Maresh, C.M.; Volek, J.S.; Denegar, C.R.; Kraemer, W.J. Cortical Activity during a Highly-Trained Resistance Exercise Movement Emphasizing Force, Power or Volume. *Brain Sci.* **2012**, *2*, 649–666. [CrossRef]
71. Falvo, M.J.; Sirevaag, E.J.; Rohrbaugh, J.W.; Earhart, G.M. Resistance training induces supraspinal adaptations: Evidence from movement-related cortical potentials. *Eur. J. Appl. Physiol.* **2010**, *109*, 923–933. [CrossRef] [PubMed]
72. Kenville, R.; Maudrich, T.; Vidaurre, C.; Maudrich, D.; Villringer, A.; Nikulin, V.V.; Ragert, P. Corticomuscular interactions during different movement periods in a multi-joint compound movement. *Sci. Rep.* **2020**, *10*, 1–13. [CrossRef] [PubMed]

73. Gronwald, T.; Ludyga, S.; Hottenrott, K. Einfluss einer intensiven Intervallbelastung auf die Beanspruchung der kortikalen Gehirnaktivität. *Schweiz. Z. Sportmed. Sporttraumatol.* **2015**, *63*, 23–28.
74. Gronwald, T.; Ludyga, S.; Hottenrott, K. Gehirnaktivität bei identischer Belastung—Eine standardisierte fahrradergometrische Laborstudie unter Normoxie und normbarer Hypoxie. *Leistungssport* **2015**, *45*, 42–47.
75. Ludyga, S.; Hottenrott, K.; Gronwald, T. Einfluss verschiedener Belastungssituationen auf die EEG-Aktivität. *Dtsch. Z. Sportmed.* **2015**, *2015*, 113–120. [CrossRef]
76. Ludyga, S.; Gronwald, T.; Hottenrott, K. Do Male and Female Cyclists' Cortical Activity Differ Before and During Cycling Exercise? *J. Sport Exerc. Psychol.* **2015**, *37*, 617–625. [CrossRef]
77. Bullock, T.; Cecotti, H.; Giesbrecht, B. Multiple stages of information processing are modulated during acute bouts of exercise. *Neuroscience* **2015**, *307*, 138–150. [CrossRef]
78. Olson, R.; Chang, Y.; Brush, C.; Kwok, A.N.; Gordon, V.X.; Alderman, B. Neurophysiological and behavioral correlates of cognitive control during low and moderate intensity exercise. *NeuroImage* **2016**, *131*, 171–180. [CrossRef]
79. Storzer, L.; Butz, M.; Hirschmann, J.; Abbasi, O.; Gratkowski, M.; Saupe, D.; Schnitzler, A.; Dalal, S. Bicycling and Walking are Associated with Different Cortical Oscillatory Dynamics. *Front. Hum. Neurosci.* **2016**, *10*, 29. [CrossRef]
80. Thompson, T.; Steffert, T.; Ros, T.; Leach, J.; Gruzelier, J. EEG applications for sport and performance. *Methods* **2008**, *45*, 279–288. [CrossRef]
81. Lloyd-Fox, S.; Blasi, A.; Elwell, C. Illuminating the developing brain: The past, present and future of functional near infrared spectroscopy. *Neurosci. Biobehav. Rev.* **2010**, *34*, 269–284. [CrossRef]
82. Park, J.; Fairweather, M.M.; Donaldson, D. Making the case for mobile cognition: EEG and sports performance. *Neurosci. Biobehav. Rev.* **2015**, *52*, 117–130. [CrossRef] [PubMed]
83. Pinti, P.; Tachtsidis, I.; Hamilton, A.; Hirsch, J.; Aichelburg, C.; Gilbert, S.; Burgess, P.W.; Pinti, P. The present and future use of functional near-infrared spectroscopy (fNIRS) for cognitive neuroscience. *Ann. N. Y. Acad. Sci.* **2020**, *1464*, 5–29. [CrossRef] [PubMed]
84. Soltanlou, M.; Sitnikova, M.A.; Nuerk, H.-C.; Dresler, T. Applications of Functional Near-Infrared Spectroscopy (fNIRS) in Studying Cognitive Development: The Case of Mathematics and Language. *Front. Psychol.* **2018**, *9*, 277. [CrossRef] [PubMed]
85. Burle, B.; Spieser, L.; Roger, C.; Casini, L.; Hasbroucq, T.; Vidal, F. Spatial and temporal resolutions of EEG: Is it really black and white? A scalp current density view. *Int. J. Psychophysiol.* **2015**, *97*, 210–220. [CrossRef] [PubMed]
86. Cutini, S.; Brigadoi, S. Unleashing the future potential of functional near-infrared spectroscopy in brain sciences. *J. Neurosci. Methods* **2014**, *232*, 152–156. [CrossRef] [PubMed]
87. A Ward, J.; Pinti, P.; Amft, O.; Van Laerhoven, K. Wearables and the Brain. *IEEE Pervasive Comput.* **2019**, *18*, 94–100. [CrossRef]
88. Maskeliūnas, R.; Damaševičius, R.; Martisius, I.; Vasiljevas, M. Consumer grade EEG devices: Are they usable for control tasks? *PeerJ* **2016**, *4*, e1746. [CrossRef]
89. Pontifex, M.B.; Hillman, C.H. Neuroelectric measurement of cognition during aerobic exercise. *Methods* **2008**, *45*, 271–278. [CrossRef]
90. Symeonidou, E.-R.; Nordin, A.D.; Hairston, W.D.; Ferris, D.P. Effects of Cable Sway, Electrode Surface Area, and Electrode Mass on Electroencephalography Signal Quality during Motion. *Sensors* **2018**, *18*, 1073. [CrossRef]
91. Smith, M. Shedding light on the adult brain: A review of the clinical applications of near-infrared spectroscopy. *Philos. Trans. R. Soc. A Math. Phys. Eng. Sci.* **2011**, *369*, 4452–4469. [CrossRef] [PubMed]
92. Ekkekakis, P. Illuminating the Black Box: Investigating Prefrontal Cortical Hemodynamics during Exercise with Near-Infrared Spectroscopy. *J. Sport Exerc. Psychol.* **2009**, *31*, 505–553. [CrossRef] [PubMed]
93. Perrey, S. Non-invasive NIR spectroscopy of human brain function during exercise. *Methods* **2008**, *45*, 289–299. [CrossRef]
94. Scarapicchia, V.; Brown, C.; Mayo, C.; Gawryluk, J. Functional Magnetic Resonance Imaging and Functional Near-Infrared Spectroscopy: Insights from Combined Recording Studies. *Front. Hum. Neurosci.* **2017**, *11*, 419. [CrossRef]

95. Quaresima, V.; Ferrari, M. Functional Near-Infrared Spectroscopy (fNIRS) for Assessing Cerebral Cortex Function During Human Behavior in Natural/Social Situations: A Concise Review. *Organ. Res. Methods* **2016**, *22*, 46–68. [CrossRef]
96. Pinti, P.; Aichelburg, C.; Gilbert, S.; Hamilton, A.; Hirsch, J.; Burgess, P.; Tachtsidis, I. A Review on the Use of Wearable Functional Near-Infrared Spectroscopy in Naturalistic Environments. *Jpn. Psychol. Res.* **2018**, *60*, 347–373. [CrossRef]
97. Zhu, Y.; Rodriguez-Paras, C.; Rhee, J.; Mehta, R.K. Methodological Approaches and Recommendations for Functional Near-Infrared Spectroscopy Applications in HF/E Research. *Hum. Factors* **2019**, *62*, 613–642. [CrossRef]
98. Gervain, J.; Mehler, J.; Werker, J.F.; Nelson, C.A.; Csibra, G.; Lloyd-Fox, S.; Shukla, M.; Aslin, R.N. Near-infrared spectroscopy: A report from the McDonnell infant methodology consortium. *Dev. Cogn. Neurosci.* **2011**, *1*, 22–46. [CrossRef]
99. Tachtsidis, I.; Scholkmann, F. False positives and false negatives in functional near-infrared spectroscopy: Issues, challenges, and the way forward. *Neurophotonics* **2016**, *3*, 30401. [CrossRef]
100. Kirilina, E.; Jelzow, A.; Heine, A.; Niessing, M.; Wabnitz, H.; Brühl, R.; Ittermann, B.; Jacobs, A.M.; Tachtsidis, I. The physiological origin of task-evoked systemic artefacts in functional near infrared spectroscopy. *NeuroImage* **2012**, *61*, 70–81. [CrossRef] [PubMed]
101. Caldwell, M.; Scholkmann, F.; Wolf, U.; Wolf, M.; Elwell, C.; Tachtsidis, I. Modelling confounding effects from extracerebral contamination and systemic factors on functional near-infrared spectroscopy. *NeuroImage* **2016**, *143*, 91–105. [CrossRef] [PubMed]
102. Kozlová, S. The Use of Near-Infrared Spectroscopy in the Sport-Scientific Context. *J. Neurol. Neurol. Disord.* **2018**, *4*, 1. [CrossRef]
103. Seidel-Marzi, O.; Ragert, P. Neurodiagnostics in Sports: Investigating the Athlete's Brain to Augment Performance and Sport-Specific Skills. *Front. Hum. Neurosci.* **2020**, *14*, 133. [CrossRef] [PubMed]
104. Carius, D.; Andrä, C.; Clauß, M.; Ragert, P.; Bunk, M.; Mehnert, J. Hemodynamic Response Alteration As a Function of Task Complexity and Expertise—An fNIRS Study in Jugglers. *Front. Hum. Neurosci.* **2016**, *10*, 1. [CrossRef]
105. Seidel, O.; Carius, D.; Kenville, R.; Ragert, P. Motor learning in a complex balance task and associated neuroplasticity: A comparison between endurance athletes and nonathletes. *J. Neurophysiol.* **2017**, *118*, 1849–1860. [CrossRef]
106. Herold, F.; Orlowski, K.; Börmel, S.; Müller, N.G. Cortical activation during balancing on a balance board. *Hum. Mov. Sci.* **2017**, *51*, 51–58. [CrossRef]
107. Fujimoto, H.; Mihara, M.; Hattori, N.; Hatakenaka, M.; Kawano, T.; Yagura, H.; Miyai, I.; Mochizuki, H. Cortical changes underlying balance recovery in patients with hemiplegic stroke. *NeuroImage* **2014**, *85*, 547–554. [CrossRef]
108. Fujimoto, H.; Mihara, M.; Hattori, N.; Hatakenaka, M.; Yagura, H.; Kawano, T.; Miyai, I.; Mochizuki, H. Neurofeedback-induced facilitation of the supplementary motor area affects postural stability. *Neurophotonics* **2017**, *4*, 1. [CrossRef]
109. Mihara, M.; Miyai, I.; Hatakenaka, M.; Kubota, K.; Sakoda, S. Role of the prefrontal cortex in human balance control. *NeuroImage* **2008**, *43*, 329–336. [CrossRef]
110. Mihara, M.; Miyai, I.; Hattori, N.; Hatakenaka, M.; Yagura, H.; Kawano, T.; Kubota, K. Cortical control of postural balance in patients with hemiplegic stroke. *NeuroReport* **2012**, *23*, 314–319. [CrossRef]
111. Herold, F.; Wiegel, P.; Scholkmann, F.; Thiers, A.; Hamacher, D.; Schega, L. Functional near-infrared spectroscopy in movement science: A systematic review on cortical activity in postural and walking tasks. *Neurophotonics* **2017**, *4*, 41403. [CrossRef]
112. Vitório, R.; Stuart, S.; Rochester, L.; Alcock, L.; Pantall, A. fNIRS response during walking—Artefact or cortical activity? A systematic review. *Neurosci. Biobehav. Rev.* **2017**, *83*, 160–172. [CrossRef] [PubMed]
113. Formenti, D.; Perpetuini, D.; Iodice, P.; Cardone, D.; Michielon, G.; Scurati, R.; Alberti, G.; Merla, A. Effects of knee extension with different speeds of movement on muscle and cerebral oxygenation. *PeerJ* **2018**, *6*, e5704. [CrossRef]
114. Borot, L.; Vergotte, G.; Perrey, S. Different Hemodynamic Responses of the Primary Motor Cortex Accompanying Eccentric and Concentric Movements: A Functional NIRS Study. *Brain Sci.* **2018**, *8*, 75. [CrossRef]

115. Kenville, R.; Maudrich, T.; Carius, D.; Ragert, P. Hemodynamic Response Alterations in Sensorimotor Areas as a Function of Barbell Load Levels during Squatting: An fNIRS Study. *Front. Hum. Neurosci.* **2017**, *11*, 268. [CrossRef] [PubMed]
116. Cavuoto, L.A.; Maikala, R.V. Role of obesity on cerebral hemodynamics and cardiorespiratory responses in healthy men during repetitive incremental lifting. *Eur. J. Appl. Physiol.* **2015**, *115*, 1905–1917. [CrossRef]
117. Ono, Y.; Noah, J.A.; Zhang, X.; Nomoto, Y.; Suzuki, T.; Shimada, S.; Tachibana, A.; Bronner, S.; Hirsch, J. Motor learning and modulation of prefrontal cortex: An fNIRS assessment. *J. Neural Eng.* **2015**, *12*, 66004. [CrossRef]
118. Noah, J.A.; Ono, Y.; Nomoto, Y.; Shimada, S.; Tachibana, A.; Zhang, X.; Bronner, S.; Hirsch, J. fMRI Validation of fNIRS Measurements During a Naturalistic Task. *J. Vis. Exp.* **2015**, *100*, e52116. [CrossRef]
119. Tachibana, A.; Noah, J.A.; Bronner, S.; Ono, Y.; Onozuka, M. Parietal and temporal activity during a multimodal dance video game: An fNIRS study. *Neurosci. Lett.* **2011**, *503*, 125–130. [CrossRef]
120. Lu, X.; Hui-Chan, C.W.-Y.; Tsang, W.W.N. Changes of heart rate variability and prefrontal oxygenation during Tai Chi practice versus arm ergometer cycling. *J. Phys. Sci.* **2016**, *28*, 3243–3248. [CrossRef]
121. Tsang, W.W.N.; Chan, K.; Cheng, C.N.; Hu, F.S.; Mak, C.T.; Wong, J.W. Tai Chi practice on prefrontal oxygenation levels in older adults: A pilot study. *Complement. Med.* **2019**, *42*, 132–136. [CrossRef] [PubMed]
122. Carius, D.; Hörnig, L.; Ragert, P.; Kaminski, E. Characterizing cortical hemodynamic changes during climbing and its relation to climbing expertise. *Neurosci. Lett.* **2019**, *715*, 134604. [CrossRef] [PubMed]
123. Jones, B.; Cooper, C.E. Near Infrared Spectroscopy (NIRS) Observation of Vastus Lateralis (Muscle) and Prefrontal Cortex (Brain) Tissue Oxygenation During Synchronised Swimming Routines in Elite Athletes. *Adv. Exp. Med. Biol.* **2018**, *1072*, 111–117. [CrossRef]
124. Balardin, J.B.; Morais, G.A.Z.; Furucho, R.A.; Trambaiolli, L.; Vanzella, P.; Biazoli, C.E.; Sato, J.R. Imaging Brain Function with Functional Near-Infrared Spectroscopy in Unconstrained Environments. *Front. Hum. Neurosci.* **2017**, *11*, 258. [CrossRef] [PubMed]
125. Santos-Concejero, J.; Billaut, F.; Grobler, L.; Oliván, J.; Noakes, T.D.; Tucker, R. Maintained cerebral oxygenation during maximal self-paced exercise in elite Kenyan runners. *J. Appl. Physiol.* **2015**, *118*, 156–162. [CrossRef] [PubMed]
126. Santos-Concejero, J.; Billaut, F.; Grobler, L.; Oliván, J.; Noakes, T.D.; Tucker, R. Brain oxygenation declines in elite Kenyan runners during a maximal interval training session. *Eur. J. Appl. Physiol.* **2017**, *117*, 1017–1024. [CrossRef]
127. Suzuki, M.; Miyai, I.; Ono, T.; Oda, I.; Konishi, I.; Kochiyama, T.; Kubota, K. Prefrontal and premotor cortices are involved in adapting walking and running speed on the treadmill: An optical imaging study. *NeuroImage* **2004**, *23*, 1020–1026. [CrossRef]
128. Seidel, O.; Carius, D.; Roediger, J.; Rumpf, S.; Ragert, P. Changes in neurovascular coupling during cycling exercise measured by multi-distance fNIRS: A comparison between endurance athletes and physically active controls. *Exp. Brain Res.* **2019**, *237*, 2957–2972. [CrossRef]
129. Tempest, G.; Parfitt, G. Self-reported tolerance influences prefrontal cortex hemodynamics and affective responses. *Cogn. Affect. Behav. Neurosci.* **2015**, *16*, 63–71. [CrossRef]
130. Tempest, G.; Davranche, K.; Brisswalter, J.; Perrey, S.; Radel, R. The differential effects of prolonged exercise upon executive function and cerebral oxygenation. *Brain Cogn.* **2017**, *113*, 133–141. [CrossRef]
131. Tempest, G.; Reiss, A.L. The Utility of Functional Near-infrared Spectroscopy for Measuring Cortical Activity during Cycling Exercise. *Med. Sci. Sports Exerc.* **2019**, *51*, 979–987. [CrossRef]
132. Ando, S.; Hatamoto, Y.; Sudo, M.; Kiyonaga, A.; Tanaka, H.; Higaki, Y. The Effects of Exercise Under Hypoxia on Cognitive Function. *PLoS ONE* **2013**, *8*, e63630. [CrossRef] [PubMed]
133. Ando, S.; Kokubu, M.; Yamada, Y.; Kimura, M. Does cerebral oxygenation affect cognitive function during exercise? *Eur. J. Appl. Physiol.* **2011**, *111*, 1973–1982. [CrossRef] [PubMed]
134. Asahara, R.; Endo, K.; Liang, N.; Matsukawa, K. An increase in prefrontal oxygenation at the start of voluntary cycling exercise was observed independently of exercise effort and muscle mass. *Eur. J. Appl. Physiol.* **2018**, *118*, 1689–1702. [CrossRef] [PubMed]
135. Asahara, R.; Matsukawa, K.; Ishii, K.; Liang, N.; Endo, K. The prefrontal oxygenation and ventilatory responses at start of one-legged cycling exercise have relation to central command. *J. Appl. Physiol.* **2016**, *121*, 1115–1126. [CrossRef]

136. Billaut, F.; Davis, J.M.; Smith, K.; Marino, F.E.; Noakes, T.D. Cerebral oxygenation decreases but does not impair performance during self-paced, strenuous exercise. *Acta Physiol.* **2010**, *198*, 477–486. [CrossRef]
137. Gayda, M.; Lapierre, G.; Dupuy, O.; Fraser, S.; Bherer, L.; Juneau, M.; Gremeaux, V.; Nigam, A. Cardiovascular and cerebral hemodynamics during exercise and recovery in obese individuals as a function of their fitness status. *Physiol. Rep.* **2017**, *5*, e13321. [CrossRef]
138. Gayda, M.; Grémeaux, V.; Bherer, L.; Juneau, M.; Drigny, J.; Dupuy, O.; Lapierre, G.; Labelle, V.; Fortier, A.; Nigam, A. Cognitive function in patients with stable coronary heart disease: Related cerebrovascular and cardiovascular responses. *PLoS ONE* **2017**, *12*, e0183791. [CrossRef]
139. Giles, G.E.; Brunyé, T.T.; Eddy, M.D.; Mahoney, C.R.; Gagnon, S.A.; Taylor, H.A.; Kanarek, R.B. Acute exercise increases oxygenated and deoxygenated hemoglobin in the prefrontal cortex. *Neuroreport* **2014**, *25*, 1320–1325. [CrossRef]
140. González-Alonso, J.; Dalsgaard, M.K.; Osada, T.; Volianitis, S.; Dawson, E.A.; Yoshiga, C.C.; Secher, N.H. Brain and central haemodynamics and oxygenation during maximal exercise in humans. *J. Physiol.* **2004**, *557*, 331–342. [CrossRef]
141. Jung, R.; Moser, M.; Baucsek, S.; Dern, S.; Schneider, S. Activation patterns of different brain areas during incremental exercise measured by near-infrared spectroscopy. *Exp. Brain Res.* **2015**, *233*, 1175–1180. [CrossRef] [PubMed]
142. Kan, B.; Speelman, C.; Nosaka, K. Cognitive demand of eccentric versus concentric cycling and its effects on post-exercise attention and vigilance. *Eur. J. Appl. Physiol.* **2019**, *119*, 1599–1610. [CrossRef] [PubMed]
143. Lin, S.-I.; Lin, P.-Y.; Chen, J.-J.J. The cortical control of cycling exercise in stroke patients: An fNIRS study. *Hum. Brain Mapp.* **2012**, *34*, 2381–2390. [CrossRef] [PubMed]
144. Ohyanagi, H.; Tsubaki, A.; Morishita, S.; Obata, H.; Qin, W.; Onishi, H. Changes in the Prefrontal Cortex Oxygenation Levels During Cycling in the Supine and Upright Positions. *Adv. Exp. Med. Biol.* **2018**, *1072*, 133–137. [CrossRef]
145. Quinn, K.; Billaut, F.; Bulmer, A.C.; Minahan, C.L. Cerebral oxygenation declines but does not impair peak oxygen uptake during incremental cycling in women using oral contraceptives. *Eur. J. Appl. Physiol.* **2018**, *118*, 2417–2427. [CrossRef] [PubMed]
146. Radel, R.; Tempest, G.; Brisswalter, J. The long and winding road: Effects of exercise intensity and type upon sustained attention. *Physiol. Behav.* **2018**, *195*, 82–89. [CrossRef] [PubMed]
147. Schmit, C.; Davranche, K.; Easthope, C.S.; Colson, S.S.; Brisswalter, J.; Radel, R. Pushing to the limits: The dynamics of cognitive control during exhausting exercise. *Neuropsychologia* **2015**, *68*, 71–81. [CrossRef] [PubMed]
148. Takehara, N.; Tsubaki, A.; Yamazaki, Y.; Kanaya, C.; Sato, D.; Morishita, S.; Onishi, H. Changes in Oxyhemoglobin Concentration in the Prefrontal Cortex and Primary Motor Cortex During Low- and Moderate-Intensity Exercise on a Cycle Ergometer. *Adv. Exp. Med. Biol.* **2017**, *977*, 241–247. [CrossRef]
149. Tsubaki, A.; Morishita, S.; Tokunaga, Y.; Sato, D.; Tamaki, H.; Yamazaki, Y.; Qin, W.; Onishi, H. Changes in Cerebral Oxyhaemoglobin Levels During and After a Single 20-Minute Bout of Moderate-Intensity Cycling. *Adv. Exp. Med. Biol.* **2018**, *1072*, 127–131. [CrossRef]
150. Tsubaki, A.; Morishita, S.; Tokunaga, Y.; Sato, D.; Qin, W.; Kojima, S.; Onishi, H. Laterality of cortical oxygenation in the prefrontal cortex during 20 min of moderate-intensity cycling exercise: A near-infrared spectroscopy study. *Ann. Phys. Rehabil. Med.* **2018**, *61*, e460. [CrossRef]
151. Tsubaki, A.; Takai, H.; Oyanagi, K.; Kojima, S.; Tokunaga, Y.; Miyaguchi, S.; Sugawara, K.; Sato, D.; Tamaki, H.; Onishi, H. Correlation Between the Cerebral Oxyhaemoglobin Signal and Physiological Signals During Cycling Exercise: A Near-Infrared Spectroscopy Study. *Adv. Exp. Med. Biol.* **2016**, *923*, 159–166. [CrossRef] [PubMed]
152. Tsubaki, A.; Takehara, N.; Sato, D.; Morishita, S.; Tokunaga, Y.; Sugawara, K.; Kojima, S.; Tamaki, H.; Yamazaki, Y.; Onishi, H. Cortical Oxyhemoglobin Elevation Persists After Moderate-Intensity Cycling Exercise: A Near-Infrared Spectroscopy Study. *Adv. Exp. Med. Biol.* **2017**, *977*, 261–268. [CrossRef]
153. Piper, S.K.; Krueger, A.; Koch, S.P.; Mehnert, J.; Habermehl, C.; Steinbrink, J.; Obrig, H.; Schmitz, C.H. A wearable multi-channel fNIRS system for brain imaging in freely moving subjects. *NeuroImage* **2013**, *85*, 64–71. [CrossRef]

154. Kojima, S.; Morishita, S.; Qin, W.; Tsubaki, A. Cerebral Oxygenation Dynamics of the Prefrontal Cortex and Motor-Related Area During Cardiopulmonary Exercise Test: A Near-Infrared Spectroscopy Study. *Adv. Exp. Med. Biol.* **2020**, *1232*, 231–237. [CrossRef] [PubMed]
155. Tsubaki, A.; Morishita, S.; Tokunaga, Y.; Sato, D.; Qin, W.; Kojima, S.; Onishi, H. Effect of Exercise Duration on Post-Exercise Persistence of Oxyhemoglobin Changes in the Premotor Cortex: A Near-Infrared Spectroscopy Study in Moderate-Intensity Cycling Exercise. *Adv. Exp. Med. Biol.* **2020**, *1232*, 193–199. [CrossRef] [PubMed]
156. Stevens, D.; Halaki, M.; Chow, C.; O'Dwyer, N. The effects of multi-stage exercise with and without concurrent cognitive performance on cardiorespiratory and cerebral haemodynamic responses. *Eur. J. Appl. Physiol.* **2018**, *118*, 2121–2132. [CrossRef] [PubMed]
157. Subudhi, A.W.; Lorenz, M.C.; Fulco, C.S.; Roach, R.C. Cerebrovascular responses to incremental exercise during hypobaric hypoxia: Effect of oxygenation on maximal performance. *Am. J. Physiol. Heart Circ. Physiol.* **2008**, *294*, H164–H171. [CrossRef]
158. Subudhi, A.W.; Miramon, B.R.; Granger, M.E.; Roach, R.C. Frontal and motor cortex oxygenation during maximal exercise in normoxia and hypoxia. *J. Appl. Physiol.* **2009**, *106*, 1153–1158. [CrossRef]
159. Subudhi, A.W.; Dimmen, A.C.; Roach, R.C. Effects of acute hypoxia on cerebral and muscle oxygenation during incremental exercise. *J. Appl. Physiol.* **2007**, *103*, 177–183. [CrossRef]
160. Cavuoto, L.A.; Maikala, R.V. Obesity and the Role of Short Duration Submaximal Work on Cardiovascular and Cerebral Hemodynamics. *PLoS ONE* **2016**, *11*, e0153826. [CrossRef]
161. Imhoff, S.; Malenfant, S.; Nadreau, É.; Poirier, P.; Bailey, D.M.; Brassard, P. Uncoupling between cerebral perfusion and oxygenation during incremental exercise in an athlete with postconcussion syndrome: A case report. *Physiol. Rep.* **2017**, *5*, e13131. [CrossRef]
162. Marillier, M.; Gruet, M.; Baillieul, S.; Wuyam, B.; Tamisier, R.; Levy, P.A.; Pépin, J.-L.; Verges, S. Impaired cerebral oxygenation and exercise tolerance in patients with severe obstructive sleep apnea syndrome. *Sleep Med.* **2018**, *51*, 37–46. [CrossRef] [PubMed]
163. Neary, J.P.; Roberts, A.D.W.; Leavins, N.; Harrison, M.F.; Croll, J.C.; Sexsmith, J.R. Prefrontal cortex oxygenation during incremental exercise in chronic fatigue syndrome. *Clin. Physiol. Funct. Imaging* **2008**, *28*, 364–372. [CrossRef] [PubMed]
164. Seifert, T.; Rasmussen, P.; Secher, N.H.; Nielsen, H.B. Cerebral oxygenation decreases during exercise in humans with beta-adrenergic blockade. *Acta Physiol.* **2009**, *196*, 295–302. [CrossRef] [PubMed]
165. Tempest, G.; Eston, R.G.; Parfitt, G. Prefrontal Cortex Haemodynamics and Affective Responses during Exercise: A Multi-Channel Near Infrared Spectroscopy Study. *PLoS ONE* **2014**, *9*, e95924. [CrossRef] [PubMed]
166. Koike, A.; Itoh, H.; Oohara, R.; Hoshimoto, M.; Tajima, A.; Aizawa, T.; Fu, L.T. Cerebral oxygenation during exercise in cardiac patients. *Chest* **2004**, *125*, 182–190. [CrossRef]
167. Huang, S.-C.; Chen, C.P.; Fu, T.-C.; Chen, Y.-J. Integration of Brain Tissue Saturation Monitoring in Cardiopulmonary Exercise Testing in Patients with Heart Failure. *J. Vis. Exp.* **2019**, *152*, e60289. [CrossRef]
168. Chen, Y.-J.; Wang, J.-S.; Hsu, C.-C.; Lin, P.-J.; Tsai, F.-C.; Wen, M.-S.; Kuo, C.-T.; Huang, S.-C. Cerebral desaturation in heart failure: Potential prognostic value and physiologic basis. *PLoS ONE* **2018**, *13*, e0196299. [CrossRef]
169. Koike, A.; Hoshimoto, M.; Tajima, A.; Nagayama, O.; Yamaguchi, K.; Goda, A.; Yamashita, T.; Sagara, K.; Itoh, H.; Aizawa, T. Critical level of cerebral oxygenation during exercise in patients with left ventricular dysfunction. *Circ. J.* **2006**, *70*, 1457–1461. [CrossRef]
170. Liao, L.-D.; Tsytsarev, V.; Delgado-Martínez, I.; Li, M.-L.; Erzurumlu, R.; Vipin, A.; Orellana, J.; Lin, Y.-R.; Lai, H.-Y.; Chen, Y.-Y.; et al. Neurovascular coupling: In vivo optical techniques for functional brain imaging. *Biomed. Eng. Online* **2013**, *12*, 38. [CrossRef]
171. Scholkmann, F.; Kleiser, S.; Metz, A.J.; Zimmermann, R.; Pavia, J.M.; Wolf, U.; Wolf, M. A review on continuous wave functional near-infrared spectroscopy and imaging instrumentation and methodology. *NeuroImage* **2014**, *85*, 6–27. [CrossRef] [PubMed]
172. Lindauer, U.; Dirnagl, U.; Füchtemeier, M.; Böttiger, C.; Offenhauser, N.; Leithner, C.; Royl, G. Pathophysiological Interference with Neurovascular Coupling—When Imaging Based on Hemoglobin Might Go Blind. *Front. Neuroenerg.* **2010**, *2*, 2. [CrossRef] [PubMed]

173. León-Carrión, J.; León-Domniguez, U. Functional Near-Infrared Spectroscopy (fNIRS): Principles and Neuroscientific Applications. In *Neuroimaging—Methods*; Bright, P., Ed.; InTech: Rijeka, Croatia, 2017; pp. 48–74. ISBN 978-953-51-0097-3.
174. Scholkmann, F.; Wolf, M. Measuring brain activity using functional near infrared spectroscopy: A short review. *Spectrosc. Eur.* **2012**, *24*, 6–10.
175. Nippert, A.R.; Biesecker, K.R.; Newman, E.A. Mechanisms Mediating Functional Hyperemia in the Brain. *Neuroscientist* **2017**, *24*, 73–83. [CrossRef] [PubMed]
176. Herold, F.; Wiegel, P.; Scholkmann, F.; Müller, N.G. Applications of Functional Near-Infrared Spectroscopy (fNIRS) Neuroimaging in Exercise–Cognition Science: A Systematic, Methodology-Focused Review. *J. Clin. Med.* **2018**, *7*, 466. [CrossRef]
177. Bunce, S.; Izzetoglu, M.; Izzetoglu, K.; Onaral, B.; Pourrezaei, K. Functional near-infrared spectroscopy. *IEEE Eng. Med. Boil. Mag.* **2006**, *25*, 54–62. [CrossRef]
178. Izzetoglu, M.; Bunce, S.C.; Izzetoglu, K.; Onaral, B.; Pourrezaei, A.K. Functional brain imaging using near-infrared technology. *IEEE Eng. Med. Boil. Mag.* **2007**, *26*, 38–46. [CrossRef]
179. Obrig, H.; Wenzel, R.; Kohl, M.; Horst, S.; Wobst, P.; Steinbrink, J.; Thomas, F.; Villringer, A. Near-infrared spectroscopy: Does it function in functional activation studies of the adult brain? *Int. J. Psychophysiol.* **2000**, *35*, 125–142. [CrossRef]
180. Rupawala, M.; Dehghani, H.; Lucas, S.J.; Tino, P.; Cruse, D. Shining a Light on Awareness: A Review of Functional Near-Infrared Spectroscopy for Prolonged Disorders of Consciousness. *Front. Neurol.* **2018**, *9*, 68. [CrossRef]
181. Delpy, D.T.; Cope, M. Quantification in tissue near-infrared spectroscopy. *Philos. Trans. R. Soc. B Boil. Sci.* **1997**, *352*, 649–659. [CrossRef]
182. Hamaoka, T.; McCully, K.K. Review of early development of near-infrared spectroscopy and recent advancement of studies on muscle oxygenation and oxidative metabolism. *J. Physiol. Sci.* **2019**, *69*, 799–811. [CrossRef]
183. Bakker, A.; Smith, B.; Ainslie, P.N.; Smith, K. Near-Infrared Spectroscopy. In *Introduction//New Directions in the Dynamic Assessment of Brain Blood Flow Regulation*; Willie, C.K., Eller, L.K., Ainslie, P.N., Eds.; INTECH Open Access Publisher: London, UK, 2012; pp. 65–88. ISBN 978-953-51-0522-0.
184. Scholkmann, F.; Metz, A.J.; Wolf, M. Measuring tissue hemodynamics and oxygenation by continuous-wave functional near-infrared spectroscopy—How robust are the different calculation methods against movement artifacts? *Physiol. Meas.* **2014**, *35*, 717–734. [CrossRef]
185. Kohl-Bareis, M. NIRS: Theoretical Background and Practical Aspects. In *Functional Neuroimaging in Exercise and Sport Sciences*; Boecker, H., Hillman, C.H., Scheef, L., Strüder, H.K., Eds.; Springer: New York, NY, USA, 2012; pp. 213–235. ISBN 978-1-4614-3292-0.
186. Almajidy, R.J.; Mankodiya, K.; Abtahi, M.; Hofmann, U.G. A Newcomer's Guide to Functional Near Infrared Spectroscopy Experiments. *IEEE Rev. Biomed. Eng.* **2020**, *13*, 292–308. [CrossRef]
187. Quaresima, V.; Bisconti, S.; Ferrari, M. A brief review on the use of functional near-infrared spectroscopy (fNIRS) for language imaging studies in human newborns and adults. *Brain Lang.* **2012**, *121*, 79–89. [CrossRef] [PubMed]
188. Ferrari, M.; Quaresima, V. A brief review on the history of human functional near-infrared spectroscopy (fNIRS) development and fields of application. *NeuroImage* **2012**, *63*, 921–935. [CrossRef]
189. Irani, F.; Platek, S.M.; Bunce, S.; Ruocco, A.C.; Chute, D. Functional Near Infrared Spectroscopy (fNIRS): An Emerging Neuroimaging Technology with Important Applications for the Study of Brain Disorders. *Clin. Neuropsychol.* **2007**, *21*, 9–37. [CrossRef] [PubMed]
190. Hoshi, Y. Functional Near-Infrared Spectroscopy: Potential and Limitations in Neuroimaging Studies. *Int. Rev. Neurobiol.* **2005**, *66*, 237–266. [CrossRef]
191. Hoshi, Y.; Yamada, Y. Overview of diffuse optical tomography and its clinical applications. *J. Biomed. Opt.* **2016**, *21*, 91312. [CrossRef]
192. Elwell, C.; Cooper, C. Making light work: Illuminating the future of biomedical optics. *Philos. Trans. A Math. Phys. Eng. Sci.* **2011**, *369*, 4358–4379. [CrossRef] [PubMed]
193. Agbangla, N.F.; Audiffren, M.; Albinet, C. Use of near-infrared spectroscopy in the investigation of brain activation during cognitive aging: A systematic review of an emerging area of research. *Ageing Res. Rev.* **2017**, *38*, 52–66. [CrossRef]

194. Shoaib, Z.; Kamran, M.A.; Mannan, M.M.N.; Jeong, M.Y. Methodologies on the Enhanced Spatial Resolution of Non-Invasive Optical Brain Imaging: A Review. *IEEE Access* **2019**, *7*, 130044–130066. [CrossRef]
195. Kumar, V.; Shivakumar, V.; Chhabra, H.; Bose, A.; Venkatasubramanian, G.; Gangadhar, B.N. Functional near infra-red spectroscopy (fNIRS) in schizophrenia: A review. *Asian J. Psychiatry* **2017**, *27*, 18–31. [CrossRef] [PubMed]
196. Strangman, G.; A Boas, D.; Sutton, J.P. Non-invasive neuroimaging using near-infrared light. *Boil. Psychiatry* **2002**, *52*, 679–693. [CrossRef]
197. Rooks, C.R.; Thom, N.J.; McCully, K.K.; Dishman, R. Effects of incremental exercise on cerebral oxygenation measured by near-infrared spectroscopy: A systematic review. *Prog. Neurobiol.* **2010**, *92*, 134–150. [CrossRef]
198. Boone, J.; Vandekerckhove, K.; Coomans, I.; Prieur, F.; Bourgois, J.G. An integrated view on the oxygenation responses to incremental exercise at the brain, the locomotor and respiratory muscles. *Eur. J. Appl. Physiol.* **2016**, *116*, 2085–2102. [CrossRef]
199. Noakes, T.D. Testing for maximum oxygen consumption has produced a brainless model of human exercise performance. *Br. J. Sports Med.* **2008**, *42*, 551–555. [CrossRef]
200. Noakes, T.D.; E Peltonen, J.; Rusko, H.K. Evidence that a central governor regulates exercise performance during acute hypoxia and hyperoxia. *J. Exp. Boil.* **2001**, *204*, 3225–3234.
201. Noakes, T.D.; St, C.; Lambert, E.V. From catastrophe to complexity: A novel model of integrative central neural regulation of effort and fatigue during exercise in humans. *Br. J. Sports Med.* **2004**, *38*, 511–514. [CrossRef]
202. Noakes, T.D.; St, C.; Lambert, E.V. From catastrophe to complexity: A novel model of integrative central neural regulation of effort and fatigue during exercise in humans: Summary and conclusions. *Br. J. Sports Med.* **2005**, *39*, 120–124. [CrossRef]
203. Noakes, T.D.; Noakes, P.T.D. The Central Governor Model of Exercise Regulation Applied to the Marathon. *Sports Med.* **2007**, *37*, 374–377. [CrossRef] [PubMed]
204. Noakes, T.D. Time to move beyond a brainless exercise physiology: The evidence for complex regulation of human exercise performance. *Appl. Physiol. Nutr. Metab.* **2011**, *36*, 23–35. [CrossRef] [PubMed]
205. Abbiss, C.R.; Laursen, P.B. Models to explain fatigue during prolonged endurance cycling. *Sports Med.* **2005**, *35*, 865–898. [CrossRef] [PubMed]
206. Robertson, C.; Marino, F.E. A role for the prefrontal cortex in exercise tolerance and termination. *J. Appl. Physiol.* **2016**, *120*, 464–466. [CrossRef] [PubMed]
207. Yamazaki, Y.; Sato, D.; Yamashiro, K.; Tsubaki, A.; Yamaguchi, Y.; Takehara, N.; Maruyama, A. Inter-individual Differences in Exercise-Induced Spatial Working Memory Improvement: A Near-Infrared Spectroscopy Study. *Adv. Exp. Med. Biol.* **2017**, *977*, 81–88. [CrossRef] [PubMed]
208. Mekari, S.; Fraser, S.; Bosquet, L.; Bonnéry, C.; Labelle, V.; Pouliot, P.; Lesage, F.; Bherer, L. The relationship between exercise intensity, cerebral oxygenation and cognitive performance in young adults. *Eur. J. Appl. Physiol.* **2015**, *115*, 2189–2197. [CrossRef]
209. Fishburn, F.; Norr, M.E.; Medvedev, A.V.; Vaidya, C.J. Sensitivity of fNIRS to cognitive state and load. *Front. Hum. Neurosci.* **2014**, *8*, 76. [CrossRef]
210. Herff, C.; Heger, D.; Fortmann, O.; Hennrich, J.; Putze, F.; Schultz, T. Mental workload during n-back task-quantified in the prefrontal cortex using fNIRS. *Front. Hum. Neurosci.* **2014**, *7*, 935. [CrossRef]
211. Causse, M.; Chua, Z.; Peysakhovich, V.; Del Campo, N.; Matton, N. Mental workload and neural efficiency quantified in the prefrontal cortex using fNIRS. *Sci. Rep.* **2017**, *7*, 5222. [CrossRef]
212. Bunce, S.C.; Izzetoglu, K.; Ayaz, H.; Shewokis, P.; Izzetoglu, M.; Pourrezaei, K.; Onaral, B. Implementation of fNIRS for Monitoring Levels of Expertise and Mental Workload. *Appl. Evol. Comput.* **2011**, *6780*, 13–22.
213. Mehta, R.K.; Parasuraman, R. Effects of Mental Fatigue on the Development of Physical Fatigue. *Hum. Factors J. Hum. Factors Erg. Soc.* **2013**, *56*, 645–656. [CrossRef]
214. Shortz, A.; Pickens, A.; Zheng, Q.; Mehta, R.K. The effect of cognitive fatigue on prefrontal cortex correlates of neuromuscular fatigue in older women. *J. Neuroeng. Rehabil.* **2015**, *12*, 115. [CrossRef] [PubMed]
215. Borragan, G.; Guerrero-Mosquera, C.; Guillaume, C.; Slama, H.; Peigneux, P. Decreased prefrontal connectivity parallels cognitive fatigue-related performance decline after sleep deprivation. An optical imaging study. *Boil. Psychol.* **2019**, *144*, 115–124. [CrossRef] [PubMed]

216. Brugnera, A.; Zarbo, C.; Adorni, R.; Gatti, A.; Compare, A.; Sakatani, K. Age-Related Changes in Physiological Reactivity to a Stress Task: A Near-Infrared Spectroscopy Study. *Adv. Exp. Med. Biol.* **2017**, *977*, 155–161. [CrossRef] [PubMed]
217. Mandrick, K.; Peysakhovich, V.; Rémy, F.; Lepron, E.; Causse, M. Neural and psychophysiological correlates of human performance under stress and high mental workload. *Boil. Psychol.* **2016**, *121*, 62–73. [CrossRef] [PubMed]
218. Mehta, R.K. Stunted PFC activity during neuromuscular control under stress with obesity. *Eur. J. Appl. Physiol.* **2015**, *116*, 319–326. [CrossRef] [PubMed]
219. Rosenbaum, D.; Hilsendegen, P.; Thomas, M.; Haeussinger, F.B.; Metzger, F.G.; Nuerk, H.-C.; Fallgatter, A.J.; Nieratschker, V.; Ehlis, A.-C. Cortical hemodynamic changes during the Trier Social Stress Test: An fNIRS study. *NeuroImage* **2017**, *171*, 107–115. [CrossRef]
220. Kalia, V.; Vishwanath, K.; Knauft, K.; Von Der Vellen, B.; Luebbe, A.; Williams, A. Acute Stress Attenuates Cognitive Flexibility in Males Only: An fNIRS Examination. *Front. Psychol.* **2018**, *9*, 9. [CrossRef]
221. Caen, K.; Vermeire, K.; Pogliaghi, S.; Moerman, A.; Niemeijer, V.; Bourgois, J.G.; Boone, J. Aerobic Interval Training Impacts Muscle and Brain Oxygenation Responses to Incremental Exercise. *Front. Physiol.* **2019**, *10*, 1195. [CrossRef]
222. Ono, Y.; Nomoto, Y.; Tanaka, S.; Sato, K.; Shimada, S.; Tachibana, A.; Bronner, S.; Noah, J.A. Frontotemporal oxyhemoglobin dynamics predict performance accuracy of dance simulation gameplay: Temporal characteristics of top-down and bottom-up cortical activities. *NeuroImage* **2014**, *85*, 461–470. [CrossRef]
223. Funahashi, S.; Andreau, J.M. Prefrontal cortex and neural mechanisms of executive function. *J. Physiol.* **2013**, *107*, 471–482. [CrossRef]
224. Miller, E.K.; Cohen, J.D. An Integrative Theory of Prefrontal Cortex Function. *Annu. Rev. Neurosci.* **2001**, *24*, 167–202. [CrossRef] [PubMed]
225. Pontifex, M.B.; McGowan, A.L.; Chandler, M.C.; Gwizdala, K.L.; Parks, A.; Fenn, K.; Kamijo, K. A primer on investigating the after effects of acute bouts of physical activity on cognition. *Psychol. Sport Exerc.* **2019**, *40*, 1–22. [CrossRef]
226. Kujach, S.; Byun, K.; Hyodo, K.; Suwabe, K.; Fukuie, T.; Laskowski, R.; Dan, I.; Soya, H. A transferable high-intensity intermittent exercise improves executive performance in association with dorsolateral prefrontal activation in young adults. *NeuroImage* **2018**, *169*, 117–125. [CrossRef] [PubMed]
227. Byun, K.; Hyodo, K.; Suwabe, K.; Ochi, G.; Sakairi, Y.; Kato, M.; Dan, I.; Soya, H. Positive effect of acute mild exercise on executive function via arousal-related prefrontal activations: An fNIRS study. *NeuroImage* **2014**, *98*, 336–345. [CrossRef]
228. Yanagisawa, H.; Dan, I.; Tsuzuki, D.; Kato, M.; Okamoto, M.; Kyutoku, Y.; Soya, H. Acute moderate exercise elicits increased dorsolateral prefrontal activation and improves cognitive performance with Stroop test. *NeuroImage* **2010**, *50*, 1702–1710. [CrossRef]
229. Hyodo, K.; Dan, I.; Suwabe, K.; Kyutoku, Y.; Yamada, Y.; Akahori, M.; Byun, K.; Kato, M.; Soya, H. Acute moderate exercise enhances compensatory brain activation in older adults. *Neurobiol. Aging* **2012**, *33*, 2621–2632. [CrossRef]
230. Morais, G.A.Z.; Scholkmann, F.; Balardin, J.B.; Furucho, R.A.; De Paula, R.C.V.; Biazoli, C.E.; Sato, J.R. Non-neuronal evoked and spontaneous hemodynamic changes in the anterior temporal region of the human head may lead to misinterpretations of functional near-infrared spectroscopy signals. *Neurophotonics* **2017**, *5*, 1. [CrossRef]
231. Matsukawa, K.; Endo, K.; Asahara, R.; Yoshikawa, M.; Kusunoki, S.; Ishida, T. Prefrontal oxygenation correlates to the responses in facial skin blood flows during exposure to pleasantly charged movie. *Physiol. Rep.* **2017**, *5*, e13488. [CrossRef]
232. Miyazawa, T.; Horiuchi, M.; Komine, H.; Sugawara, J.; Fadel, P.J.; Ogoh, S. Skin blood flow influences cerebral oxygenation measured by near-infrared spectroscopy during dynamic exercise. *Eur. J. Appl. Physiol.* **2013**, *113*, 2841–2848. [CrossRef]
233. Nasseri, N.; Caicedo, A.; Scholkmann, F.; Zohdi, H.; Wolf, U. Impact of Changes in Systemic Physiology on fNIRS/NIRS Signals: Analysis Based on Oblique Subspace Projections Decomposition. *Adv. Exp. Med. Biol.* **2018**, *1072*, 119–125. [CrossRef]

234. Takahashi, T.; Takikawa, Y.; Kawagoe, R.; Shibuya, S.; Iwano, T.; Kitazawa, S. Influence of skin blood flow on near-infrared spectroscopy signals measured on the forehead during a verbal fluency task. *NeuroImage* **2011**, *57*, 991–1002. [CrossRef] [PubMed]
235. Fantini, S.; Ruesch, A.; Kainerstorfer, J.M. Noninvasive Optical Studies of the Brain. *Neurophotonics Biomed. Spectrosc.* **2019**, 25–52. [CrossRef]
236. Fantini, S.; Frederick, B.D.; Sassaroli, A. Perspective: Prospects of non-invasive sensing of the human brain with diffuse optical imaging. *APL Photonics* **2018**, *3*, 110901. [CrossRef] [PubMed]
237. Von Lühmann, A.; Li, X.; Müller, K.-R.; Boas, D.A.; Yücel, M.A. Improved physiological noise regression in fNIRS: A multimodal extension of the General Linear Model using temporally embedded Canonical Correlation Analysis. *NeuroImage* **2020**, *208*, 116472. [CrossRef] [PubMed]
238. Al-Rawi, P.G.; Smieleweski, P.; Kirkpatrick, P.J. Evaluation of a Near-Infrared Spectrometer (NIRO 300) for the Detection of Intracranial Oxygenation Changes in the Adult Head. *Stroke* **2001**, *32*, 2492–2500. [CrossRef]
239. Metz, A.J.; Klein, S.D.; Scholkmann, F.; Wolf, U. Continuous coloured light altered human brain haemodynamics and oxygenation assessed by systemic physiology augmented functional near-infrared spectroscopy. *Sci. Rep.* **2017**, *7*, 10027. [CrossRef]
240. Scholkmann, F.; Hafner, T.; Metz, A.J.; Wolf, M.; Wolf, U. Effect of short-term colored-light exposure on cerebral hemodynamics and oxygenation, and systemic physiological activity. *Neurophotonics* **2017**, *4*, 1. [CrossRef]
241. Durantin, G.; Gagnon, J.-F.; Tremblay, S.; Dehais, F. Using near infrared spectroscopy and heart rate variability to detect mental overload. *Behav. Brain Res.* **2014**, *259*, 16–23. [CrossRef]
242. Borresen, J.; I Lambert, M. Autonomic control of heart rate during and after exercise: Measurements and implications for monitoring training status. *Sports Med.* **2008**, *38*, 633–646. [CrossRef]
243. Hottenrott, K.; Hoos, O.; Esperer, H.D. Herzfrequenzvariabilität und Sport. *Herz* **2006**, *31*, 544–552. [CrossRef]
244. Plews, D.J.; Laursen, P.B.; Stanley, J.; Kilding, A.E.; Buchheit, M. Training Adaptation and Heart Rate Variability in Elite Endurance Athletes: Opening the Door to Effective Monitoring. *Sports Med.* **2013**, *43*, 773–781. [CrossRef] [PubMed]
245. Massaro, S.; Pecchia, L. Heart Rate Variability (HRV) Analysis: A Methodology for Organizational Neuroscience. *Organ. Res. Methods* **2016**, *22*, 354–393. [CrossRef]
246. Sen, J.; McGill, D. Fractal analysis of heart rate variability as a predictor of mortality: A systematic review and meta-analysis. *Chaos* **2018**, *28*, 072101. [CrossRef] [PubMed]
247. Thayer, J.F.; Åhs, F.; Fredrikson, M.; Sollers, J.J.; Wager, T.D. A meta-analysis of heart rate variability and neuroimaging studies: Implications for heart rate variability as a marker of stress and health. *Neurosci. Biobehav. Rev.* **2012**, *36*, 747–756. [CrossRef]
248. Thayer, J.F.; Yamamoto, S.S.; Brosschot, J. The relationship of autonomic imbalance, heart rate variability and cardiovascular disease risk factors. *Int. J. Cardiol.* **2010**, *141*, 122–131. [CrossRef]
249. Shaffer, F.; Ginsberg, J. An Overview of Heart Rate Variability Metrics and Norms. *Front. Public Health* **2017**, *5*, 258. [CrossRef]
250. Castaldo, R.; Melillo, P.; Bracale, U.; Caserta, M.; Triassi, M.; Pecchia, L. Acute mental stress assessment via short term HRV analysis in healthy adults: A systematic review with meta-analysis. *Biomed. Signal Process. Control* **2015**, *18*, 370–377. [CrossRef]
251. Vesterinen, V.; Nummela, A.T.; Heikura, I.; Laine, T.; Hynynen, E.; Botella, J.; Häkkinen, K. Individual Endurance Training Prescription with Heart Rate Variability. *Med. Sci. Sports Exerc.* **2016**, *48*, 1347–1354. [CrossRef]
252. Gronwald, T.; Schulze, S.; Ludyga, S.; Hottenrott, K. Evaluierung individueller Trainingsvorgaben auf Basis der Herzfrequenzvariabilität für ein Lauftraining im Freizeit-und Gesundheitssport. *Praxis* **2016**, *105*, 1065–1070. [CrossRef]
253. Vesterinen, V.; Häkkinen, K.; Hynynen, E.; Mikkola, J.; Hokka, L.; Nummela, A. Heart rate variability in prediction of individual adaptation to endurance training in recreational endurance runners. *Scand. J. Med. Sci. Sports* **2011**, *23*, 171–180. [CrossRef]
254. Hottenrott, K. HRV Regenerationsmanagement: State of Art. *Sportärztezeitung* **2019**, *1*, 2–6.
255. Bellenger, C.R.; Fuller, J.T.; Thomson, R.L.; Davison, K.; Robertson, E.Y.; Buckley, J.D. Monitoring Athletic Training Status Through Autonomic Heart Rate Regulation: A Systematic Review and Meta-Analysis. *Sports Med.* **2016**, *46*, 1461–1486. [CrossRef] [PubMed]

256. Gronwald, T.; Hoos, O.; Ludyga, S.; Hottenrott, K. Non-linear dynamics of heart rate variability during incremental cycling exercise. *Res. Sports Med.* **2018**, *27*, 88–98. [CrossRef] [PubMed]
257. Gronwald, T.; Hoos, O.; Hottenrott, K. Effects of Acute Normobaric Hypoxia on Non-linear Dynamics of Cardiac Autonomic Activity During Constant Workload Cycling Exercise. *Front. Physiol.* **2019**, *10*, 999. [CrossRef]
258. Gronwald, T.; Hoos, O.; Hottenrott, K. Effects of a Short-Term Cycling Interval Session and Active Recovery on Non-Linear Dynamics of Cardiac Autonomic Activity in Endurance Trained Cyclists. *J. Clin. Med.* **2019**, *8*, 194. [CrossRef]
259. Gronwald, T.; Hoos, O. Correlation properties of heart rate variability during endurance exercise: A systematic review. *Ann. Noninvasive Electrocardiol.* **2019**, *25*, e12697. [CrossRef]
260. Gronwald, T.; Hoos, O.; Hottenrott, K. Influence of Performance Level of Male Runners on Non-linear Dynamics of Heart Rate Variability During a 10Km Race. *Int. J. Perform. Anal. Sport* **2020**, 1–15. [CrossRef]
261. De Godoy, M.F. Nonlinear Analysis of Heart Rate Variability: A Comprehensive Review. *J. Cardiol.* **2016**, *3*, 528–533. [CrossRef]
262. Voss, A.; Schulz, S.; Schroeder, R.; Baumert, M.; Caminal, P. Methods derived from nonlinear dynamics for analysing heart rate variability. *Philos. Trans. A Math. Phys. Eng. Sci.* **2008**, *367*, 277–296. [CrossRef]
263. Huikuri, H.V.; Mäkikallio, T.H.; Perkiömäki, J. Measurement of heart rate variability by methods based on nonlinear dynamics. *J. Electrocardiol.* **2003**, *36*, 95–99. [CrossRef]
264. Colzato, L.S.; Jongkees, B.J.; De Wit, M.; Van Der Molen, M.J.W.; Steenbergen, L. Variable heart rate and a flexible mind: Higher resting-state heart rate variability predicts better task-switching. *Cogn. Affect. Behav. Neurosci.* **2018**, *18*, 730–738. [CrossRef] [PubMed]
265. Frewen, J.; Finucane, C.; Savva, G.M.; Boyle, G.; Coen, R.F.; Kenny, R.A. Cognitive function is associated with impaired heart rate variability in ageing adults: The Irish longitudinal study on ageing wave one results. *Clin. Auton. Res.* **2013**, *23*, 313–323. [CrossRef] [PubMed]
266. Gillie, B.L.; Vasey, M.W.; Thayer, J.F. Heart Rate Variability Predicts Control Over Memory Retrieval. *Psychol. Sci.* **2013**, *25*, 458–465. [CrossRef] [PubMed]
267. Hansen, A.L.; Johnsen, B.H.; Thayer, J.F. Vagal influence on working memory and attention. *Int. J. Psychophysiol.* **2003**, *48*, 263–274. [CrossRef]
268. Al Hazzouri, A.Z.; Haan, M.N.; Deng, Y.; Neuhaus, J.; Yaffe, K. Reduced heart rate variability is associated with worse cognitive performance in elderly Mexican Americans. *Hypertension* **2013**, *63*, 181–187. [CrossRef] [PubMed]
269. Ranchet, M.; Morgan, J.C.; Akinwuntan, A.E.; Devos, H. Cognitive workload across the spectrum of cognitive impairments: A systematic review of physiological measures. *Neurosci. Biobehav. Rev.* **2017**, *80*, 516–537. [CrossRef]
270. Forte, G.; Favieri, F.; Casagrande, M. Heart Rate Variability and Cognitive Function: A Systematic Review. *Front. Mol. Neurosci.* **2019**, *13*, 710. [CrossRef]
271. Matos, F.D.O.; Vido, A.; Garcia, W.F.; Lopes, W.A.; Pereira, A. A Neurovisceral Integrative Study on Cognition, Heart Rate Variability, and Fitness in the Elderly. *Front. Aging Neurosci.* **2020**, *12*, 51. [CrossRef]
272. Siennicka, A.; Quintana, D.; Fedurek, P.; Wijata, A.; Paleczny, B.; Ponikowska, B.; Danel, D. Resting heart rate variability, attention and attention maintenance in young adults. *Int. J. Psychophysiol.* **2019**, *143*, 126–131. [CrossRef]
273. Grässler, B.; Hökelmann, A.; Cabral, R.H. Resting heart rate variability as a possible marker of cognitive decline. *Kinesiology* **2020**, *52*, 72–84. [CrossRef]
274. Mather, M.; Thayer, J.F. How heart rate variability affects emotion regulation brain networks. *Curr. Opin. Behav. Sci.* **2018**, *19*, 98–104. [CrossRef] [PubMed]
275. Smith, R.; Thayer, J.F.; Khalsa, S.S.; Lane, R.D. The hierarchical basis of neurovisceral integration. *Neurosci. Biobehav. Rev.* **2017**, *75*, 274–296. [CrossRef] [PubMed]
276. Thayer, J.F.; Hansen, A.L.; Saus-Rose, E.; Johnsen, B.H. Heart Rate Variability, Prefrontal Neural Function, and Cognitive Performance: The Neurovisceral Integration Perspective on Self-regulation, Adaptation, and Health. *Ann. Behav. Med.* **2009**, *37*, 141–153. [CrossRef] [PubMed]
277. Thayer, J.F.; Lane, R.D. Claude Bernard and the heart-brain connection: Further elaboration of a model of neurovisceral integration. *Neurosci. Biobehav. Rev.* **2009**, *33*, 81–88. [CrossRef]

278. Thayer, J.F.; Lane, R.D. A model of neurovisceral integration in emotion regulation and dysregulation. *J. Affect. Disord.* **2000**, *61*, 201–216. [CrossRef]
279. Park, G.; Thayer, J.F. From the heart to the mind: Cardiac vagal tone modulates top-down and bottom-up visual perception and attention to emotional stimuli. *Front. Psychol.* **2014**, *5*, 278. [CrossRef]
280. Thayer, J. A Neurovisceral Integration Model of Heart Rate Variability. In *Reference Module in Neuroscience and Biobehavioral Psychology*; Elsevier BV: Amsterdam, The Netherlands, 2017.
281. Javaloyes, A.; Sarabia, J.M.; Lamberts, R.P.; Moya-Ramón, M. Training Prescription Guided by Heart-Rate Variability in Cycling. *Int. J. Sports Physiol. Perform.* **2019**, *14*, 23–32. [CrossRef]
282. Kiviniemi, A.; Hautala, A.J.; Kinnunen, H.; Tulppo, M. Endurance training guided individually by daily heart rate variability measurements. *Eur. J. Appl. Physiol.* **2007**, *101*, 743–751. [CrossRef]
283. Da Silva, D.F.; Ferraro, Z.M.; Adamo, K.B.; Machado, F.A. Endurance Running Training Individually Guided by HRV in Untrained Women. *J. Strength Cond. Res.* **2019**, *33*, 736–746. [CrossRef]
284. Scholkmann, F.; Wolf, U. The Pulse-Respiration Quotient: A Powerful but Untapped Parameter for Modern Studies About Human Physiology and Pathophysiology. *Front. Physiol.* **2019**, *10*, 371. [CrossRef]
285. Scholkmann, F.; Zohdi, H.; Wolf, U. The resting-state pulse-respiration quotient of humans: Lognormally distributed and centred around a value of four. *Physiol. Res.* **2019**, *68*, 1027–1032. [CrossRef] [PubMed]

© 2020 by the authors. Licensee MDPI, Basel, Switzerland. This article is an open access article distributed under the terms and conditions of the Creative Commons Attribution (CC BY) license (http://creativecommons.org/licenses/by/4.0/).

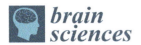

Article

Shedding Light on the Effects of Moderate Acute Exercise on Working Memory Performance in Healthy Older Adults: An fNIRS Study

Katharina Stute [1], Nicole Hudl [1], Robert Stojan [1,2] and Claudia Voelcker-Rehage [1,2,*]

1 Institute of Human Movement Science and Health, Chemnitz University of Technology, 09126 Chemnitz, Germany; katharina.stute@hsw.tu-chemnitz.de (K.S.); nicole.hudl@hsw.tu-chemnitz.de (N.H.); robert.stojan@uni-muenster.de (R.S.)
2 Department of Neuromotor Behavior and Exercise, Institute of Sport and Exercise Sciences, University of Muenster, 48149 Muenster, Germany
* Correspondence: claudia.voelcker-rehage@uni-muenster.de; Tel.: +49-251-83-32461

Received: 29 September 2020; Accepted: 16 October 2020; Published: 3 November 2020

Abstract: Numerous studies have reported the beneficial effects of acute exercise on executive functions. Less is known, however, about the effects of exercise on working memory as one subcomponent of executive functions and about its effects on older adults. We investigated the effects of acute moderate-intensity exercise on working memory performance, the respective cortical hemodynamic activation patterns, and the development and persistence of such effects in healthy older adults. Forty-four participants (*M*: 69.18 years ± 3.92; 21 females) performed a letter 2-back task before and at three time points after (post 15 min, post 30 min, and post 45 min) either listening to an audiobook or exercising (15 min; 50% VO_2-peak). Functional near-infrared spectroscopy (fNIRS) was used to assess cortical hemodynamic activation and brain-behavior correlations in the fronto-parietal working memory network. Overall, we found no group differences for working memory performance. However, only within the experimental group, 2-back performance was enhanced 15 min and 45 min post-exercise. Furthermore, 15 min post-exercise frontal activation predicted working memory performance, regardless of group. In sum, our results indicate slight beneficial effects of acute moderate-intensity exercise on working memory performance in healthy older adults. Findings are discussed in light of the cognitive aging process and moderators affecting the exercise-cognition relationship.

Keywords: aging; cardiovascular exercise; cognition; executive functions; fronto-parietal network; neuroimaging

1. Introduction

Numerous studies in the field of sport and exercise sciences have focused on the human aging process and examined the relationship between chronic exercise and cognition from a neuroscientific perspective [1,2]. More recently, researchers have become increasingly interested in how and to what extent a single bout of exercise (also referred to as acute exercise) affects cognitive performance in executive control tasks. Executive control is a concept that encompasses a number of processes, such as updating of information, shifting between tasks, and inhibiting responses and/or information [3,4]. The premise underlying acute exercise-executive control research is that physiological changes (e.g., increased cerebral blood flow) induced by acute exercise have the potential to improve executive control [5].

Meta-analytic evidence suggests that acute exercise might be particularly beneficial for older adults [6,7], probably due to compromised cognitive reserve and frontal lobe functioning and they thus have greater capacity for improvement in response to exercise compared to young adults [8]. Yet, age-related changes differ noticeably both inter- and intra-individually and across cognitive domains [9,10], and hence it is probably also the case with the effects of exercise. One executive function particularly sensitive to age-related decline is working memory [11–13]. Working memory is an important component underlying higher-level cognitive processes [9], such as language comprehension, learning, and reasoning, which requires simultaneous storage and processing of information [3]. Working memory performance decreases with age due to neural changes of the underlying brain networks [14,15]. Verbal working memory tasks (e.g., the letter n-back task) have been typically associated with a frontal left dominant neural activation pattern in young adults [16–18]. Yet, bilateral hemispheric recruitment of the prefrontal cortex (PFC) has been described to occur as an age-independent domain-general strategy to master increasing task demands [19]. Typically, older adults show a hemispheric asymmetry reduction of prefrontal activation, which is generally referred to as the hemispheric asymmetry reduction in older adults (HAROLD) model [20]. In addition to frontal brain regions, parietal brain regions are likewise involved in the human working memory network. Within the fronto-parietal working memory network [21], frontal regions are associated with the executive processing components [22]. These processing components have been reported to be more affected by the human aging process than the temporary storage components associated with parietal brain regions [18,23], where the integration of visuo-spatial and associative information takes place [24]. Similarly, evidence from neuroimaging studies supports the hypothesis that older adults show a relative reduction in occipital activity, accompanied by a relative increase in frontal activity [25,26], which is discussed as a posterior-anterior shift in aging (PASA) [27]. Further, working memory performance decrements in older adults seem to be associated with structural alterations [28,29] in cerebral microcirculation, which implies age-related decline in microvascular density, thereby contributing to a reduction in cerebral blood flow [30,31]. This, in turn, is likely to reduce metabolic support for neural signaling, especially when levels of neural activity are high, thus contributing to a decline in cognitive performance [30].

One method to investigate the different cortical hemodynamic activation patterns during cognitive testing is functional near-infrared spectroscopy (fNIRS). fNIRS is an optical neuroimaging method that allows for measuring brain tissue concentration changes of oxygenated (O_2Hb) and deoxygenated hemoglobin (HHb) in the cortex, based on the different absorption spectra of the two chromophores in the near-infrared wavelength range [32]. By shining near-infrared light (650–950 nm) on the scalp and placing a detector a few centimeters apart, changes in the amount of diffuse light reaching the detector provide a measure of changes in cerebral hemoglobin concentrations [33]. Moreover, fNIRS is a non-invasive, safe, portable, and relatively low-cost brain imaging method that is especially well-suited for exercise-cognition research, as it is fairly robust against motion artifacts and has a relatively short preparation time [33–35]. Cognitively demanding tasks, such as the n-back task [36], typically lead to an increase of O_2Hb and an anticorrelated decrease of HHb (i.e., the hemodynamic response function) in the blood because of changes in cerebral blood flow due to neurovascular coupling [37,38]. This is interpreted as an indicator of functional brain activity [39–41]. The benefit of applying functional neuroimaging methods, such as fNIRS, in the field of acute exercise-cognition research is that it allows investigating to what extent exercise-induced changes in neural processes underly behavioral outcomes [5].

So far, only three studies have investigated the effects of acute exercise on executive functions in healthy older adults using fNIRS out of which one investigated working memory performance [42] and two inhibitory control [43,44]. In older adults, benefits on working memory performance following an acute bout of light intensity exercise have been found to be accompanied by increased cerebral blood flow in the left PFC while performing a delayed match-to-sample task [42], whereas benefits on inhibitory control (i.e., the Stroop task) have been reported to be accompanied by increased activation bilaterally in the dorsolateral prefrontal cortex (DLPFC), ventrolateral prefrontal cortex (VLPFC) [44], and right frontopolar area [43] following an acute bout of moderate-intensity exercise. This has been interpreted as a compensatory process in light of the HAROLD model [20]. Due to limited evidence from studies with older adults, studies with younger adults might serve to narrow down possible acute exercise effects in older adults. In young adults, benefits on working memory performance following an acute bout of light-intensity exercise were accompanied by increased cerebral blood flow in the right VLPFC at low levels of task demands in a spatial working memory task [45]. Conversely, a supramaximal intensity (i.e., Wingate anaerobic test) showed no beneficial effect on 2-back task performance despite higher prefrontal oxygenation in both hemispheres in young adults [46]. Most fNIRS studies that assessed acute exercise-induced effects in young adults, however, have been conducted in the domain of inhibitory control [47–51]. These studies revealed a beneficial effect of an acute bout of exercise on inhibitory control (i.e., Stroop [47–50] and Go-/No-Go task performance [51]). This was shown particularly for acute moderate [48,49,51], but also for acute light [43] and high-intensity intermittent exercise [50]. In young adults, these performance increments were accompanied by increased cerebral blood flow either in the left DLPFC [49,50], the left DLPFC and FPA [47], or bilaterally in the DLPFC [48] for the Stroop task. For the Go/No-Go task, decreased cortical activation bilaterally in the DLPFC and in the supplementary motor area was associated with better performance in young adults [51]. Taken together, the beneficial effects of acute exercise seem to be independent of age, but the cortical hemodynamic activation patterns related to improved task performance appear to depend on the executive control task and differ between younger and older adults.

Another influencing factor on the exercise-cognition relationship is the time point of cognitive task assessment post-exercise [5,6]. Overall, studies with both young [44–51] and older adults [42–44] either looked at the immediate effects (up to 5 min post-exercise) of acute exercise [44,51] or were restricted to a time window ranging from 5 min [45–48], 10 min [42], 15 min [43,49,50], up to 30 min [45] post-exercise and investigated inhibitory control [43,44,47–51] or working memory performance [42,45,46]. However, systematic investigations of the persistence of acute exercise effects are missing. As a result, little is known about the development and persistence of acute exercise effects over time after exercise cessation. This, however, can be seen as a prerequisite regarding the practical relevance of acute exercise (e.g., active work breaks) or the design of exercise programs in clinical settings (e.g., stroke rehabilitation).

To sum up, past studies with older adults suggest a positive link between acute moderate-intensity exercise and inhibitory control [43,44], but evidence on exercise-induced changes on working memory remains scarce [42]. Moreover, investigations have been restricted to the immediate effects within a time window of 30 min post-exercise in young adults and 15 min post-exercise in older adults. Also, the underlying cortical hemodynamic activation patterns need further investigation. Therefore, the aim of this study was threefold. First, we aimed to investigate how an acute bout of moderate-intensity exercise (50% VO$_2$-peak) affects working memory performance at three time points after exercise cessation (i.e., post 15 min, post 30 min, and post 45 min) in a sample of healthy older adults. Secondly, we applied multichannel fNIRS to examine exercise-induced changes in cortical hemodynamic activation patterns. Thirdly, we assessed how changes on the behavioral level (i.e., 2-back task performance) were related to exercise-induced changes in cerebral blood flow in task-relevant regions, mainly the fronto-parietal working memory network. Based on the current literature on inhibitory control and working memory in young and older adults, we hypothesized that an acute bout of moderate-intensity exercise improves working memory performance, as assessed by the 2-back task and that these performance improvements would persist at least up to 15 min after exercise cessation. With regard to cortical hemodynamic activation patterns, we expected higher cortical activation in frontal, compared to parietal brain regions in both groups. Within frontal brain regions, we expected the experimental group (EG) to show higher cortical activation than the control group (CG) at least up to 15 min post-exercise. Further, we expected the exercise-induced increase in cerebral blood flow in left frontal brain regions to be positively related to 2-back task performance.

2. Materials and Methods

2.1. Participants

Forty-four healthy, right-handed [52] older adults between 64 and 79 years of age (mean age: 69.18 years ± 3.92; 21 females) participated in this study. Participants were re-recruited as part of a study within the DFG (German Research Foundation, Bonn, Germany) Priority Program SPP 1772 "Multitasking". Participants were recruited from the participant pool of the Cognition, Brain and Movement Lab of Chemnitz University of Technology (Chemnitz, Germany), newspaper articles and radio announcements by the press office and cross media department of the university, and in person during university lectures for older adults. All participants took part voluntarily in the study and provided written informed consent. Further, they provided medical clearance from a cardiologist to participate in the cardiovascular fitness test (VO_2-peak).

Participants received no monetary compensation. The study was approved by the local ethics commission of the faculty of Behavioral and Social Sciences of Chemnitz University of Technology, Germany (V-280-17-CVR-Multitasking-29062018) and was conducted in accordance with the latest version of the Declaration of Helsinki. Interested volunteers were screened for the following exclusion criteria in an initial telephone interview: (a) Age range violations (<65 and >80 years; an exception was made for one participant aged 64 as the spouse was already enrolled in the study), (b) use of walking aids, (c) former or current health impairments (severe cardiovascular diseases, such as heart attacks, neurological diseases, stroke; and motor impairments limiting the participant to walk uninterrupted for 30 min, vision impairments or current relevant injuries), (d) obesity (Body Mass Index (BMI) cut-off: BMI > 30), and (e) left-handedness. All interested eligible participants were sent a comprehensive questionnaire concerning demographics, health status, and physical activity level (adopted version of the Baecke Physical Activity Questionnaire) [53], which they were asked to bring with them on their first testing day. Further exclusion tests were applied based on participants' first laboratory test day: (a) Screening for hand dominance [52], (right handers only), (b) Mini Mental State Examination (MMSE) cut-off: <27 [54], and (c) abnormalities in the Freiburg Visual Acuity Test (FrACT; version 3.9.0) [55]. No participant had to be excluded based on these tests. After screening and exercise testing, participants were matched with respect to age, cardiovascular fitness level, and gender (cf. Table 1) and either assigned to an EG or a CG. Sample size was calculated using G*Power [56]. We assumed a small to moderate effect size of $f^2 = 0.20$ (alpha = 0.05, $1 - p = 0.80$, numerator df = 1, number of groups = 2, number of measurements = 4) based on a previous study by Hyodo and colleagues [43]. A total sample of $N = 36$ was estimated to achieve sufficient statistical power to detect differences between the two groups. Taking attrition of typically 20% into account, we recruited a total sample of $N = 44$ older adults. Data from two participants were excluded from all analyses due to a lack of understanding of the cognitive task. The characteristics of the remaining 42 participants are summarized in Table 1. We had to exclude another seven participants from the fNIRS ANOVA as their fNIRS data were incomplete, either for technical reasons ($n = 3$), insufficient fNIRS signal quality ($n = 3$) at one time-point, or due to physical discomfort of the participant ($n = 1$), resulting in a sample of $n = 35$ for the fNIRS ANOVA (cf. Table S1).

Table 1. Participant characteristics of the experimental (EG) and control group (CG).

Variable	EG (n = 19)	CG (n = 23)	p
Age (range)	68.26 ± 3.31 (65 – 79)	69.7 ± 4.23 (64 – 79)	0.226
Gender (f|m)	10|9	10|13	0.779
BMI (kg/m^2)	24.47 ± 2.23	24.91 ± 2.39	0.539
Education (years)	15.66 ± 2.36	15.85 ± 2.31	0.795
MMSE (sum score)	29.28 ± 0.11	29.09 ± 1.16	0.568
VO$_2$-peak (mL/kg/min)	25.48 ± 5.98	24.52 ± 6.29	0.617
Heat rate (bpm) at VO$_2$-peak	138.55 ± 18.27	135.40 ± 16.94	0.569
Watt (W) at VO$_2$-peak	135.84 ± 30.29	139.09 ± 39.61	0.767
Borg score (RPE) at VO$_2$-peak	12.30 ± 1.29	12.39 ± 1.83	0.862

Note. All values are given as mean (*M*) ± standard deviation (*SD*). Age = age in years; Gender = female|male; BMI = Body Mass Index expressed in kg/m^2; Education = years of formal education; MMSE = sum score of the Mini Mental State Examination; VO$_2$-peak = peak oxygen uptake during the cardiovascular fitness test expressed in mL/kg/min; bpm = beats per minute; RPE = rate of perceived exertion according to Borg's 6–20 RPE scale.

2.2. Behavioral Measurements

2.2.1. Working Memory Task

Working memory performance was assessed by use of a letter n-back task. Stimuli consisted of white letters in Arial font with a stimulus object size of 180 pixels, which were presented in the center of a screen on a black background (24 inch monitor (IIYAMA G-Master GB2488HSU-B2, IIYAMA CORPORATION, HA Hoofddorp, The Netherlands, screen resolution of 1920 × 1080 pixels)). The software, Presentation, version 20.3, Build 02.25.19 (NeuroBehavioral Systems, Inc., Berkeley, CA, USA) was used for stimulus presentation and behavioral recordings (reaction time (RT) and accuracy (ACC)). Each stimulus was presented for 500 ms followed by a response interval of 1500 ms in which a white fixation cross was displayed instead of the stimulus, resulting in a total response window of 2000 ms. A randomized stimulus onset jitter between 800–1200 ms (on average 1000 ms) was implemented, resulting in an averaged total trial time of 3000 ms. The participants' task was to decide whether the displayed letter matched the letter in the previous trial (1-back condition) or two trials before (2-back condition). In the 0-back condition, the letter "X" served as the target, whereas in the 1-back and 2-back condition, the target was randomly selected out of a set of 20 consonants. All conditions were presented randomly in two blocks of 15 trials, of which five were target trials. Every condition was followed by a rest period of 27 s, during the last 5 s of which the instructions for the next trial were displayed. Every block had a duration of 45 s. For each trial, participants indicated whether the stimulus was a target (= match) trial by pressing a green button with their index finger (right arrow key), or a non-target (= non-match) trial by pressing a red button with their middle finger (down arrow key) installed on a German keyboard. Before the experiment started, all participants performed either one or two practice blocks per condition (15–30 trials) to familiarize themselves with the task. The total duration of the n-back task was 6:45 min. Participants were seated comfortably in a quiet, dimly lit room at a viewing distance of approximately 90 cm from the screen. Participants were instructed to respond as fast and as accurately as possible.

2.2.2. Perceived Difficulty of the Working Memory Task

As cognitive load has a crucial impact on behavioral performance, participants were asked to indicate the perceived difficulty of each load condition and the control condition of the n-back task on Borg's 6–20 RPE scale [57] for each time point.

2.2.3. Behavioral Data Preprocessing

Behavioral data of the n-back task were preprocessed using R 3.6.3 [58] and RStudio 1.2.5033 [59], with speed (RT) and ACC as outcome measures for behavioral performance. The first two trials from every block for each load condition were discarded from analysis, since in the 2-back condition the first two trials are necessarily non-match trials, resulting in 26 trials per condition and time point. In case of a premature response (RT < 200 ms) [60], or a response omission (RT > 2000 ms) [61], a trial was counted as an error, resulting in a response window between 200 ms and 2000 ms after stimulus onset. N-back task performance was included if a participant reached at least 73% correct responses corresponding to 19 out of 26 trials (99% quantile of the binomial distribution with $N = 26$ and $p = 0.5$) in the 1-back condition at pretest (exclusion of $n = 1$ participant). Further, standardized z-scores were used to identify and discard extreme values ($|z| > 3.29$) in the rate-correct score (cf. below) across all participants for each combination of load condition and time point (exclusion of $n = 1$ participant). Further, we combined RT and ACC into a single performance measure to control for speed–accuracy trade-offs [62], by use of the rate-correct score (RCS) as an index of response speed adjusted for errors [63]. For statistical analysis, the RCS was computed for each condition for all time points as participants' number of correct responses divided by the sum of RTs for all responses (both correct and incorrect). The RCS can be interpreted directly as correct responses per time unit (seconds in our case). A higher RCS represents better overall performance on the n-back task.

2.3. fNIRS Measurements

Concentration changes in the amount of oxygenated (O$_2$Hb), deoxygenated (HHb), and total hemoglobin (HbT) in the cortex were recorded by use of two portable, continuous-wave fNIRS optical tomography systems (NIRSport 88, NIRx Medical Technologies LLC, New York, NY, USA) in a single-subject tandem setup. The montage setup consisted of 16 illuminating sources (LED; time multiplexing) and 16 detectors (silicon photodiode), arranged at an inter-optode distance of approximately 3 cm, providing an adequate compromise between depth sensitivity and signal-to-noise ratio [64]. The NIRScaps for optode placement (EASYCAP GmbH, Herrsching, Germany) were available in four different sizes (head circumferences of 54 cm, 56 cm, 58 cm, and 60 cm) and suitable for all participants. The center of the NIRScap was placed according to the international 10-20 system over the vertex (Cz), by marking the halfway point between nasion and inion and the left and right preauricular points [65]. A retaining overcap (EASYCAP GmbH, Herrsching, Germany) was attached on top of the NIRScap to ensure that no ambient light from other sources (e.g., sunlight, room light) than the fNIRS device could interfere with the fNIRS signal. All data sets were recorded using the acquisition software NIRStar 15.2 (NIRx Medical Technologies LLC, New York, NY, USA) at a sampling rate of 3.47 Hz and two wavelengths of near-infrared light (760 nm for HHb and 850 nm for O$_2$Hb). Each recording was preceded by an automatic calibration process, as implemented in the acquisition software NIRStar 15.2 (NIRx Medical Technologies LLC, New York, NY, USA) to determine an optimum amplification factor of 0.4–4.0 V for each channel (i.e., source-detector combination). Participants were asked to avoid head movements, frowning, jaw clenching, or talking during the experiment to minimize extracerebral contamination of the fNIRS signal.

2.3.1. fNIRS Probe Placement and Region of Interest (ROI) Definition

We used the automated anatomical labeling atlas Brodman [66], as implemented in the fNIRS Optodes' Location Decider (fOLD) to assign cortical hemodynamic changes during the 2-back task to specific brain regions [67]. For the frontal cortex, we set the fNIRS probes to cover the left (channel 1–4) and right (channel 14, 15, 17, 18) DLPFC (BA 9/46) and the left (channel 5–9) and right (channel 10–13, 16) VLPFC (BA 44/45). For the parietal cortex, we set the fNIRS probes to cover the left (channel 19, 21–23, 25) and right (channel 29, 31–33, 35) inferior parietal lobe (IPL; BA 39/40) and the left (channel 20, 24) and right (channel 30, 34) superior parietal lobe (SPL; BA 7) (cf. Figure 1a). Based on this assumption, we excluded all channels from further analysis which did not cover our ROI, namely the fronto-parietal network, that were channels 26 (S11-D12), 27 (S12-D11), and 28 (S12-D12) on the left hemisphere, and channels 36 (S15-D16), 37 (S16-D15), and 38 (S16-D16) on the right hemisphere. Overall, this procedure led to a montage setup with 18 channels covering the bilateral DLPFC and VLPFC, and 14 channels covering the bilateral IPL and SPL. An overview of the spatial organization and the sensitivity profile of the fNIRS optode placement is shown in Figure 1. A detailed overview of all channels and their respective international 10–20 system position [68] and corresponding ROI can be found in the supplements (cf. Table S2). The probabilistic path of photon migration through the head for the sensitivity profile was estimated using the Monte-Carlo photon transport software tMCimg via the Atlas Viewer from HomER2 [69,70] (cf. Figure 1b).

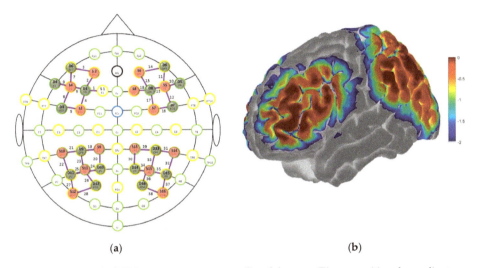

Figure 1. (a) For the fNIRS measurements, sources (S) and detectors (D) were positioned according to the international 10–20 system; (b) results of the Monte-Carlo simulation based on 1×10^{-7} photons (per optode) over the frontal and parietal cortex from a lateral view; the colorbar unit represents the spatial sensitivity of the fNIRS measurements. It is expressed in mm^{-1} and values range from 0.01 to 1 in log10 units: −2 to 0.

2.3.2. fNIRS Data Preprocessing

Preprocessing was performed in Matlab R2018a (The MathWorks, Natick, MA, USA) and by use of additional scripts from the HomER2 toolbox, version 2.3 [69]. First, the raw optical intensity time series data were converted to changes in optical density (OD) using the hmrIntensity2OD function [71]. We plotted the power spectrum of every O_2Hb time series to assess the quality of the fNIRS signal. Since a frequency peak of the cardiac activity around 1 Hz in the O_2Hb signal indicates good contact between the optical probe and the scalp [72], every channel that did not match this criterion was excluded from further analysis. Following this procedure, 11.43% of the data across all participants and time points were removed from further analysis. Correction for motion artifacts was performed using wavelet filtering, which has been described as a promising approach to reduce the influence of motion artifacts [71]. We used an algorithm described by Molavi and Dumont [73], as implemented in the HomER2 hmrMotionCorrectWavelet filtering function. The algorithm applies a probability threshold for removing outlying wavelet coefficients, which were assumed to correspond to motion artifacts. We used a threshold of 0.1 times the inter-quartile range, as recommended [73]. We then applied a band-pass filter (third-order low-pass and fifth-order high-pass Butterworth filter) with cut-off frequencies of 0.01–0.08 Hz to remove physiological noise like cardiac frequency, respiratory frequency, Mayer waves, and very low-frequency oscillations [39]. Then, the OD time-series data were converted into concentration changes expressed in units of molar $\times 10^{-8}$ of O_2Hb, HHb, and HbT using the modified Beer-Lambert law [74], that included an age-dependent differential path length factor (DPF) using the following formula: $DPF_{807} = 4.99 + 0.067 \times A^{0.814}$, where DPF is the DPF measured at 807 nm and A is age in years [75]. All trials related to the same condition and time point were block averaged (time window: −2 to 45 s) using the HomER2 hmrBlockAvg function to recover the mean hemodynamic response. Finally, to remove remaining outliers, we standardized the range of each condition for each time point across all channels by use of standardized z-scores and excluded all channels outside the range of |3.29| (99.95% quantile of the standard normal distribution). Based on this approach, 1.58% of the data were removed from further analysis. For statistical analysis, we combined O_2Hb and HHb into a single measure of cortical activation by use of hemoglobin difference (HBdiff = O_2Hb − HHb) which represents oxygen supply (saturation as measured by O_2Hb) versus demand (extraction as measured by HHb) [76].

2.4. Cardiovascular Fitness Test

Cardiovascular fitness was assessed by spiroergometry (ZAN600 CPET, nSpire Health, Oberthulba, Germany) on a stationary bicycle (Lode Corival cpet, Groningen, The Netherlands) by use of a ramp protocol to determine participants' peak oxygen consumption (VO_2-peak). A ramp protocol with a progressively increasing load of 15 W/min, starting with 10 W, was used for women and a progressively increasing load of 20 W/min, starting with 20 W, was used for men. Participants were told to keep their revolutions per minute (rpm) between 60 and 80. All tests were supervised by an experienced sports scientist. Electrocardiography (recorded with a twelve-lead ECG fully digital stress system; Kiss, GE Healthcare, Munich, Germany), breath-by-breath respiration, heart rate, and blood pressure were monitored continuously. Every two minutes, participants were asked to indicate their rate of perceived exertion (RPE) on Borg's 6–20 RPE scale [57]. The scale ranged from 6 = "very easy" to 20 = "extremely difficult".

All spiroergometry protocols started with a 3 min rest period and finished with a 5 min cool-down period (1 min initial load and then no load). Tests were terminated due to volitional exhaustion, or (at the latest) by reaching a respiratory exchange ratio of ≥1.05–1.10 for more than 30 s. Further, protocols were terminated if the maximum age-predicted heart rate was reached (approximately >(220−age)) or a risk factor occurred (i.e., systolic blood pressure ≥230/115 mmHg, abnormal ECG response). Participants' VO_2-peak was determined by the average of the last five values of the last fully completed load level (approximately 10 s). The watt level corresponding to 50% of the individual participants' VO_2-peak was used to determine the individual intensity of the acute exercise intervention. We opted against a maximal graded exercise test, since raising the exercise intensity to the level of VO_2-max was considered unsafe for older adults due to medical concerns. Participants were asked to avoid any vigorous exercise and consumption of caffeine and alcohol for at least 12 h before exercise testing.

2.5. Exercise Intervention

All participants assigned to the EG cycled at 50% of their individual VO_2-peak for a duration of 15 min on a stationary bicycle (Lode Corival cpet, Groningen, the Netherlands) with a cadence between 60 and 80 rpm. Participants were fitted with a Polar A300 heart rate (HR) monitor (Polar Electro Oy, Kempele, Finland) with an H7 HR sensor (Polar Electro Oy, Kempele, Finland) to measure their HR during the exercise intervention, just before commencement (pre) and during the n-back task at multiple time points post-exercise (i.e., post 15 min, post 30 min, and post 45 min). Further, participants were asked to indicate their rate of perceived exertion (RPE) by pointing with their index finger on Borg's 6–20 RPE scale [57], just before the start, every 2 min during, and at the end of the exercise intervention as an indicator of physiological arousal and to control for exercise intensity.

We chose a moderate intensity corresponding to 50% of participants' VO_2-peak and lasting for 15 min, since the largest benefits for executive control tasks have been associated with moderate-intensity exercise and a duration of 10–20 min [6,77]. Additionally, cerebral blood flow has been reported to increase between low and moderate exercise intensities, to remain stable from moderate-to-hard intensities and then to decline at very hard or maximal intensities to oxygenation values similar to those observed during low-intensity exercise [78].

The watt level during the exercise intervention ranged from 40 W to 104 W, with a mean of 68.11 W ± 15.23 (cf. Table 1 for VO$_2$-peak values). At the end of the acute exercise intervention, average heart rate and RPE were 119.84 ± 17.90 beats per minute (bpm) (cf. Figure 2) and 13.63 ± 2.14 points on Borg's 6–20 RPE scale [57], respectively, which corresponds to moderate-intensity exercise according to the guidelines of the American College of Sports Medicine [79]. At the start of the first n-back task after the exercise intervention (i.e., post 15 min), participants' HR was, on average, 77.42 bpm (*SD* = 13.26), that is 11.57% higher (*SD* = 9.08) than their average HR at rest. After 45 min, the averaged HR was 70.11 bpm (*SD* = 11.43), that is 1.28% higher (*SD* = 8.53) than the average HR at rest; thus, HR values returned to baseline approximately at the start of the last follow-up measurement (i.e., post 45 min).

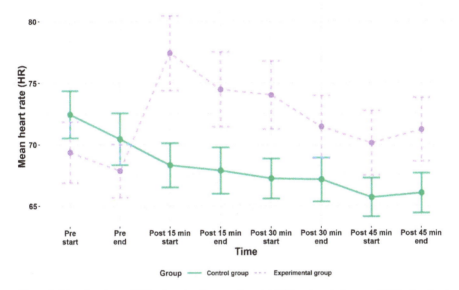

Figure 2. Mean heart rate (HR) values for the experimental (EG) and control group (CG) before (pre) and post-exercise (follow-up measurements) for the beginning (start) and the end of each n-back task. All values are given as mean (*M*); error bars represent one standard error (*SE*) of the mean.

As expected, the HR values of the CG remained relatively stable from time point pre to post 45 min. All HR values before (pre) and post-exercise (follow-up measurements) for the beginning (start) and the end of each n-back task can be found in the Supplementary Materials (cf. Table S3).

2.6. Design and Testing Procedures

This study was designed as a between-subjects pre- and post-test comparison. Participants visited the laboratory twice. On their first visit, they returned the questionnaires concerning demographics, health status, and physical activity level which they had filled out at home. In addition, all participants performed the cardiovascular fitness test (spiroergometry). During their second visit, all participants assigned to the EG performed the n-back task (cf. Figure 3b) before exercising at 50% of their VO$_2$-peak for 15 min on a stationary bicycle (Lode Corival cpet, Groningen, The Netherlands), as well as 15 min, 30 min, and 45 min after exercise cessation (cf. Figure 3a). Participants in the CG listened to an audiobook for 15 min instead of exercising. fNIRS data were recorded before exercise and post 15 min, post 30 min, and post 45 min, but not during exercise or while listening to the audiobook in the control condition, respectively.

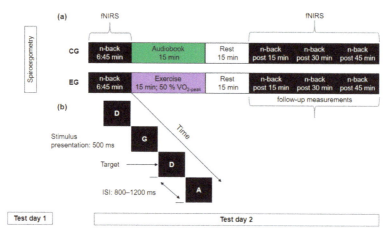

Figure 3. (**a**) Schematic illustration of the design and testing procedures consisting of two test days for the experimental (EG) and control group (CG). Using functional near-infrared spectroscopy (fNIRS), cortical hemodynamic activation was measured while participants performed the letter n-back task. (**b**) Schematic illustration of the 2-back condition of the n-back task. Stimulus presentation time was 500 ms, inter stimulus interval (ISI) was 800–1200 ms (on average 1000 ms). Participants were allowed to respond up to 2000 ms.

2.7. Statistical Analysis

All statistical analyses were performed using R 3.6.3 [58] and RStudio 1.2.5033 [59]. The additional packages "ez" [80] and "emmeans" [81], were used for the mixed repeated measures analysis of variance (ANOVA) and post-hoc comparisons. Plots were created with the "ggplot2" package [82]. Perceived difficulty of the n-back task was analyzed by a 2 (group: Experimental, control) × 4 (time: Pre, post 15 min, post 30 min, post 45 min) × 3 (load condition: 0-back, 1-back, 2-back) mixed repeated measures ANOVA, with group as the between-subjects factor and time and load condition as within-subjects factors. Due to ceiling effects in the control condition (0-back) and in the low-working memory load condition (1-back) in terms of ACC and as cognitive load has a crucial impact both on behavioral performance and neural effort, we limited our analysis to the 2-back condition.

Behavioral data (RCS) were analyzed with a 2 (group: Experimental, control) × 4 (time: Pre, post 15 min, post 30 min, post 45 min) mixed repeated measures ANOVA with group as between-subjects factor and time as within-subjects factor under the highest cognitive load condition (i.e., 2-back). Further, to test our hypothesis that acute exercise effects would persist at least up to 15 min after exercise cessation and to assess performance improvements over the course of the experiment within each group, we used planned contrasts to calculate differences between time point pre and the three follow-up measurement time points for each group.

For the hemodynamic data, HBdiff for the DLPFC and VLPFC were strongly correlated ($r = 0.78$, $p < 0.001$ for left hemisphere; $r = 0.83$, $p < 0.001$ for right hemisphere) and did not differ significantly. Likewise, the IPL and SPL data were strongly correlated ($r = 0.92$, $p < 0.001$ for left hemisphere; $r = 0.87$, $p < 0.001$ for right hemisphere). Further, HBdiff for the averaged right and left DLPFC and VLPFC data ($r = 0.81$, $p < 0.001$ for frontal cortex), as well as the averaged right and left IPL and SPL data ($r = 0.91$, $p < 0.001$ for parietal cortex) were strongly correlated, as well as the frontal and parietal data within each hemisphere ($r = 0.73$, $p < 0.001$ for left hemisphere and $r = 0.84$, $p < 0.001$ for right hemisphere). We therefore pooled and averaged the DLPFC and VLPFC to "frontal" and the IPL and SPL data to "parietal" by hemisphere. Likewise, the frontal and parietal data were pooled and averaged by hemisphere to the "left" and "right" hemispheres, respectively. fNIRS data (HBdiff) were analyzed with a 2 (group: Experimental, control) × 4 (time: Pre, post 15 min, post 30 min, post 45 min)

× 2 (region: Frontal, parietal) × 2 (hemisphere: Left, right) repeated measures ANOVA with group as between-subjects factor and time, region, and hemisphere as within-subjects factors under the highest cognitive load condition (i.e., 2-back). Further, to test our hypothesis that HBdiff values were higher in ROI frontal left compared to the parietal brain regions, we calculated planned contrasts. Additionally, planned contrasts were calculated similarly to the behavioral data, for time point pre compared to the three follow-up measurement time points for each group.

All planned contrasts were corrected according to the Bonferroni procedure, if necessary. If sphericity was violated (using Mauchly's test), the data were Greenhouse-Geisser-corrected. For all analyses, p-values < 0.05 were regarded as significant. Effect sizes were calculated for significant results by generalized eta squared (η_{ges}^2). Post-hoc testing was carried out using Welch's t-test for pairwise comparisons of estimated marginal means (emmeans) with Bonferroni-adjusted alpha levels to determine pre- to post-measurement changes. EG and CG were statistically similar to one another on measures of age, gender, BMI, years of formal education, MMSE, and cardiovascular fitness level, as determined by paired t-tests and a chi-square test for gender (cf. Table 1). Consequently, we abstained from including covariates.

To assess the relation between behavioral and neurophysiological data, correlation and multiple regression analyses via the forced entry procedure were computed for each time point with group and HBdiff for each ROI (frontal left and right, parietal left and right) as predictors for behavioral performance (RCS) under the highest cognitive load condition (i.e., 2-back) in the regression models. We abstained from including BMI in the correlational analysis, as all participants had normal weight. From the remaining factors, only the MMSE revealed a significant correlation coefficient, which was then included into the regression models.

3. Results

3.1. Behavioral Results—Rate-Correct Score (RCS)

As shown in Figure 4, working memory performance improved in both groups from time point pre to post 15 min at which performance differences between the two groups were most pronounced in favor of the EG. This is evidenced by a higher RCS, indicating better overall performance on the 2-back task. For RCS data, the repeated-measures ANOVA revealed a main effect of time, $F(2.75, 110.05) = 6.54$, $p = 0.001$, $\eta_{ges}^2 = 0.03$, indicating that performance improved over time.

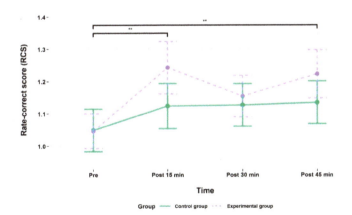

Figure 4. 2-back task performance as measured by the rate-correct score (RCS) for the experimental (EG) and control group (CG) at time point pre (baseline) and at the follow-up measurements after the acute exercise intervention (EG) or listening to the audiobook (CG), respectively. All values are given as mean (*M*); error bars represent one standard error (*SE*) of the mean. ** $p < 0.01$.

For time, a priori planned contrasts revealed for the EG a significant difference in 2-back task performance between time points pre (*M*: 1.05, *SE*: 0.05) and post 15 min (*M*: 1.24, *SE*: 0.08; $p \leq 0.001$), and also post 45 min (*M*: 1.22, *SE*: 0.07; $p = 0.001$), indicating significant performance improvements with reference to the time point pre. For the CG, no such differences were found in any contrast. All behavioral results (RCS, perceived difficulty) and the values that were used to calculate the RCS (RT, ACC) are summarized in Table 2. The corresponding values for these parameters for the control condition (0-back) and the low-working memory load condition (1-back) can be found in the Supplementary Materials (cf. Tables S4 and S5).

Table 2. Time course of 2-back task performance for the experimental (EG) and control group (CG).

	Time Point	EG (*n* = 19)	CG (*n* = 23)
		2-back	2-back
RT per trial (ms)	Pre	837.34 ± 37.65	885.07 ± 57.39
	Post 15 min	788.38 ± 47.22	857.52 ± 57.18
	Post 30 min	809.00 ± 43.07	847.58 ± 49.49
	Post 45 min	796.57 ± 46.10	846.37 ± 51.21
ACC (%)	Pre	84.62 ± 2.39	86.62 ± 2.56
	Post 15 min	91.70 ± 1.84	88.46 ± 1.98
	Post 30 min	88.87 ± 1.74	88.80 ± 1.23
	Post 45 min	91.70 ± 1.67	89.30 ± 1.69
RCS	Pre	1.05 ± 0.05	1.05 ± 0.07
	Post 15 min	1.24 ± 0.08	1.12 ± 0.07
	Post 30 min	1.15 ± 0.06	1.13 ± 0.07
	Post 45 min	1.22 ± 0.07	1.13 ± 0.07
Perceived difficulty	Pre	14.26 ± 0.42	13.91 ± 0.37
	Post 15 min	13.42 ± 0.50	12.96 ± 0.37
	Post 30 min	13.37 ± 0.52	13.17 ± 0.36
	Post 45 min	13.58 ± 0.51	12.91 ± 0.43

Note. All values are given as mean (*M*) ± one standard error (*SE*) of the mean; RT = reaction time; ACC = accuracy; RCS = rate–correct score.

3.2. Behavioral Results—Perceived Diffifulty

Perceived difficulty of the n-back task increased as a function of cognitive load from the control condition (0-back) up to the high working memory load condition (2-back) in both groups (cf. Figure 5). This was confirmed by a main effect of condition, $F(1.54, 61.48) = 187.45$, $p < 0.001$, $\eta_{ges}^2 = 0.53$. Further, the main effect of time, $F(2.17, 86.81) = 6.64$, $p = 0.002$, $\eta_{ges}^2 = 0.02$, was statistically significant, indicating that perceived difficulty declined over time. All interaction effects were non-significant (cf. Table S6). Post-hoc analyses indicated that perceived difficulty increased as a function of condition (i.e., cognitive load) from 0-back (*M*: 8.55, *SE*: 0.13) to 1 back (*M*: 10.15, *SE*: 0.14), as well as from 0-back to 2-back (*M*: 13.41, *SE*: 0.14) and from 1-back to 2-back. Further, the "pre" time point (*M*: 11.29, *SE*: 0.24) was perceived as significantly more difficult compared to all other time points: post 15 min (*M*: 10.54, *SE*: 0.24), post 30 min (*M*: 10.50, *SE*: 0.25), and post 45 min (*M*: 10.62, *SE*: 0.26). However, none of the other time points varied in perceived difficulty.

3.3. fNIRS Results

Overall, mean cortical hemodynamic activation, as measured by HBdiff, was higher in the parietal than the frontal brain regions in both groups and was similar for both hemispheres. When comparing the activation between both groups, the CG showed higher values in both regions (frontal, parietal) and hemispheres (left, right) at almost all time points (cf. Figure 6 and Table S7). The ANOVA confirmed a main effect of region, $F(1, 33) = 4.59$, $p = 0.040$, $\eta_{ges}^2 = 0.012$, with higher values for the parietal (*M*: 1.99, *SE*: 0.24) than frontal (*M*: 1.14, *SE*: 0.21) brain regions. All other main and interaction effects yielded non-significant results (cf. Table S8). The planned contrasts between the ROI frontal left and parietal brain regions for each group, as well as between time point pre and the three follow-up measurement time points for each group were non-significant (all $p > 0.05$).

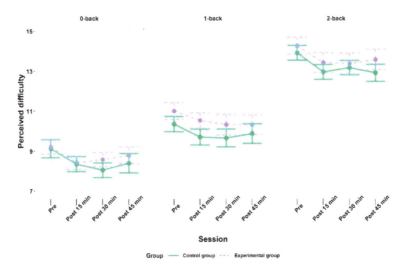

Figure 5. Perceived difficulty of the n-back task indicated by the experimental (EG) and control group (CG) at time point pre (baseline) and at the follow-up measurements after the acute exercise intervention (EG) or listening to the audiobook (CG), respectively. All values are given as mean (M); error bars represent one standard error (SE) of the mean.

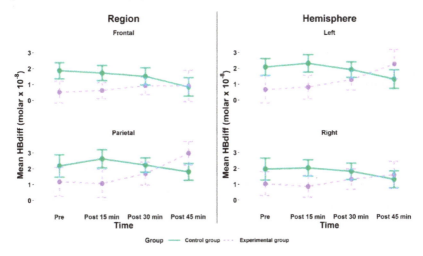

Figure 6. Mean cortical hemodynamic activity as measured by HBdiff in region (frontal, parietal) and hemisphere (**left, right**) during the 2-back task for the experimental (EG) and control group (CG) at time point pre (baseline) and at the follow-up measurements after the acute exercise intervention (EG) or listening to the audiobook (CG), respectively. All values are given as mean (M); error bars represent one standard error (SE) of the mean.

Figure 7 reveals the cortical activation patterns across the 45 s measurement time of the 2-back task. Both groups demonstrated an almost similar time course of activation (i.e., initial increase followed by a peak with a subsequent decrease) with nearly identical magnitude of activation while performing the 2-back task.

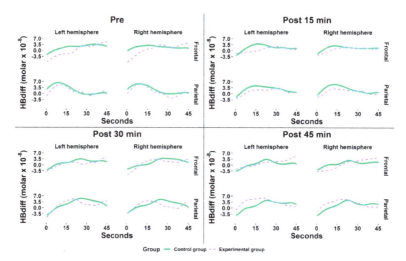

Figure 7. Mean cortical hemodynamic activity as measured by HBdiff during the 2-back task for the experimental (EG) and control group (CG) at the time point pre (baseline) and at the follow-up measurements after the acute exercise intervention (EG) or listening to the audiobook (CG), respectively. All values are given as mean (*M*); the colored frames on the curves correspond to one standard error (*SE*) of the mean.

3.4. Interrelation of HBdiff and Behavioral Performance

We performed correlation and regression analyses to further examine the relationship between HBdiff and 2-back task performance over time (cf. Table 3).

Table 3. Results of the multiple regression analysis with rate-correct score (RCS) as criterion and group, HBdiff for each ROI (frontal left and right, parietal left and right), and MMSE as predictors for each time point.

		Regression Coefficients				F Statistic			
Time Point	Effect	B	β	T	p	F	df	p	adjR²
Pre	Group: EG	0.00	0.00	−0.02	0.986	2.93	6,30	0.023	0.24
	MMSE	0.10	0.38	2.53	0.017				
	Frontal (left)	0.04	0.50	1.51	0.141				
	Frontal (right)	−0.05	−0.74	−1.88	0.069				
	Parietal (left)	0.04	0.60	1.28	0.211				
	Parietal (right)	0.00	−0.08	−0.18	0.857				
Post 15 min	Group: EG	0.18	0.26	1.62	0.116	2.10	6,29	0.083	0.16
	MMSE	0.10	0.31	1.70	0.100				
	Frontal (left)	0.08	0.65	2.64	0.013				
	Frontal (right)	−0.08	−0.62	−2.05	0.049				
	Parietal (left)	0.00	−0.01	−0.01	0.994				
	Parietal (right)	0.04	0.41	0.59	0.563				
Post 30 min	Group: EG	0.06	0.10	0.62	0.540	1.27	6,32	0.299	0.04
	MMSE	0.08	0.30	1.70	0.098				
	Frontal (left)	0.01	0.09	0.25	0.803				
	Frontal (right)	−0.05	−0.67	−1.72	0.095				
	Parietal (left)	0.03	0.35	0.76	0.453				
	Parietal (right)	0.02	0.28	0.58	0.565				
Post 45 min	Group: EG	0.04	0.07	0.42	0.679	1.10	6,31	0.383	0.02
	MMSE	0.06	0.20	1.18	0.246				
	Frontal (left)	0.03	0.47	1.38	0.176				
	Frontal (right)	−0.04	−0.47	−1.42	0.164				
	Parietal (left)	0.01	0.12	0.28	0.783				
	Parietal (right)	0.01	0.11	0.24	0.811				

Note. B = non-standardized coefficients; T = t-test value; EG = experimental group; MMSE = Mini Mental State Examination. For the categorical variable group, the control group (CG) serves as reference category.

There was a significant correlation between the participants' MMSE score and RCS performance at time point pre only ($r = 0.20$, $p < 0.001$). No significant association was found between RCS performance and gender, age, education, and VO_2-peak. Thus, we abstained from including these variables in the regression models. Overall, the regression model with group, HBdiff for each ROI (frontal left and right, parietal left and right), and MMSE as predictors for RCS performance was significant for time point pre ($p = 0.023$). The ROI frontal left significantly predicted RCS performance at time point post 15 min ($B = 0.08$, $p = 0.013$). Hence, if HBdiff in the frontal left ROI increases by 1 (expressed in units of molar $\times 10^{-8}$ of HBdiff), the RCS is estimated to increase by 0.08. All other predictors did not significantly explain variance (cf. Table 3).

4. Discussion

The present study was designed to examine the effects of a 15 min acute bout of moderate-intensity exercise on working memory performance. In order to advance knowledge about acute exercise effects from a neuro-cognitive perspective, cortical hemodynamic activity was assessed during cognitive testing before and at three time points post-exercise (i.e., post 15 min, post 30 min, and post 45 min). We found a significant time effect for working memory performance, but no interaction with the group. Yet, within the exercise group, 2-back task performance was significantly enhanced 15 min and 45 min post-exercise, indicating that exercise might have at least slight effects on working memory performance. Regardless of group, higher cortical activation in the working memory core network (i.e., left frontal) was associated with higher working memory performance at time point post 15 min.

4.1. Effects of Moderate-Intensity Exercise on Behavioral Performance

When interpreting the main effects, behavioral performance analysis did not point to a significant influence of group allocation or measurement time point on 2-back task performance, as measured by the RCS. Thus, we need to assume that the acute exercise intervention did not enhance executive performance compared to the control condition (i.e., listening to an audiobook). However, on the descriptive level and on the level of a priori planned contrasts, the behavioral data suggest an improvement of 2-back task performance due to an acute bout of moderate-intensity exercise, especially 15 min and 45 min post-exercise, thereby providing slight evidence for the beneficial effects of moderate-intensity exercise on working memory performance in older adults. This is in line with previous studies which investigated the effects of acute moderate-intensity exercise on working memory [42,45] and inhibitory control [43,49], by use of a comparable exercise protocol or high-intensity intermittent exercise [50]. However, due to missing interaction effects, the results need to be interpreted with caution.

Despite task familiarization prior to the start of the experiment, practice effects in both groups may have occurred. This is supported by the higher subjective difficulty rating of the first 2-back task run compared to all follow-up measurement time points. One explanation for this might lie in successful strategy use [83] and a less demanding stimulus-response relation due to more automatic motor responses, namely the process of rule learning over time [84]. One option to lower the influence of practice on task performance might have lain in increasing task demands. However, we abstained from including a 3-back condition in our final experimental design as our pilot study had resulted in participants partly performing at chance level.

When investigating the development and persistence of acute moderate-intensity exercise over time, lower intensities have been shown to benefit cognitive performance immediately after exercise, whereas higher exercise intensities have been associated with benefits in cognitive performance with a delay [6]. Therefore, we assumed moderate-intensity exercise (i.e., 50% of participants VO_2-peak) to induce improvements in working memory performance at least up to 15 min post-exercise, as has been shown for inhibitory control tasks in young [49] and older adults [43]. This hypothesis was partly confirmed by planned contrasts within the EG, but not by group differences 15 min post-exercise. One explanation might be that the intensity we used was not strenuous enough to induce more distinct cognitive improvements 15 min post-exercise and beyond. On the other hand, studies with young adults comparing the effects of different exercise intensities either during [85,86], or following an acute bout of exercise [48] point to impairments in cognitive functioning when the physical load becomes too heavy, especially in lower fit individuals [86].

Interestingly, studies investigating moderate-intensity exercise effects on inhibitory control in older adults found significant effects [43,44,49,51]. These divergent findings for inhibitory control and working memory suggest that although inhibition and working memory have a close interrelation and share neural networks [87], acute moderate-intensity exercise might exert differential effects depending on the degree of involvement of each executive function in the task. Further, studies reported only weak to moderate correlations between Stroop and 2-back task performance [88–90]. Compared to the Stroop task [91], as a classical measure of inhibitory control, the letter n-back task is more vulnerable to aging effects due to its manifold cognitive processing efforts [83,92]. Especially in older adults, mainly attentional and verbal memory capacities seem to play a crucial role in the n-back task [92]. In comparison to the n-back task, we understand the Stroop task as a rather pure inhibitory control task, since color-word reading per se is a more automatic process that has to be voluntarily suppressed by ink color naming. Thus, even though the naming condition of the Stroop task is of higher attentional demand and in particular need of control, it might be less cognitively demanding than the 2-back task. In this context, the unique components of inhibition and working memory might need to be disentangled to further our understanding of why acute exercise might exert differential effects on different executive functions.

Even though meta-analytic evidence generally supports the positive effect of acute exercise across several aspects of cognition [6,7,93,94], one may keep in mind that only a few cognitive functions have been studied in the context of exercise-cognition research (predominantly inhibition) and that mainly young adults have been studied [5]. Our results support the assumption that moderate acute exercise does not necessarily improve cognitive performance [5,6]. It is most likely that rather diverse moderators, such as exercise intensity, duration, modality, the cognitive task applied, and the time point of the post-exercise assessment can potentially influence the extent to which acute exercise may have an enhancing effect on cognition [5,6]. Whether the slight effects of acute moderate intensity exercise on working memory performance in our study are due to exercise intensity, duration, or the cognitive task applied remains speculative.

4.2. Effects of Acute Moderate-Intensity Exercise on Cortical Hemodynamic Activation Patterns and Its Relation to Behavioral Performance

This is the first study which investigated the influence of an acute bout of moderate-intensity exercise on working memory performance before and at three time points after exercise cessation (i.e., post 15 min, post 30 min, and post 45 min) in a sample of healthy older adults. Furthermore, we addressed the underlying neural mechanisms by measuring cortical hemodynamic activation patterns using fNIRS. Brain activity was registered in the frontal (DLPFC/VLPFC) and parietal (IPL/SPL) brain regions, while participants performed a letter n-back task to assess the development and persistence of acute moderate-intensity exercise effects over time. Additionally, the relationship between cortical hemodynamic activation patterns and working memory performance was investigated. Overall, we expected cortical hemodynamic activation to be higher in frontal, as compared to parietal brain regions, as described by the PASA model [27] for both groups. Further, we expected cortical hemodynamic activity to be even more pronounced in the EG as a result of an acute exercise-induced increase in cerebral blood flow. Drawing on the results of acute moderate-intensity exercise on working memory [42] and inhibition in older adults [43,44], we expected the EG to show even higher HBdiff values in frontal brain regions compared to the CG at least up to 15 min post-exercise.

Even though there is still some doubt as to whether the recruitment of additional neural resources from anterior regions (e.g., PFC) contributes to the maintenance of cognitive performance in older adults [10,27,95], one potential compensatory mechanism is higher prefrontal activation through upregulation (i.e., an age-related increase in brain activity directly correlated with better performance) [89]. A related hypothesis which might explain the phenomenon of higher cortical activation in frontal, compared to parietal brain regions in older adults is that increases in PFC activity rather reflect reduced neural efficiency or specificity as a result of age-related structural and neurochemical changes [96–99]. From this point of view, enhanced frontal brain activity does not necessarily contribute to the maintenance of working memory performance in older adults. Even though it is difficult to adjudicate between explanatory approaches based on average activity levels within brain regions, recent evidence suggests that increased PFC activation accompanied by high cognitive task performance reflects compensatory mechanisms. In contrast, increased PFC activation accompanied by lower task performance reflects reduced efficiency or specificity, rather than compensation [90,100,101].

Contrary to our expectations, overall, our results revealed higher cortical activation as measured by HBdiff in parietal, compared to frontal brain regions. Thus, our data do not point to the proposed age-related shift of activation from parietal to frontal brain regions, as supposed by the PASA model [10,27]. Given that parietal activation is related to the storage component of working memory [23] and cortical activation positively relates to the amount of stored items [18], our findings might show that the 2-back task relied more than expected on the storage components of working memory, leading to higher cortical activation in the parietal cortex that superimposed the typical pattern described by the PASA model. To assess how cortical hemodynamic activation patterns are linked to working memory performance over time, we ran a multiple regression analysis for each time point. Our results yielded no significant correlation between the RCS and HBdiff in any ROI at baseline and the follow-up measurements at post 30 min and post 45 min for both groups. Interestingly, the regression model for the time point post 15 min showed a positive effect of left-lateralized brain activation, whereas right-lateralized brain activation was negatively related to RCS performance. This negative effect of right frontal activation, accompanied by a positive effect of left frontal activation, which is related to increased cognitive performance, might suggest that acute exercise does not facilitate compensational reorganization, as assumed by the HAROLD model [20]. Rather, this points to enhanced processing within the working memory core network (i.e., left frontal). This, in turn, is in line with the assumption that compensatory neural networks are less efficient than the original task networks, and thus, in order to establish long-lasting beneficial effects (e.g., more efficient processing), processing within the core network should be maintained or reinforced [95].

Therefore, our results are in contrast to a comparable study by Hyodo and colleagues [43], who report greater bilateral activation, that is, broader activation in line with the HAROLD model [20], during a Stroop task following an acute bout of moderate-intensity exercise. Additionally, planned contrast within the EG between the pre-test and time point post 15 min showed improved RCS performance. Thus, one might speculate that acute moderate-intensity exercise affects the executive processing and attention component of working memory in the frontal cortex [22], to a greater extent than the storage component located in the parietal cortex [18,23,24].

5. Limitations

The human aging process is characterized by highly individual trajectories in brain structure and function [102]. Age-related cerebral atrophy (e.g., structural shrinkage) is discussed as one factor that diminishes the sensitivity of the fNIRS measurement. Therefore, the distance between the cortex and the surface of the scalp (where the fNIRS sources and detectors are positioned) increases and measured activation may underestimate the actual cortex activation [103,104]. However, all participants of our sample reported good health with no former or current history of neurological diseases, indicating at least no pathological changes. Yet, by integrating our study results into previous, comparable studies, explanatory power remains a general problem of studies with older adults. Although we used a high-density fNIRS setup by use of a single-subject tandem setup covering frontal and parietal brain regions, the fNIRS montage set-up did not include short separation channels. Instead, all sources and detectors were arranged at an inter-optode distance of approximately 3 cm. Thus, the fNIRS signal might be biased, due to acute exercise evoked systemic changes (e.g., skin blood flow, respiration, blood pressure, sympathetic nervous system activity) in the extracerebral compartment, which might lead to false-positive results [102]. However, we started the post-exercise fNIRS measurements 15 min after exercise cessation and cerebral artery mean blood flow velocities and skin blood flow have been reported to return to values similar to those observed during rest within 15 min after acute moderate intensity exercise [43,49]. Thus, we are confident in assuming that changes in systemic physiology did not influence our results.

6. Outlook

Future studies will have to systematically address the extent to which the after-effects of acute exercise depend on moderators such as exercise intensity, duration and modality, the cognitive task applied, and its time point of assessment post-exercise [5,6] to examine the (design) characteristics that facilitate the enhancing effect of acute exercise on cognition. With regard to cortical hemodynamic activation patterns underlying behavioral outcomes, our findings by use of an fNIRS measurement set-up covering both frontal and parietal brain regions highlight the need for whole-head measurement set-ups. The conclusions which can be drawn from the widely used set-ups restricted to the PFC are necessarily limited due to the involvement of frontal and parietal brain regions in executive control tasks. Therefore, further studies in the field of exercise-cognition research are needed, which focus on age-related changes in whole brain cortical hemodynamic activation patterns following different exercise-intensities (moderate vs. high-intensity) and exercise protocols (continuous vs. interval) and executive control tasks. Further, as indicated by the considerable variability in our behavioral and fNIRS data, future research will have to investigate inter-individual differences in response to acute exercise. Ultimately, the human cognitive aging process is characterized by high inter- and intra-individual variability leading to substantial variability within and between participants.

7. Conclusions

This study investigated the effects of an acute bout of moderate-intensity exercise (15 min; 50% VO_2-peak) on working memory performance (i.e., n-back task) in a sample of healthy older adults compared to a resting control condition (i.e., listening to an audiobook). Additionally, we addressed the development and persistence of acute exercise effects and the underlying neural mechanisms by measuring cortical hemodynamic activation patterns using fNIRS during cognitive testing before and at multiple follow-up measurement time points (i.e., post 15 min, post 30 min, and post 45 min). Only within the exercise group, 2-back task performance was significantly enhanced 15 min and 45 min post-exercise, indicating that exercise might have at least slight effects on working memory performance and that effects last up to 45 min. Regardless of group, higher cortical activation in the working memory core network (i.e., left frontal) was associated with better overall n-back task performance at the time point post 15 min. Results support the practical relevance of short active breaks to enhance cognitive performance and might be also transferred to clinical settings in future studies.

Supplementary Materials: The following are available online at http://www.mdpi.com/2076-3425/10/11/813/s1, Table S1: Participant characteristics of the Experimental (EG) and control group (CG) for the fNIRS ANOVA, Table S2: Overview of all channels (i.e., source-detector combination) and their respective international 10–20 system position and corresponding ROI, Table S3: Average heart rate values for the experimental (EG) and control group (CG) at the start and end of each n-back task at time point pre (baseline) and follow-up measurements (post 15 min to post 45 min), Table S4: Time course of 0-back task performance for the experimental (EG) and control group (CG), Table S5: Time course of 1-back task performance for the experimental (EG) and control group (CG), Table S6: Repeated-measures ANOVA statistics for perceived difficulty, Table S7: Mean values and standard errors of cortical hemodynamic activity as measured by HBdiff in region (frontal, parietal) and hemisphere (left, right) during the 2-back task for the experimental (EG) and control group (CG), Table S8: Repeated-measures ANOVA statistics for fNIRS data.

Author Contributions: Conceptualization, K.S. and C.V.-R.; Data curation, K.S.; Formal analysis, K.S.; Funding acquisition, C.V.-R.; Investigation, K.S.; Methodology, K.S., R.S. and C.V.-R.; Project administration, K.S., N.H. and C.V.-R.; Resources, C.V.-R. Software, K.S. and R.S.; Supervision, C.V.-R.; Visualization, K.S.; Writing—Original draft, K.S.; Writing—Review & editing, N.H., R.S. and C.V.-R. All authors have read and agreed to the published version of the manuscript.

Funding: This research was supported by a grant within the Priority Program, SPP 1772 from the German Research Foundation (Deutsche Forschungsgemeinschaft, DFG), grant number VO 1432/22-1 and by a doctoral scholarship grant of the European Social Fund (Europäischer Sozialfond, ESF) and the Free State of Saxony, grant number 100342331 to R.S. The publication of this article was funded by Chemnitz University of Technology.

Acknowledgments: We thank Karen Mersiovsky for proofreading the manuscript.

Conflicts of Interest: The authors declare no conflict of interest. The funders had no role in the design of the study; in the collection, analyses, or interpretation of data; in the writing of the manuscript, or in the decision to publish the results.

References

1. Bherer, L.; Erickson, K.I.; Liu-Ambrose, T. A review of the effects of physical activity and exercise on cognitive and brain functions in older adults. *J. Aging Res.* **2013**, *2013*, 1–8. [CrossRef] [PubMed]
2. Gomez-Pinilla, F.; Hillman, C. The influence of exercise on cognitive abilities. *Compr. Physiol.* **2013**, *3*, 403–428. [CrossRef] [PubMed]
3. Diamond, A. Executive functions. *Annu. Rev. Psychol.* **2013**, *64*, 135–168. [CrossRef] [PubMed]
4. Miyake, A.; Friedman, N.P.; Emerson, M.J.; Witzki, A.H.; Howerter, A.; Wager, T.D. The unity and diversity of executive functions and their contributions to complex "frontal lobe" tasks: A latent variable analysis. *Cogn. Psychol.* **2000**, *41*, 49–100. [CrossRef] [PubMed]
5. Pontifex, M.B.; McGowan, A.L.; Chandler, M.C.; Gwizdala, K.L.; Parks, A.C.; Fenn, K.; Kamijo, K. A primer on investigating the after effects of acute bouts of physical activity on cognition. *Psychol. Sport Exerc.* **2019**, *40*, 1–22. [CrossRef]
6. Chang, Y.K.; Labban, J.D.; Gapin, J.I.; Etnier, J.L. The effects of acute exercise on cognitive performance: A meta-analysis. *Brain Res.* **2012**, *1453*, 87–101. [CrossRef] [PubMed]
7. Ludyga, S.; Gerber, M.; Brand, S.; Holsboer-Trachsler, E.; Pühse, U. Acute effects of moderate aerobic exercise on specific aspects of executive function in different age and fitness groups: A meta-analysis. *Psychophysiology* **2016**, *53*, 1611–1626. [CrossRef]
8. Etnier, J.L.; Drollette, E.S.; Slutsky, A.B. Physical activity and cognition: A narrative review of the evidence for older adults. *Psychol. Sport Exerc.* **2019**, *42*, 156–166. [CrossRef]
9. Glisky, E.L. Changes in cognitive function in human aging. In *Brain Aging: Models, Methods, and Mechanisms*; Riddle, D.R., Ed.; CRC Press; Taylor & Francis: Boca Raton, FL, USA, 2007; pp. 3–20.
10. Grady, C. The cognitive neuroscience of ageing. *Nat. Rev. Neurosci.* **2012**, *13*, 491–505. [CrossRef]
11. Baddeley, A. Working memory. *Science* **1992**, *255*, 556–559. [CrossRef]
12. Park, D.C.; Bischof, G.N. The aging mind: Neuroplasticity in response to cognitive training. *Dialogues Clin. Neurosci.* **2013**, *15*, 109–119. [PubMed]
13. Park, D.C.; Lautenschlager, G.; Hedden, T.; Davidson, N.S.; Smith, A.D.; Smith, P.K. Models of visuospatial and verbal memory across the adult life span. *Psychol. Aging* **2002**, *17*, 299–320. [CrossRef]
14. Grady, C.L.; Craik, F.I. Changes in memory processing with age. *Curr. Opin. Neurol.* **2000**, *10*, 224–231. [CrossRef]
15. Miyake, A.; Shah, P. Models of working memory: An introduction. In *Models of Working Memory: Mechanisms of Active Maintenance and Executive Control*; Miyake, A., Shah, P., Eds.; Cambridge University Press: New York, NY, USA, 1999; pp. 1–27. [CrossRef]
16. Reuter-Lorenz, P.A.; Jonides, J.; Smith, E.E.; Hartley, A.; Miller, A.; Marshuetz, C.; Koeppe, R.A. Age differences in the frontal lateralization of verbal and spatial working memory revealed by pet. *J. Cogn. Neurosci.* **2000**, *12*, 174–187. [CrossRef]
17. Reuter-Lorenz, P.A.; Lustig, C. Brain aging: Reorganizing discoveries about the aging mind. *Curr. Opin. Neurol.* **2005**, *15*, 245–251. [CrossRef]
18. Eriksson, J.; Vogel, E.K.; Lansner, A.; Bergström, F.; Nyberg, L. Neurocognitive architecture of working memory. *Neuron* **2015**, *88*, 33–46. [CrossRef]

19. Höller-Wallscheid, M.S.; Thier, P.; Pomper, J.K.; Lindner, A. Bilateral recruitment of prefrontal cortex in working memory is associated with task demand but not with age. *Proc. Natl. Acad. Sci. USA* **2017**, *114*, E830–E839. [CrossRef]
20. Cabeza, R. Hemispheric asymmetry reduction in older adults: The harold model. *Psychol. Aging* **2002**, *17*, 85–100. [CrossRef]
21. Rypma, B. A neural efficiency hypothesis of age-related changes in human working memory performance. In *The Cognitive Neuroscience of Working Memory*; Osaka, N., Logie, R.H., D'Esposito, M., Eds.; Oxford University Press: Oxford, UK, 2007; pp. 281–302. [CrossRef]
22. Osaka, M. Neural bases of focusing attention in working memory: An fmri study based on individual differences. In *The Cognitive Neuroscience of Working Memory*; Osaka, N., Logie, R.H., D'Esposito, M., Eds.; Oxford University Press: Oxford, UK, 2007; pp. 99–117. [CrossRef]
23. Smith, E.E.; Jonides, J. Working memory: A view from neuroimaging. *Cogn. Psychol.* **1997**, *33*, 5–42. [CrossRef]
24. Salthouse, T.A. The processing-speed theory of adult age differences in cognition. *Psychol. Rev.* **1996**, *103*, 403–428. [CrossRef]
25. Rypma, B.; D'Esposito, M. Isolating the neural mechanisms of age-related changes in human working memory. *Nat. Neurosci.* **2000**, *3*, 509–515. [CrossRef]
26. Grossman, M.; Cooke, A.; DeVita, C.; Alsop, D.; Detre, J.; Chen, W.; Gee, J. Age-related changes in working memory during sentence comprehension: An fmri study. *NeuroImage* **2002**, *15*, 302–317. [CrossRef]
27. Davis, S.W.; Dennis, N.A.; Daselaar, S.M.; Fleck, M.S.; Cabeza, R. Que pasa? The posterior-anterior shift in aging. *Cereb. Cortex* **2008**, *18*, 1201–1209. [CrossRef]
28. Antonenko, D.; Flöel, A. Healthy aging by staying selectively connected: A mini-review. *Gerontology* **2014**, *60*, 3–9. [CrossRef] [PubMed]
29. Jagust, W. Vulnerable neural systems and the borderland of brain aging and neurodegeneration. *Neuron* **2013**, *77*, 219–234. [CrossRef] [PubMed]
30. Riddle, D.R.; Sonntag, W.E.; Lichtenwalner, R.J. Microvascular plasticity in aging. *Ageing Res. Rev.* **2003**, *2*, 149–168. [CrossRef]
31. Deak, F.; Freeman, W.M.; Ungvari, Z.; Csiszar, A.; Sonntag, W.E. Recent developments in understanding brain aging: Implications for alzheimer's disease and vascular cognitive impairment. *J. Gerontol. A Biol. Sci. Med. Sci.* **2016**, *71*, 13–20. [CrossRef]
32. Pinti, P.; Tachtsidis, I.; Hamilton, A.; Hirsch, J.; Aichelburg, C.; Gilbert, S.; Burgess, P.W. The present and future use of functional near-infrared spectroscopy (fnirs) for cognitive neuroscience. *Ann. N. Y. Acad. Sci.* **2020**, *1464*, 5–29. [CrossRef]
33. Yücel, M.A.; Selb, J.J.; Huppert, T.J.; Franceschini, M.A.; Boas, D.A. Functional near infrared spectroscopy: Enabling routine functional brain imaging. *Curr. Opin. Biomed. Eng.* **2017**, *4*, 78–86. [CrossRef]
34. Piper, S.K.; Krueger, A.; Koch, S.P.; Mehnert, J.; Habermehl, C.; Steinbrink, J.; Obrig, H.; Schmitz, C.H. A wearable multi-channel fnirs system for brain imaging in freely moving subjects. *NeuroImage* **2014**, *85*, 64–71. [CrossRef]
35. Herold, F.; Wiegel, P.; Scholkmann, F.; Müller, N.G. Applications of functional near-infrared spectroscopy (fnirs) neuroimaging in exercise-cognition science: A systematic, methodology-focused review. *J. Clin. Med.* **2018**, *7*, 466. [CrossRef]
36. Kirchner, W.K. Age differences in short-term retention of rapidly changing information. *J. Exp. Psychol.* **1958**, *55*, 352–358. [CrossRef]
37. Owen, A.M.; McMillan, K.M.; Laird, A.R.; Bullmore, E. N-back working memory paradigm: A meta-analysis of normative functional neuroimaging studies. *Hum. Brain Mapp.* **2005**, *25*, 46–59. [CrossRef]
38. Sorond, F.A.; Schnyer, D.M.; Serrador, J.M.; Milberg, W.P.; Lipsitz, L.A. Cerebral blood flow regulation during cognitive tasks: Effects of healthy aging. *Cortex* **2008**, *44*, 179–184. [CrossRef] [PubMed]
39. Scholkmann, F.; Kleiser, S.; Metz, A.J.; Zimmermann, R.; Mata Pavia, J.; Wolf, U.; Wolf, M. A review on continuous wave functional near-infrared spectroscopy and imaging instrumentation and methodology. *NeuroImage* **2014**, *85*, 6–27. [CrossRef] [PubMed]
40. Villringer, A.; Planck, J.; Hock, C.; Schleinkofer, L.; Dirnagl, U. Near infrared spectroscopy (nirs): A new tool to study hemodynamic changes during activation of brain function in human adults. *Neurosci. Lett.* **1993**, *154*, 101–104. [CrossRef]

41. Ferrari, M.; Quaresima, V. A brief review on the history of human functional near-infrared spectroscopy (fnirs) development and fields of application. *NeuroImage* **2012**, *63*, 921–935. [CrossRef]
42. Tsujii, T.; Komatsu, K.; Sakatani, K. Acute effects of physical exercise on prefrontal cortex activity in older adults: A functional near-infrared spectroscopy study. In *Oxygen Transport to Tissue Xxxix. Advances in Experimental Medicine and Biology*; Halpern, H., LaManna, J., Harrison, D., Epel, B., Eds.; Springer: Cham, Germany, 2013; Volume 765, pp. 293–298. [CrossRef]
43. Hyodo, K.; Dan, I.; Suwabe, K.; Kyutoku, Y.; Yamada, Y.; Akahori, M.; Byun, K.; Kato, M.; Soya, H. Acute moderate exercise enhances compensatory brain activation in older adults. *Neurobiol. Aging* **2012**, *33*, 2621–2632. [CrossRef] [PubMed]
44. Ji, Z.; Feng, T.; Mei, L.; Li, A.; Zhang, C. Influence of acute combined physical and cognitive exercise on cognitive function: An nirs study. *PeerJ* **2019**, *7*, e7418. [CrossRef]
45. Yamazaki, Y.; Sato, D.; Yamashiro, K.; Tsubaki, A.; Yamaguchi, Y.; Takehara, N.; Maruyama, A. Inter-individual differences in exercise-induced spatial working memory improvement: A near-infrared spectroscopy study. In *Oxygen Transport to Tissue Xxxix. Advances in Experimental Medicine and Biology*; Halpern, H., LaManna, J., Harrison, D., Epel, B., Eds.; Springer: Cham, Germany, 2017; Volume 977, pp. 81–88. [CrossRef]
46. Bediz, C.S.; Oniz, A.; Guducu, C.; Ural Demirci, E.; Ogut, H.; Gunay, E.; Cetinkaya, C.; Ozgoren, M. Acute supramaximal exercise increases the brain oxygenation in relation to cognitive workload. *Front. Hum. Neurosci.* **2016**, *10*, 174. [CrossRef]
47. Byun, K.; Hyodo, K.; Suwabe, K.; Ochi, G.; Sakairi, Y.; Kato, M.; Dan, I.; Soya, H. Positive effect of acute mild exercise on executive function via arousal-related prefrontal activations: An fnirs study. *NeuroImage* **2014**, *98*, 336–345. [CrossRef]
48. Endo, K.; Matsukawa, K.; Liang, N.; Nakatsuka, C.; Tsuchimochi, H.; Okamura, H.; Hamaoka, T. Dynamic exercise improves cognitive function in association with increased prefrontal oxygenation. *J. Physiol. Sci.* **2013**, *63*, 287–298. [CrossRef]
49. Yanagisawa, H.; Dan, I.; Tsuzuki, D.; Kato, M.; Okamoto, M.; Kyutoku, Y.; Soya, H. Acute moderate exercise elicits increased dorsolateral prefrontal activation and improves cognitive performance with stroop test. *NeuroImage* **2010**, *50*, 1702–1710. [CrossRef]
50. Kujach, S.; Byun, K.; Hyodo, K.; Suwabe, K.; Fukuie, T.; Laskowski, R.; Dan, I.; Soya, H. A transferable high-intensity intermittent exercise improves executive performance in association with dorsolateral prefrontal activation in young adults. *NeuroImage* **2018**, *169*, 117–125. [CrossRef]
51. Murata, Y.; Watanabe, T.; Terasawa, S.; Nakajima, K.; Kobayashi, T.; Nakade, K.; Terasawa, K.; Maruo, S.K. Moderate exercise improves cognitive performance and decreases cortical activation in go/no-go task. *BAOJ Med. Nurs.* **2015**, *1*, 1–7. [CrossRef]
52. Oldfield, R.C. The assessment and analysis of handedness: The edinburgh inventory. *Neuropsychologia* **1971**, *9*, 97–113. [CrossRef]
53. Baecke, J.A.; Burema, J.; Frijters, J.E. A short questionnaire for the measurement of habitual physical activity in epidemiological studies. *Am. J. Clin. Nutr.* **1982**, *36*, 936–942. [CrossRef] [PubMed]
54. Folstein, M.F.; Folstein, S.E.; McHugh, P.R. "Mini-mental state": A practical method for grading the cognitive state of patients for the clinician. *J. Psychiatr. Res.* **1975**, *12*, 189–198. [CrossRef]
55. Bach, M. The freiburg visual acuity test–automatic measurement of visual acuity. *Optom. Vis. Sci.* **1996**, *73*, 49–53. [CrossRef]
56. Faul, F.; Erdfelder, E.; Lang, A.G.; Buchner, A. G*power 3: A flexible statistical power analysis program for the social, behavioral, and biomedical sciences. *Behav. Res. Methods* **2007**, *39*, 175–191. [CrossRef] [PubMed]
57. Borg, G.A. Psychophysical bases of perceived exertion. *Med. Sci. Sports Exerc.* **1982**, *14*, 377–381. [CrossRef] [PubMed]
58. R Core Team. *R: A Language and Environment for Statistical Computing*; R Foundation for Statistical Computing: Vienna, Austria, 2020.
59. RStudio Team. *Rstudio: Integrated Development for R*; RStudio, Inc.: Boston, MA, USA, 2019.
60. Frtusova, J.B.; Phillips, N.A. The auditory-visual speech benefit on working memory in older adults with hearing impairment. *Front. Psychol.* **2016**, *7*, 490. [CrossRef]
61. Bock, O.; Haeger, M.; Voelcker-Rehage, C. Structure of executive functions in young and in older persons. *PLoS ONE* **2019**, *14*, e0216149. [CrossRef]

62. Liesefeld, H.R.; Janczyk, M. Combining speed and accuracy to control for speed-accuracy trade-offs(?). *Behav. Res. Methods* **2019**, *51*, 40–60. [CrossRef]
63. Woltz, D.J.; Was, C.A. Availability of related long-term memory during and after attention focus in working memory. *Mem. Cogn.* **2006**, *34*, 668–684. [CrossRef]
64. Strangman, G.E.; Li, Z.; Zhang, Q. Depth sensitivity and source-detector separations for near infrared spectroscopy based on the colin27 brain template. *PLoS ONE* **2013**, *8*, e66319. [CrossRef] [PubMed]
65. Jurcak, V.; Tsuzuki, D.; Dan, I. 10/20, 10/10, and 10/5 systems revisited: Their validity as relative head-surface-based positioning systems. *NeuroImage* **2007**, *34*, 1600–1611. [CrossRef]
66. Rorden, C.; Brett, M. Stereotaxic display of brain lesions. *Behav. Neurol.* **2000**, *12*, 191–200. [CrossRef]
67. Zimeo Morais, G.A.; Balardin, J.B.; Sato, J.R. Fnirs optodes' location decider (fold): A toolbox for probe arrangement guided by brain regions-of-interest. *Sci. Rep.* **2018**, *8*, 3341. [CrossRef]
68. Jasper, H.H. Report of the committee on methods of clinical examination in electroencephalography: 1957. *Electroencephalogr. Clin. Neurophysiol.* **1958**, *10*, 370–375. [CrossRef]
69. Huppert, T.J.; Diamond, S.G.; Franceschini, M.A.; Boas, D.A. Homer: A review of time-series analysis methods for near-infrared spectroscopy of the brain. *Appl. Opt.* **2009**, *48*, D280–D298. [CrossRef] [PubMed]
70. Aasted, C.M.; Yücel, M.A.; Cooper, R.J.; Dubb, J.; Tsuzuki, D.; Becerra, L.; Petkov, M.P.; Borsook, D.; Dan, I.; Boas, D.A. Anatomical guidance for functional near-infrared spectroscopy: Atlasviewer tutorial. *Neurophotonics* **2015**, *2*, 020801. [CrossRef]
71. Brigadoi, S.; Ceccherini, L.; Cutini, S.; Scarpa, F.; Scatturin, P.; Selb, J.; Gagnon, L.; Boas, D.A.; Cooper, R.J. Motion artifacts in functional near-infrared spectroscopy: A comparison of motion correction techniques applied to real cognitive data. *NeuroImage* **2014**, *85*, 181–191. [CrossRef]
72. Themelis, G.; D'Arceuil, H.; Diamond, S.G.; Thaker, S.; Huppert, T.J.; Boas, D.A.; Franceschini, M.A. Near-infrared spectroscopy measurement of the pulsatile component of cerebral blood flow and volume from arterial oscillations. *J. Biomed. Opt.* **2007**, *12*, 014033. [CrossRef] [PubMed]
73. Molavi, B.; Dumont, G.A. Wavelet-based motion artifact removal for functional near-infrared spectroscopy. *Physiol. Meas.* **2012**, *33*, 259–270. [CrossRef]
74. Delpy, D.T.; Cope, M.; van der Zee, P.; Arridge, S.; Wray, S.; Wyatt, J. Estimation of optical pathlength through tissue from direct time of flight measurement. *Phys. Med. Biol.* **1988**, *33*, 1433–1442. [CrossRef]
75. Duncan, A.; Meek, J.H.; Clemence, M.; Elwell, C.E.; Fallon, P.; Tyszczuk, L.; Cope, M.; Delpy, D.T. Measurement of cranial optical path length as a function of age using phase resolved near infrared spectroscopy. *Pediatr. Res.* **1996**, *39*, 889–894. [CrossRef]
76. Tempest, G.D.; Eston, R.G.; Parfitt, G. Prefrontal cortex haemodynamics and affective responses during exercise: A multi-channel near infrared spectroscopy study. *PLoS ONE* **2014**, *9*, e95924. [CrossRef]
77. Brisswalter, J.; Collardeau, M.; René, A. Effects of acute physical exercise characteristics on cognitive performance. *Sports Med.* **2002**, *32*, 555–566. [CrossRef]
78. Rooks, C.R.; Thom, N.J.; McCully, K.K.; Dishman, R.K. Effects of incremental exercise on cerebral oxygenation measured by near-infrared spectroscopy: A systematic review. *Prog. Neurobiol.* **2010**, *92*, 134–150. [CrossRef] [PubMed]
79. American College of Sports Medicine. *Acsm's Guidelines for Exercise Testing and Prescription*, 10th ed.; Wolters Kluwer Health: Philadelphia, PA, USA, 2018.
80. Lawrence, M.A. Ez: Easy Analysis and Visualization of Factorial Experiments; R Package Version 4.4-0; 2016. Available online: https://cran.r-project.org/package=ez (accessed on 3 June 2020).
81. Lenth, R. Emmeans: Estimated Marginal Means, Aka Least-Squares Means; R package version 1.4.7; 2020. Available online: https://CRAN.R-project.org/package=emmeans (accessed on 3 June 2020).
82. Wickham, H. *Ggplot2: Elegant Graphics for Data Analysis*, 2nd ed.; Springer: New York, NY, USA, 2016. [CrossRef]
83. McElree, B. Working memory and focal attention. *J. Exp. Psychol. Learn. Mem. Cogn.* **2001**, *27*, 817–835. [CrossRef]
84. Boettiger, C.A.; D'Esposito, M. Frontal networks for learning and executing arbitrary stimulus-response associations. *J. Neurosci.* **2005**, *25*, 2723–2732. [CrossRef] [PubMed]
85. Mekari, S.; Fraser, S.; Bosquet, L.; Bonnéry, C.; Labelle, V.; Pouliot, P.; Lesage, F.; Bherer, L. The relationship between exercise intensity, cerebral oxygenation and cognitive performance in young adults. *Eur. J. Appl. Physiol.* **2015**, *115*, 2189–2197. [CrossRef] [PubMed]

86. Labelle, V.; Bosquet, L.; Mekary, S.; Bherer, L. Decline in executive control during acute bouts of exercise as a function of exercise intensity and fitness level. *Brain Cogn.* **2013**, *81*, 10–17. [CrossRef]
87. McNab, F.; Leroux, G.; Strand, F.; Thorell, L.; Bergman, S.; Klingberg, T. Common and unique components of inhibition and working memory: An fmri, within-subjects investigation. *Neuropsychologia* **2008**, *46*, 2668–2682. [CrossRef]
88. Friedman, N.P.; Miyake, A.; Corley, R.P.; Young, S.E.; Defries, J.C.; Hewitt, J.K. Not all executive functions are related to intelligence. *Psychol. Sci.* **2006**, *17*, 172–179. [CrossRef]
89. Friedman, N.P.; Miyake, A.; Young, S.E.; DeFries, J.C.; Corley, R.P.; Hewitt, J.K. Individual differences in executive functions are almost entirely genetic in origin. *J. Exp. Psychol. Gen.* **2008**, *137*, 201–225. [CrossRef] [PubMed]
90. Miller, K.M.; Price, C.C.; Okun, M.S.; Montijo, H.; Bowers, D. Is the n-back task a valid neuropsychological measure for assessing working memory? *Arch. Clin. Neuropsychol.* **2009**, *24*, 711–717. [CrossRef]
91. Stroop, J.R. Studies of interference in serial verbal reactions. *J. Exp. Psychol. Gen.* **1992**, *121*, 15–23. [CrossRef]
92. Gajewski, P.D.; Hanisch, E.; Falkenstein, M.; Thönes, S.; Wascher, E. What does the n-back task measure as we get older? Relations between working-memory measures and other cognitive functions across the lifespan. *Front. Psychol.* **2018**, *9*, 2208. [CrossRef]
93. Lambourne, K.; Tomporowski, P. The effect of exercise-induced arousal on cognitive task performance: A meta-regression analysis. *Brain Res.* **2010**, *1341*, 12–24. [CrossRef]
94. Etnier, J.L.; Salazar, W.; Landers, D.M.; Petruzzello, S.J.; Han, M.; Nowell, P. The influence of physical fitness and exercise upon cognitive functioning: A meta-analysis. *J. Sport Exerc. Psychol.* **1997**, *19*, 249–277. [CrossRef]
95. Park, D.C.; Reuter-Lorenz, P. The adaptive brain: Aging and neurocognitive scaffolding. *Annu. Rev. Psychol.* **2009**, *60*, 173–196. [CrossRef]
96. West, R.L. An application of prefrontal cortex function theory to cognitive aging. *Psychol. Bull.* **1996**, *120*, 272–292. [CrossRef] [PubMed]
97. Park, D.C.; Polk, T.A.; Park, R.; Minear, M.; Savage, A.; Smith, M.R. Aging reduces neural specialization in ventral visual cortex. *Proc. Natl. Acad. Sci. USA* **2004**, *101*, 13091–13095. [CrossRef]
98. Raz, N.; Rodrigue, K.M. Differential aging of the brain: Patterns, cognitive correlates and modifiers. *Neurosci. Biobehav. Rev.* **2006**, *30*, 730–748. [CrossRef] [PubMed]
99. Nyberg, L.; Lövdén, M.; Riklund, K.; Lindenberger, U.; Bäckman, L. Memory aging and brain maintenance. *Trends Cogn. Sci.* **2012**, *16*, 292–305. [CrossRef]
100. Morcom, A.M.; Henson, R.N.A. Increased prefrontal activity with aging reflects nonspecific neural responses rather than compensation. *J. Neurosci.* **2018**, *38*, 7303–7313. [CrossRef]
101. Reuter-Lorenz, P.A.; Cappell, K.A. Neurocognitive aging and the compensation hypothesis. *Curr. Dir. Psychol. Sci.* **2008**, *17*, 177–182. [CrossRef]
102. Cabeza, R.; Albert, M.; Belleville, S.; Craik, F.I.M.; Duarte, A.; Grady, C.L.; Lindenberger, U.; Nyberg, L.; Park, D.C.; Reuter-Lorenz, P.A.; et al. Maintenance, reserve and compensation: The cognitive neuroscience of healthy ageing. *Nat. Rev. Neurosci.* **2018**, *19*, 701–710. [CrossRef] [PubMed]
103. Fjell, A.M.; Walhovd, K.B.; Fennema-Notestine, C.; McEvoy, L.K.; Hagler, D.J.; Holland, D.; Brewer, J.B.; Dale, A.M. One-year brain atrophy evident in healthy aging. *J. Neurosci.* **2009**, *29*, 15223–15231. [CrossRef] [PubMed]
104. Bonnéry, C.; Leclerc, P.O.; Desjardins, M.; Hoge, R.; Bherer, L.; Pouliot, P.; Lesage, F. Changes in diffusion path length with old age in diffuse optical tomography. *J. Biomed. Opt.* **2012**, *17*, 056002. [CrossRef] [PubMed]

Publisher's Note: MDPI stays neutral with regard to jurisdictional claims in published maps and institutional affiliations.

© 2020 by the authors. Licensee MDPI, Basel, Switzerland. This article is an open access article distributed under the terms and conditions of the Creative Commons Attribution (CC BY) license (http://creativecommons.org/licenses/by/4.0/).

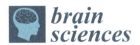

Article

On Your Mark, Get Set, Self-Control, Go: A Differentiated View on the Cortical Hemodynamics of Self-Control during Sprint Start

Kim-Marie Stadler [1], Wanja Wolff [1,2] and Julia Schüler [1,*]

1. Department of Sport Science, University of Konstanz, 78464 Konstanz, Germany; kim-marie.stadler@uni-konstanz.de (K.-M.S.); wanja.wolff@uni-konstanz.de (W.W.)
2. Department of Educational Psychology, University of Bern, 3012 Bern, Switzerland
* Correspondence: julia.schueler@uni-konstanz.de; Tel.: +49-7531-88-2629

Received: 30 June 2020; Accepted: 27 July 2020; Published: 29 July 2020

Abstract: Most sports are self-control demanding. For example, during a sprint start, athletes have to respond as fast as possible to the start signal (action initiation) while suppressing the urge to start too early (action inhibition). Here, we examined the cortical hemodynamic response to these demands by measuring activity in the two lateral prefrontal cortices (lPFC), a central area for self-control processes. We analyzed activity within subregions of the lPFC, while subjects performed a sprint start, and we assessed if activation varied as a function of hemisphere and gender. In a counterbalanced within-subject design, 39 participants (age: mean (M) = 22.44, standard deviation (SD) = 5.28, 22 women) completed four sprint start conditions (blocks). In each block, participants focused on inhibition (avoid false start), initiation (start fast), no start (do not start) and a combined condition (start fast; avoid false start). We show that oxyhemoglobin in the lPFC increased after the set signal and this increase did not differ between experimental conditions. Increased activation was primarily observed in ventral areas of the lPFC, but only in males, and this increase did not vary between hemispheres. This study provides further support for the involvement of the ventral lPFC during a sprint start, while highlighting gender differences in the processing of sprint start-induced self-control demands.

Keywords: sprint start; self-control; cerebral oxygenation; ventral-lateral-prefrontal-cortex

1. Introduction

Winning or losing in a sprint race is determined by milliseconds and is highly dependent on a perfect start [1–4]. The sprint start contributes 5% of the overall 100 m race time [5]. Also, in other sports, the start plays a decisive role for the overall performance. For example, in the shortest swimming races (50 m), the start accounts for 33% of the total race time, making it even more important for the overall result [6]. Taken together, in many different sports, a fast and excellent race start plays a central role in determining the race outcome [7–9].

Start performance hinges on a diverse set of variables. For example, start position [5,10], force rate [2,11], reaction time and acceleration [4,12], they all affect how well an athlete is able to start. However, cognitive processes also contribute to a good sprint start. For example, an external attentional focus has been shown to be more effective for the start reaction time than an internal attentional focus [13]. Moreover, agility (i.e., the capacity for rapid movement changes during a sprint) is dependent on effective information processing [13,14]. To illustrate, during a sprint start, the athlete needs to recognize and process the acoustic start signal, make the decision to initiate the start and enact this decision by producing the required movement. Thus, the athlete is required to inhibit the urge to start until a signal indicates otherwise (i.e., action inhibition) and then initiate a movement as fast as possible (action initiation).

Action inhibition and initiation are two processes that rely on self-control [15,16]. Self-control is defined as the ability to regulate and alter "one's own inner states, processes and responses (..), including (..) actions, thoughts, feelings, desires and performances" [17] (pp. 6–7) to achieve a specific goal. Self-control is conducive to a plethora of positive short- and long-term outcomes [18–21].

Exerting self-control is, however, not easy, and is associated with negative experiences. People often fail to apply the amount of self-control that would be required [20]. For example, we often do not manage to resist a short-term temptation (e.g., snacking) that would be at odds with a long-term goal (lose weight). Exerting self-control is experienced as effortful and aversive [22–25] and therefore, people tend to avoid exerting self-control if possible [24]. In line with this, most theories on self-control suggest that applying self-control produces costs, and is therefore invested sparingly [22–24,26]. For example, it has been suggested that the effort one experiences while applying self-control serves as a signal to indicate the costs of one's current action and serves as a prompt to withhold further effort [26]. In line with this, a large body of research on the ego-depletion effect has shown that prior self-control exertion leads to impaired subsequent performance in non-sporting [27] as well as in sporting tasks [28,29]. For example, Englert and Bertrams [30] showed that participants who had completed a self-control-demanding task prior to a basketball free-throw test performed worse than participants who had not worked on a self-control-demanding task. More importantly for the present paper, research has shown that participants who had completed a self-control-demanding task prior to a sprint start displayed worse reaction times and more false starts in subsequent sprint starts [31,32]. In sum, a large body of research shows that self-control is important for sports performance in general [29] and emerging research has found support for the proposed importance of self-control for sprint starts, too [31,32].

2. Cortical Underpinnings of Self-Control

In light of its importance for goal-directed behavior, a large body of neuroscientific research has focused on understanding the neuroscience of self-control [24,33–35]. Much evidence points to an executive control network that governs self-controlled, top-down processing [24,34–36]. According to this approach, self-control can be broken down into the three components, namely, specification, regulation and monitoring [37]. Thus, self-control consists of a continuous loop in which control signals are specified, applied and the outcome is monitored to assess whether the control signal needs to be adjusted. It has been proposed that the specification and monitoring components of control are performed by the dorsal Anterior Cingulate Cortex (dACC), whereas regulation is primarily executed by the lateral prefrontal cortex (lPFC) [37]. Thus, research suggests that the actual process of applying self-control, for example to control the impulse to start too early in a sprint race, is executed by the lPFC. Additional support for the proposed role of lPFC in self-control processes comes from clinical research, where, for example, patients who suffer from attention deficit hyperactivity disorder have been shown to display lower activation in lPFC during control-demanding tasks [38]. Depending on the specific control function that is required in a situation, different areas of the lPFC are engaged in the control process. For example, dorsolateral areas seem to govern top-down attention control, whereas ventrolateral areas seem important for response inhibition [39].

The cortical underpinnings of self-control in sports—and for sprint starts specifically—are less well understood. In line with research and theorizing from cognitive neuroscience, self-control demands in sports covary with lPFC activation [40]. While a number of studies has already investigated lPFC activity during endurance performance [41,42], only one study has assessed lPFC activation during a sprint start [43]. In a within-subject repeated measures design, male participants performed three sprint start sequences while lPFC activity was measured with functional near-infrared spectroscopy (fNIRS) [43]. A significant increase in lPFC oxygenation prior to the start signal indicated high self-control demands during a sprint start. In this study, exploratory analyses indicated that different subareas of the lPFC were active in conditions that differed in regard to the self-control demands they supposedly imposed: if participants only had to avoid producing a false start (i.e., action inhibition), this was accompanied by a strong increase in ventral parts of lPFC and a less pronounced increase in anterior parts of the lPFC, compared to when participants had to focus on avoiding a false start, while also producing a maximally fast start (action initiation). In addition, no activation changes in posterior parts of the lPFC were observed, irrespective of condition. Hence, preliminary empirical evidence supports the presumed role of lPFC during sprint starts. It is our research goal to better understand how the lPFC covaries with the self-control demands of a sprint start. Thus, the present study takes up the results of Wolff et al. [43] and tests them within the framework of a previously formulated hypothesis.

3. Present Study

In this study, we aim to replicate and extend prior research on the lPFC involvement during sprint starts [43]. Specifically, we use fNIRS to capture cortical oxygenation changes during a sprint start sequence that consists of the prompts "On your marks", "Set" and "Go". Aiming at replicating Wolff et al. [43], we test if lPFC oxygenation increases in the time interval between Set and Go. Extending their work on a general level, we assess if lPFC oxygenation increases differ as a function of participant gender. This is an important extension because research points towards sex differences in self-control performance [44,45]. In addition, some research points towards a differential involvement of left and right hemispheres in self-control [46,47]. Thus, as a second extension, we test if lPFC oxygenation changes differ between the left and the right hemisphere.

In addition, we test if the facets of self-control demands (action initiation, action inhibition), that we aim to trigger using different instructions for the sprint start, cause specific changes in the lPFC. Our different start conditions were developed in order to emphasize the self-control demands for action inhibition and action initiation: Participants either had to focus on action inhibition (avoid a false start), on a fast action initiation (start as soon as possible), on both (start as soon as possible and avoid a false start) or did not start at all (no start), which was expected to increase the demand for action inhibition. Since all conditions impose self-control demands, we test the hypothesis that lPFC activation would significantly increase in all four sprint start conditions (action inhibition, action initiation, combined, no-start). However, since the no-start condition only imposes the self-control demand to inhibit any start action on accident, we expect the lPFC activation to be the lowest in this condition.

Finally, we a priori tested the activation differences of specific regions of the lPFC to follow up on the explorative findings by Wolff et al. [43]. Specifically, Wolff et al. [43] used fNIRS to monitor oxygenation changes over different parts of the lPFC and found that specific parts of their montage according to the international 5/10 system responded with increased activation during the sprint start (anterior: F6–AF8, AF4–AF8, AF3–AF7, F5–AF7; ventral: F6–F8, F6–FC6, F5–FC5, F5–F7), whereas no activation changes were observed for the other parts (F6–F4, AF4–F4, FC4–FC6, FC4–F4, F2–F4, F1–F3, AF3–F3, FC3–F3, FC3–FC5, F5–F3). Thus, we test the hypothesis that ventral and anterior parts of the lPFC show significantly higher activation in all four start conditions than the remaining parts of the chosen lPFC montage.

4. Methods

4.1. Design

The study was conducted in the Sport Psychology Lab of the authors' University and was based on an experimental, randomized within-subject design. Thus, each subject participated in all four start conditions.

4.2. Participants

We recruited a sample of $n = 60$ participants (27 male, 33 female; mean (M) M_{age} = 22.44, standard deviation (SD) SD_{age} = 5.28). The majority of the participants studied psychology ($n = 33$) or sport science ($n = 6$). The requirements for study participation were German language skills, age between 18 and 30 years to minimize age-dependent differences in cortical oxygenation and no extensive experience with sprint starts but doing sport regularly. Participants reported to be physically active for three to four times a week ($M_{weeklysport}$ = 3.25, $SD_{weeklysport}$ = 2.11), with one exercise session lasting on average 67.67 min ($SD_{minutes}$ = 31.64). The main sport activities were running, weight-lifting and dancing. They received 15 EUR for participation. Due to recording errors and missing trigger definitions in the raw data, only $n = 39$ (22 women) of the full dataset remained for statistical analyses. The study was conducted in agreement with the declaration of Helsinki and does not fall within the remit of the Ethics Committee of the University.

4.3. Procedure

The testing session lasted approximately 90 min and study sessions were conducted whenever participants were available. Participants were welcomed, received and signed a written informed consent form and completed a demographic questionnaire. They were asked whether they followed the instructions (no caffeine and alcohol consumption and no exercise 24 h prior to the experiment, and no caffeine two hours before) as requested prior to the testing session. The experimenter explained the task and all four start conditions carefully. Sprint starts were carried out in a standing position. Participants were given time to practice the sprint start sequence until they felt confident in starting with the experiment. This was not standardized but participants chose freely how much practice they needed before starting. Next, fNIRS equipment was prepared and set up. After calibrating and optimizing the signal, participants wore the fNIRS recorder in a backpack. Hemodynamic changes were recorded in real-time and transferred via Team Viewer® to an external computer and signal quality was monitored constantly. Then, the sprint start procedure started.

The sprint start sequence was the same as in the study of Wolff et al. [43]. The same consecutive start signals ("On your marks", "Set", "Go") were vocally presented to the participants for all start conditions. The instructions for the sprint starts, which represent the experimental manipulation (see below), were presented by a computerized voice to avoid possible biases by the experimenter and to ensure the same inter stimulus interval (see Figure 1).

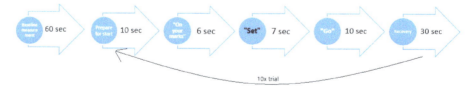

Figure 1. Procedure of a sprint start sequence. Structure and timeframe are the same for all four sprint start conditions. Conditions differ only by task instruction.

Participants completed four blocks (i.e., start conditions). Participants either had to focus on false start inhibition (Action inhibition start condition, "Avoid a false start!"), on action initiation (Action initiation start condition, "Start as fast as possible!"), on both (combined start condition, "Start as fast as possible and avoid a false start!") or did not start at all (no-start condition, "Don't start!"). Each block consisted of 10 trials. Each block started with a 60 s baseline measurement of the prefrontal activity in a standing position while participants fixated on a black cross on the floor. Then, the instructions about the upcoming start condition followed. On the signal "On your marks", subjects placed their supporting leg behind the starting line, which was marked by black tape on the floor. The other foot was placed on a start mat (rectangular mat on the floor). On the signal "Set", which followed six seconds later, participants bent their knees and hip to shift their weight onto the front leg. Seven seconds after the "Set" signal, the "Start" signal was given, and in the action inhibition, action initiation and combined start condition participants started. In the no-start condition, no response was required. Subjects ended their sprint at a "stop" line five meters after the start line. Each trial was followed by a 30 s break to ensure that oxygenation changes returned to baseline level [48]. The order of conditions was counterbalanced to prevent order effects. After the experiment, participants were asked to answer follow-up questions (motivation, perceived task difficulty, momentary exhaustion). Finally, they were debriefed, paid and thanked for their participation.

4.4. Measures

fNIRS measurement: A multichannel continuous wave fNIRS imaging system (NIRSport, NIRx Medical Technologies LLC, Los Angeles, NY, USA) was used to measure hemodynamic changes during the sprint start. fNIRS is non-invasive and can be used during active sport exercises (e.g., cycle ergometry, treadmill walking, running) [49–52]. fNIRS measures changes in oxygenated (HbO) and de-oxygenated (HbR) hemoglobin in the cerebral cortex using NIR light [53]. 8 × 8 (8 Sources + 8 Detectors) optodes were placed bilaterally (two 4 sources + 4 detectors) according to the international 5/10 system [54]. We used the same montage of optodes as described in Wolff et al. [43] (Figure 2).

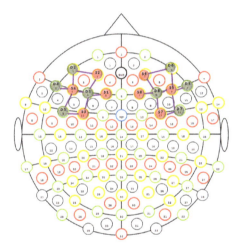

Figure 2. 8 Sources and 8 detectors were placed according to the international 5/10 system: E1 at F1, E2 at AF3, E3 at FC3, E4 at F5, D1 at F3, D2 at AF7, D3 at FC5, D4 at F7, E5 at F6, E6 at AF4, E7 at FC4, E8 at F2, D5 at F8, D6 at AF8, D7 at FC6, and D8 at F4.

The cap was set up and fixed so that CV-point 14 was placed in the middle of the head (half-length distance between both ears and half-length distance between nasion and inion). Furthermore, an overcap was put over the probe holder cap to secure and improve optode contact and to minimize the impact from ambient light.

Hemodynamic changes in the lPFC were measured 2 s before the set signal (baseline) and 5 to 7 s after the set signal (response to set signal).

Follow-up questions: On a 7-point Likert scale (1 = not at all, 7 = very much), participant's motivation to execute the sprint starts as fast as possible was assessed. In addition, participants were asked to indicate (open answer field) which sprint start condition was the most difficult for them (no-start, action inhibition start, action initiation start, combined start). Finally, momentary exhaustion was assessed on a 7-point Likert scale (1 = not at all, 7 = very much): "How exhausted do you fell right now?"

4.5. Preprocessing

fNIRS preprocessing: To preprocess raw fNIRS data, Homer2 was used [55]. First, channels (source-detector combinations) with too high or too low optical density were removed using the enPruneChannels function with the following function arguments: $dRange(1) = 1e^{-2}$; $dRange(2) = 3e$; $SNRthresh = 2$; $SDrange(1) = 0.0$; $SDrange(2) = 45.0$, $reset = 0$. Secondly, by taking the logarithm of the signal, raw optical intensity data was converted into changes in optical density (OD). To correct motion artifacts, we used the Wavelet_Motion_Correction function with an IQR of 1.5, which is known to be efficient in recovering the hemodynamic response function [56–58]. Remaining motion artifacts were removed using the *hmrMotionArtifact* function with the following arguments: $tMotion = 0.5$; $tMask = 1.0$; $STDEVthresh = 10.0$; $AMPthresh = 1.00$. If a Set or Start signal was within a time range of −3 to 10 s of a detected-motion artifact, this trial was removed from further analysis. Following Wolff et al. [43], the corrected data were low-pass-filtered using a cut-off frequency at 0.5 Hz and converted into oxygenated (HbO) and de-oxygenated (HbR) hemoglobin concentration changes using the modified Beer–Lambert law [59]. Finally, referring to Essenpreis, Cope, Elwell, Arridge, van der Zee & Delpy [60], path length factors were chosen differently for the two wavelengths (7.3 for 760 nm and 6.4 for 850 nm) and the *hmBlockAvg* function was applied to obtain corrected group averaged oxygenation values [55].

Channel selection: After preprocessing the data, time interval plots (−2 s before the Set signal to 7 s after Start signal) of averaged hemodynamic changes, for each sprint start condition, were illustrated in Homer2. Explorative findings of Wolff et al. [43] identified some channels (source–detector combinations) as relevant, as these showed a high hemodynamic response during self-control execution while other channels did not respond to the experimental demands. To test the robustness of these findings, we grouped the channels as separate regions of interest (ROIs) following Wolff et al. [43]. We grouped two anterior channels on the right hemisphere (F6–AF8, AF4–AF8) and two anterior channels on the left hemisphere (AF3–AF7, F5–AF7) as anterior parts of the lPFC. Two ventral channels on the right hemisphere (F6–F8, F6–FC6) and two ventral channels on the left hemisphere (F5–FC5, F5–F7) were grouped as ventral parts of the lPFC. The five remaining channels on the right hemisphere (F6–F4, AF4–F4, FC4–FC6, FC4–F4, F2–F4) and the five remaining channels on the left hemisphere (F1–F3, AF3–F3, FC3–F3, FC3–FC5, F5–F3) were summarized as other parts of the lPFC. Hence, we analyzed them (anterior, ventral, others) as three ROIs.

5. Results

5.1. Manipulation Check

Motivation during the experiment and fatigue level after the experiment were measured on a 7-point Likert scale (1 = not at all, 7 = very much). Participants were generally motivated to perform well (M = 5.865; SD = 0.905; Range = 4–7) and were not very exhausted directly after the experiment (M = 2.919, SD = 1.937, Range = 1–7). Contrary to our expectations, 33.3% (n = 12) of the participants rated the no-start condition as being the most difficult, compared with 25% (n = 9) who perceived the action initiation start condition, 16.7% (n = 6) the combined start condition and 8.3% (n = 3) the action inhibition start condition as the most difficult. Six participants did not answer the question, but were still included in subsequent analyses.

5.2. Cortical Activity during Sprint Start

Data was restructured and merged using Matlab (R2016a; Natick, Massachusetts: The MathWorks Inc.). To test if lPFC oxygenation increases in the time-interval between Set and Go, we conducted a three-way repeated measures analysis of variance (ANOVA), having three within factors: The first factor was Time (Baseline vs. Set), comparing the lPFC activation 2 s before the start (baseline) and 5 to 7 s after the set signal (response to set signal). The second factor was Condition (no-start, action inhibition start, action initiation start, combined start), and the third factor was region of interest (ROI) (Anterior, Ventral, Others). Oxygenated hemoglobin (HbO) concentration was analyzed as the dependent variable. De-oxygenated hemoglobin (HbR) concentration was not analyzed. To assess differences between factor levels, Bonferroni-corrected post-hoc t-tests were computed. Statistical analyses were executed in R (3.5.1; R Core Team, Vienna, Austria, 2018). The assumption of sphericity was met for all repeated measure ANOVAs. We set statistical significance at $\alpha = 0.05$. We calculated partial η^2 as effect-size estimates [61].

No significant three-way interaction between Time, Condition and ROI was found, F (4,168) = 0.346, $p = 0.864$, $\eta^2 = 0.009$. A significant main effect for Time was found, F (1,38) = 7.290, $p = 0.010$, $\eta^2 = 0.161$. Hence, oxygenated hemoglobin significantly increased from 2 s before the Set signal to 7 s after the Set signal. Furthermore, a significant main effect was found for ROI (F(2,65) = 9.431, $p < 0.001$, $\eta^2 = 0.199$), but no main effect for Condition (F (3,98) = 0.695, $p = 0.537$ $\eta^2 = 0.018$) was found. Hence, oxygenation increase differs as a function of subareas of the lPFC (ROI), but not as a function of start condition (Condition) (see Figure 3 and Table A1). A significant ROI × Time interaction (F (2,65) = 9.431, $p < 0.001$, $\eta^2 = 0.199$), but no significant ROI × Condition interaction (F (4,168) = 0.346, $p = 0.864$, $\eta^2 = 0.009$) was found. Thus, oxygenation differences in subareas of the lPFC (ROI) covaried with the time (Baseline vs. Set), but not with start conditions. No significant Condition × Time interaction (F (3,98) = 0.695, $p = 0.537$, $\eta^2 = 0.018$) was found. Hence, start condition did not covary with time (Baseline vs. Set).

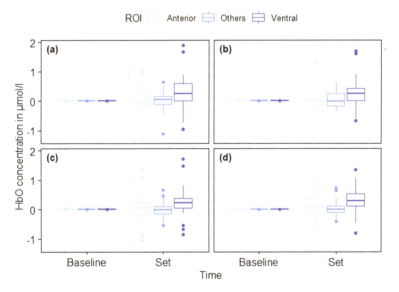

Figure 3. Boxplots of oxygenated hemoglobin (HbO) concentrations (in µmol/L) grouped in regions of interest (ROIs) (anterior, ventral, others) for all four sprint start conditions (action inhibition start (**a**), action initiation start (**b**), combined start (**c**), no-start (**d**)) 2 s before the set signal (baseline) and 5 to 7 s after the set signal (response to set signal). Middle lines inside each box represent the median scores, top lines of each box indicate the upper quartiles, bottom lines of each box indicate lower quartiles, upper and lower vertical lines indicate upper and lower whiskers and dots represent outliers.

Bonferroni-corrected post-hoc pairwise comparison indicated that cortical activity significantly increased from 2 s before the Set signal to 7 s after the Set signal in anterior parts ($p = 0.016$) and ventral parts ($p < 0.001$), but not in other parts ($p = 0.452$) of the lPFC.

As we could not find a condition effect for the different sprint start sequences (no-start, action inhibition start, action initiation start, combined start), we summarized all four averaged hemodynamic changes to increase the statistical power of the subsequent analyses.

5.3. Regions of Interest (ROIs), Laterality and Gender Effects

We conducted a three-way mixed measures ANOVA having Gender (Male vs. Female) as a between factor and two within factors: ROI (ventral, anterior, others) to compare activity differences in specific subareas of the lPFC and Laterality (right vs. left) to compare hemispheric activity differences. Only lPFC activation 5 to 7 s after the set signal (response to set signal) was taken into account. We computed Bonferroni-corrected post hoc t-tests to assess differences between specific factor levels.

No statistically significant three-way interaction between Gender, ROI and Laterality was found, $F(2,70) = 0.691$, $p = 0.505$, $\eta^2 = 0.019$. A large significant main effect emerged for ROI ($F(2,70) = 14.856$, $p < 0.001$, $\eta^2 = 0.298$), but not for Gender ($F(1,35) = 1.373$, $p = 0.249$, $\eta^2 = 0.038$) and Laterality ($F(1,35) = 0.305$, $p = 0.584$, $\eta^2 = 0.009$). Hence, oxygenation changes were pronounced significantly stronger in specific subareas of the lPFC, but did not differ as a function of participants' gender or between the left and right hemisphere (see Table 1 and Figure 4).

Table 1. Values of oxygenated hemoglobin (HbO) concentration.

Regions of Interest (ROIs)	Laterality	Male n	Male M (SD)	Female n	Female M (SD)	Mean Differences
Ventral	Right Hemisphere	17	0.492 (0.514)	21	0.070 (0.425)	0.422
	Left Hemisphere	17	0.503 (0.485)	21	0.135 (0.432)	0.368
Anterior	Right Hemisphere	16	0.014 (0.396)	22	0.060 (0.496)	−0.046
	Left Hemisphere	17	0.147 (0.345)	22	0.083 (0.379)	0.064
Others	Right Hemisphere	17	0.004 (0.243)	22	0.035 (0.300)	−0.031
	Left Hemisphere	17	−0.024 (0.237)	22	0.027 (0.288)	−0.051

Note. n = number of persons; M = mean value; SD = standard deviation.

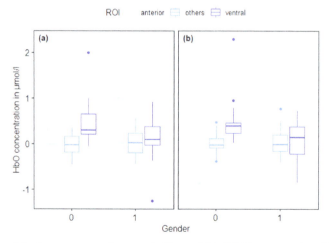

Figure 4. Boxplots of group averaged oxygenated hemoglobin (HbO) concentrations (in µmol/L) 5 to 7 s after set signal differentiated for regions of interest (ROIs) (anterior, others, ventral), Gender (Male = 0, Female = 1) and for Laterality (left (**a**) and right (**b**) hemisphere). Middle lines inside each box represent the median scores, top lines of each box indicate the upper quartiles, bottom lines of each box indicate lower quartiles, upper and lower vertical lines indicate upper and lower whiskers and dots represent outliers.

Furthermore, the three-way repeated measures ANOVA revealed a significant strong interaction Gender × ROI effect ($F(2,70) = 10.042$, $p < 0.001$, $\eta^2 = 0.223$), but no significant Gender × Laterality ($F(1,35) = 0.094$, $p = 0.761$, $\eta^2 = 0.003$) and ROI × Laterality ($F(2,70) = 0.852$, $p = 0.431$, $\eta^2 = 0.024$) effect. Thus, oxygenation differences in subareas of the lPFC covaried with participants' gender, but not with laterality.

Bonferroni-corrected post-hoc multiple pairwise comparisons indicated that oxygenation increases were significantly higher in ventral compared to anterior parts of the lPFC ($p = 0.003$) and in ventral compared to other parts of the lPFC ($p < 0.001$). For male participants, cortical activity was significantly higher in ventral parts compared to anterior parts of the lPFC ($p < 0.001$) and in ventral parts compared to other parts of the lPFC ($p < 0.001$). Thus, oxygenation changes in male participants are significantly magnified in ventral parts of the lPFC. No significant cortical activity differences were found for female participants ($p > 0.95$). Thus, lPFC oxygenation increases in female participants did not differ between subareas of the lPFC.

6. Discussion

In this study, we aimed to explore the cortical underpinnings of the required self-control during sprint start execution. We replicated and extended the study of Wolff et al. [43] on oxygenation changes in the lPFC during a self-control-demanding sprint start. In line with previous research, we observed a significant increase in cortical activity in the lPFC in the timeframe between the Set and Start signal of a sprint start sequence. In contrast to previous findings [43], oxygenation did not differ between experimental conditions that were designed to vary the level of task-induced self-control demands. Replicating previous research [43], the increase in lPFC oxygenation was particularly pronounced in ventral parts, whereas no oxygenation change was observed in other subareas of the lPFC. Extending previous research, we observed that the substantial increase in oxygenation in the ventral parts of the lPFC occurred in male but not in female participants. Finally, we did not find evidence for oxygenation differences between the right and left hemisphere. Taken together, our results provide further evidence for a robust involvement of the lPFC´s more ventral parts during a sprint start, but, interestingly, this effect was only found in males and it did not vary between hemispheres. We believe these findings to be important for the following three reasons.

First, our results show that only the most ventral parts of the lPFC (optodes, according to the international 5/10 system: F6–F8, F6–FC6, F5–FC5, F5–F7) responded to the self-control demands of readying oneself for an imminent sprint start with an increase in cerebral oxygenation. Herewith, we confirmed what the exploratory analyses in Wolff et al. [43] suggested. Importantly, this finding is also in accordance with research from cognitive neuroscience that different self-regulatory processes are governed by different subregions of the lPFC [39]. For example, the ventral lPFC has been shown to be responsible for response inhibition, whereas the dorsolateral PFC has been linked to top-down attention control [39], and anterior regions of the PFC have been ascribed a role in cognitive branching [62]. In the context of the self-control demands a sprint start imposes, the pronounced involvement of the ventral lPFC as the prime structure for response inhibition makes intuitive sense. Effective response inhibition in the timeframe between Set and Go might be particularly difficult for participants that do not have a background in sprint running (as is the case with the participants in this study). Indeed, research shows that prior self-control exertion increases the number of false starts in athletes with no sprint start experience [32], whereas athletes with track and field experience showed delayed starting but not more false starts if they had exerted self-control in a previous task [31]. Further tentative support for the need to control the impulse to start prematurely comes from our observation that the magnitude of the increase in ventral lPFC oxygenation did not differ between experimental conditions. This finding was surprising, as the no-start condition was expected to require less self-control demands. However, our manipulation check indicated that participants actually perceived the no start condition as being the most challenging condition. Thus, conditions that were expected to increase the demands for action initiation and/or action inhibition (action inhibition start, action initiation start, combined start) were neither perceived as being more challenging, nor did they covary with a more pronounced cortical hemodynamic response. The requirement of not starting (no-start condition) appeared to have been the most challenging.

Second, our findings shed some light on gender differences in the cortical processing of the self-control demands of a sprint start. Research from basic neuroscience points towards gender differences in the magnitude of activation changes in cortical and subcortical brain regions, such as medial frontal cingulate cortices, globus pallidus, thalamus and parahippocampal gyrus, indicating greater neural activation in men than in women [63]. In line with this, we observed a stronger oxygenation change in the ventral lPFC in men than in women. Thus, while we found robust evidence for the stronger involvement of ventral lPFC between the Set and Go signal in males, this area does not respond with a significant increase in females. One reason for our failure to observe this effect in females could be due to variations in neuroanatomy between females and males, which can lead to differences in neural activity [63] and behavioral differences [64]. However, as our fNIRS montage covered the lPFC very broadly, one might expect to see a more pronounced oxygenation increase in other channels for females. However, this was not the case. Also, in previous research, no cortical and subcortical brain regions demonstrated greater activation in women than in men during a self-control task [63]. Thus, we believe our findings are more in line with research on gender differences in regard to self-control. Indeed, research indicates that females outperform males in behavioral control tasks [44,45,65]. Importantly, females show better behavioral inhibitory control than males during a two-choice oddball task in which subjects need to respond to standard and deviant stimuli [45]. Thus, results indicate that females have advantages concerning the control of inhibitory processes. In line with this, Li et al. [63] showed that females needed less cortical and subcortical activation to achieve similar reaction times and accuracy rates in a stop signal task than males. In different words, men may require more neural resources to control their behavior. Going back to sprint starts, females might be able to deal more efficiently with the self-control demands of a sprint start. Interestingly, this interpretation is in line with data from the 2008 Bejing Olympics, where female sprinters produced only four false starts (in 387 races), compared to 25 false starts that where produced by male sprinters (in 439 races) [66].

Third, it is still an ongoing debate whether self-control demands are processed more in the right or left hemisphere or if there is no hemispheric difference in lPFC activity. Previous studies showed that self-control tasks, such as go/no-go activation, are accompanied by more activity in the left hemispheric prefrontal cortex [46,47]. Our results indicate no lateralization patterns. Cortical activity of the lPFC was not significantly higher in the right or in the left hemisphere. Also, no two-way interaction effects with gender or ROI were found. Hence, we did not find evidence for hemispheric differences in oxygenation in different subareas of the lPFC or as a function of participants' gender.

7. Limitations

Against our expectations, the magnitude of cortical activation did not differ as a function of start condition. Hence, cortical activity was not significantly lower for the no-start condition compared to the other three start conditions (promotion, prevention, optimal). Thus, manipulations that supposedly added different self-control demands (impulse control and action initiation) did not lead to higher cortical activation in contrast to a singular self-control demand (impulse control). These findings do not support our hypothesis and previous conclusions [43]. Possibly, our manipulation was not successful, as indicated by the manipulation check: The no-start condition was perceived as the most difficult one. This was unexpected because compared to the other three sprint start conditions, the no-start condition only imposes impulse control (to not start). As the application of self-control produces costs and is invested sparingly [22–24], less complex self-control demands (only impulse control) should be perceived as less aversive and difficult. However, given that responding to the go signal might be a very strong behavioral impulse, it is conceivable that the intensity of the required control signal needs to be comparably high to control this almost automatic impulse.

Perceived subjective difficulty is frequently used as a marker to assess perceived self-control investment and costs. Maybe more individually challenging start conditions might lead to higher cortical activation and higher demand of self-control. Therefore, subjective difficulty of sprint start conditions need to be measured in a more differentiated way (e.g., 7 point Likert-Scale), to allow for a comparison between conditions in more absolute terms. Additionally, physical and psychological variables like perceived effort, frustration, fatigue or cognitive overload might also contribute to the processing of control demands, and it would be interesting to also assess such variables. However, our manipulation check showed that participants were generally motivated to perform well and were not extremely exhausted.

8. Future Research

In the current study, we did not examine to what extent activity in the ventral lPFC is related to the actual start performance. Evaluating behavioral performance in a sprint start task could be operationalized by measuring the reaction time. McEwan, Ginis & Bray [67] demonstrated in a dart-throw task that effective self-control increases reaction time of movement initiation and accuracy of throwing motion. More importantly, Englert et al. [31,32] showed that participants who had completed a self-control-demanding task prior to a sprint start displayed worse reaction times. We believe it would be an important question for future research to unravel the relationship between the cortical response after the Set signal and the resultant reaction time.

Differences in behavioral performance (here: reaction time) can also arise in consequence to experience differences: elite sprinters differentiate from well-trained sprinters due to significantly faster starts in 60 and 100 m races [12]. Englert et al. [32] showed that prior self-control exertion leads to worse starting times in elite sprinters, but no increase in the number of false starts, whereas the number of false starts increases in athletes with no sprint start experiences. Linking these findings, it is highly interesting and promising for future research to investigate oxygenation and behavioral differences (e.g., reaction time, false start rate and start technique) between novice and professional sprinters. Referring to the findings of Lipps et al. [66], which show a lower false start rate for women than for men, it is a fascinating research question to compare these behavioral differences between female and male sprinters and assess how they covary with changes in lPFC activation changes. Further variables of interest for future research are how difficult participants perceive the task to be and how they feel during the testing session. Thus, it might be instructive to assess these variables with the Profile of Mood States (POMS) [68] questionnaire and Borg Scale [69] before and after the sprint start in future studies.

9. Conclusions

It is well established that self-control is indispensable for an optimal sport performance, such as sprint start execution [31,32,43]. In line with previous research, we observed a significant increase in cortical activity in the lPFC during sprint start preparation. Additionally, we showed that particularly ventral parts of the lPFC are activated prior to the Go signal of a sprint start. Hence, exploratory findings [43] concerning the importance of ventral parts of lPFC for self-control execution during sprint starts could be replicated. In extension to this, we observed that a significant increase in cortical activity in the ventral parts of the lPFC did not occur in females, but only in male participants. No lateralization patterns were found. This study transfers findings from basic neuroscience to sports and facilitates the understanding of the cortical processing of sport-specific self-control demands.

Author Contributions: Conceptualization, W.W.; methodology, W.W. and K.-M.S.; software, W.W. and K.-M.S.; validation, W.W. and K.-M.S.; formal analysis, K.-M.S.; investigation, K.-M.S. and M.K.; resources, W.W. and J.S.; data curation, K.-M.S.; writing—original draft preparation, K.-M.S.; writing—review and editing, W.W. and J.S.; visualization, K.-M.S.; supervision, W.W. and J.S.; project administration, W.W.; funding acquisition, J.S. All authors have read and agreed to the published version of the manuscript.

Funding: This research received no external funding.

Acknowledgments: We thank Magdalena Kusserow for assistance with data collection.

Conflicts of Interest: The authors declare no conflict of interest.

Appendix A

Table A1. Values of oxygenated hemoglobin (HbO) concentration.

Regions of Interest (ROIs)	Start Condition	Baseline n	Baseline M (SD)	Set n	Set M (SD)
Ventral	Action inhibition start	39	0.00 (0.00)	39	0.289 (0.538)
	Action initiation start	39	0.00 (0.00)	39	0.256 (0.503)
	Combined start	39	0.00 (0.00)	39	0.237 (0.455)
	No-Start	39	0.00 (0.00)	39	0.309 (0.416)
Anterior	Action inhibition start	39	0.00 (0.00)	39	0.076 (0.436)
	Action initiation start	39	0.00 (0.00)	39	0.092 (0.448)
	Combined start	39	0.00 (0.00)	39	0.064 (0.493)
	No-Start	39	0.00 (0.00)	39	0.113 (0.399)
Others	Action inhibition start	39	0.00 (0.00)	39	0.028 (0.298)
	Action initiation start	39	0.00 (0.00)	39	0.028 (0.274)
	Combined start	39	0.00 (0.00)	39	−0.021 (0.282)
	No-Start	39	0.00 (0.00)	39	0.032 (0.240)

Note. n = number of persons; M = mean value; SD = standard deviation. As all values were normalized, all baseline values are zero.

References

1. Brown, T.D.; Vescovi, J.D. Maximum speed: Misconceptions of sprinting. *Strength Cond. J.* **2012**, *34*, 37–41. [CrossRef]
2. Helmick, K. Biomechanical analysis of sprint start positioning. *Track Coach* **2003**, *163*, 5209–5214.
3. Majumdar, A.S.; Robergs, R.A. The science of speed: Determinants of performance in the 100 m sprint. *Int. J. Sports Sci. Coach.* **2011**, *6*, 479–493. [CrossRef]
4. Salo, A.; Bezodis, I. Which starting style is faster in sprint running standing or crouch start? *Sports Biomech.* **2004**, *3*, 43–53. [CrossRef] [PubMed]
5. Harland, M.J.; Steele, J.R. Biomechanics of the Sprint Start. *Sports Med.* **1997**, *23*, 11–20. [CrossRef] [PubMed]
6. West, D.J.; Owen, N.J.; Cunningham, D.J.; Cook, C.J.; Kilduff, L.P. Strength and power predictors of swimming starts in international sprint swimmers. *J. Strength Cond. Res.* **2011**, *25*, 950–955. [CrossRef] [PubMed]
7. Cossor, J.M.; Mason, B.R. Swim start performances at the Sydney 2000 Olympic Games. In *XIXth Symposium on Biomechanics in Sports*; Blackwell, J., Ed.; University of California: San Francisco, CA, USA, 2001; pp. 70–74.
8. Brüggemann, G.P.; Morlock, M.; Zatsiorsky, V.M. Analysis of the Bobsled and Men's Luge Events at the XVII Olympic Winter Games in Lillehammer. *J. Appl. Biomech.* **1997**, *13*, 98–108. [CrossRef]
9. Zanoletti, C.; La Torre, A.; Merati, G.; Rampinini, E.; Impellizzeri, F.M. Relationship between push phase and final race time in skeleton performance. *J. Strength Cond. Res.* **2006**, *20*, 579–583.
10. Eikenberry, A.; McAuliffe, J.; Welsh, T.N.; Zerpa, C.; McPherson, M.; Newhouse, I. Starting with the "right" foot minimizes sprint start time. *Acta Psychol.* **2008**, *127*, 495–500. [CrossRef]
11. Mero, A. Force-time characteristics and running velocity of male sprinters during the acceleration phase of sprinting. *Res. Q. Exerc. Sport* **1988**, *59*, 94–98. [CrossRef]
12. Slawinski, J.; Bonnefoy, A.; Levêque, J.-M.; Ontanon, G.; Riquet, A.; Dumas, R.; Chèze, L. Kinematic and kinetic comparisons of elite and well-trained sprinters during sprint start. *J. Strength Cond. Res.* **2010**, *24*, 896–905. [CrossRef] [PubMed]
13. Ille, A.; Selin, I.; Do, M.-C.; Thon, B. Attentional focus effects on sprint start performance as a function of skill level. *J. Sports Sci.* **2013**, *31*, 1705–1712. [CrossRef] [PubMed]
14. Sheppard, J.M.; Young, W.B. Agility literature review: Classifications, training and testing. *J. Sport Sci.* **2006**, *24*, 915–932. [CrossRef] [PubMed]
15. Brass, M.; Haggard, P. To do or not to do: The neural signature of self-control. *J. Neurosci.* **2007**, *27*, 9141–9145. [CrossRef]

16. de Ridder, D.T.D.; Lensvelt-Mulders, G.; Finkenauer, C.; Stok, F.; Baumeister, R.F. Taking stock of self-control: A meta-analysis of how trait self-control relates to a wide range of behaviors. *Personal. Soc. Psychol. Rev.* **2012**, *16*, 76–99. [CrossRef]
17. Baumeister, R.F.; Heatherton, T.F.; Tice, D.M. *Losing Control: How and Why People Fail at Self-Regulation*; Academic Press: San Diego, CA, USA, 1994.
18. Baumeister, R.F.; Vohs, K.D.; Tice, D.M. The strength model of self-control. *Curr. Dir. Psychol. Sci.* **2007**, *16*, 351–355. [CrossRef]
19. Blain, B.; Hollard, G.; Pessiglione, M. Neural mechanisms underlying the impact of daylong cognitive work on economic decisions. *Proc. Natl. Acad. Sci. USA* **2016**, *113*, 6967–6972. [CrossRef]
20. Mischel, W.; Shoda, Y.; Rodriguez, M.L. Delay of gratification in children. *Science* **1989**, *244*, 933–938. [CrossRef]
21. Muraven, M.; Tice, D.M.; Baumeister, R.F. Self-control as a limited resource: Regulatory depletion patterns. *J. Personal. Soc. Psychol.* **1998**, *74*, 774–789. [CrossRef]
22. Dixon, M.L.; Christoff, K. The decision to engage cognitive control is driven by expected reward-value. Neural and behavioral evidence. *PLoS ONE* **2012**, *7*, e51637. [CrossRef]
23. Kool, W.; Botvinick, M. A labor/leisure tradeoff in cognitive control. *J. Exp. Psychol. Gen.* **2014**, *143*, 131–141. [CrossRef]
24. Shenhav, A.; Musslick, S.; Lieder, F.; Kool, W.; Griffiths, T.L.; Cohen, J.D.; Botvinick, M.M. Toward a rational and mechanistic account of mental effort. *Annu. Rev. Neurosci.* **2017**, *40*, 99–124. [CrossRef] [PubMed]
25. Wolff, W.; Sieber, V.; Bieleke, M.; Englert, C. Task duration and task order do not matter: No effect on self-control performance. *Psychol. Res.* **2019**, 1–11. [CrossRef]
26. Wolff, W.; Martarelli, C.S. Bored into depletion? Towards a tentative integration of perceived self-control exertion and boredom as guiding signals for goal-directed behavior. *Perspect. Psychol. Sci.* **2020**. [CrossRef] [PubMed]
27. Hagger, M.S.; Wood, C.; Stiff, C.; Chatzisarantis, N.L.D. Ego depletion and the strength model of self-control: A meta-analysis. *Psychol. Bull.* **2010**, *136*, 495–525. [CrossRef] [PubMed]
28. Brown, D.M.Y.; Graham, J.D.; Innes, K.I.; Harris, S.; Flemington, A.; Bray, S.R. Effects of prior cognitive exertion on physical performance: A systematic review and meta-analysis. *Sports Med.* **2020**, *50*, 497–529. [CrossRef] [PubMed]
29. Giboin, L.-S.; Wolff, W. The effect of ego depletion or mental fatigue on subsequent physical endurance performance: A meta-analysis. *Perform. Enhanc. Health* **2019**, *7*, 100150. [CrossRef]
30. Englert, C.; Bertrams, A. Anxiety, ego depletion, and sports performance. *J. Sport Exerc. Psychol.* **2012**, *34*, 580–599. [CrossRef]
31. Englert, C.; Bertrams, A. The Effect of ego depletion on sprint start reaction time. *J. Sport Exerc. Psychol.* **2014**, *36*, 506–515. [CrossRef]
32. Englert, C.; Persaud, B.N.; Oudejans, R.R.D.; Bertrams, A. The influence of ego depletion on sprint start performance in athletes without track and field experience. *Front. Psychol.* **2015**, *6*, 1–16. [CrossRef]
33. Botvinick, M.; Braver, T. Motivation and cognitive control: From behavior to neural mechanism. *Annu. Rev. Psychol.* **2015**, *66*, 83–113. [CrossRef]
34. Carter, C.S.; van Veen, V. Anterior cingulate cortex and conflict detection. An update of theory and data. *Cogn. Affect. Behav. Neurosci.* **2007**, *7*, 367–379. [CrossRef]
35. Cohen, J.; Lieberman, M.D. The common neural basis of exerting self-control in multiple domains. In *Self Control Insociety, Mind, and Brain*; Hassin, R.R., Ochsner, K.N., Trope, Y., Eds.; Oxford University Press: New York, NY, USA, 2010; pp. 141–160. [CrossRef]
36. Miller, E.K.; Cohen, J.D. An integrative theory of prefrontal cortex function. *Annu. Rev. Neurosci.* **2001**, *24*, 167–202. [CrossRef] [PubMed]
37. Shenhav, A.; Botvinick, M.M.; Cohen, J.D. The expected value of control: An integrative theory of anterior cingulate cortex function. *Neuroscience* **2013**, *79*, 217–240. [CrossRef] [PubMed]
38. Hart, H.; Radua, J.; Nakao, T.; Mataix-Cols, D.; Rubia, K. Meta-analysis of functional magnetic resonance imaging studies of inhibition and attention in attention-deficit/hyperactivity disorder: Exploring task-specific, stimulant medication, and age effects. *JAMA Psychiatry* **2013**, *70*, 185–198. [CrossRef]
39. Dubin, M.J.; Maia, T.V.; Peterson, B.S. Cognitive Control in the Service of Self-Regulation. In *The Encyclopedia of Behavioral Neuroscience*; Koob, G.F., le Moal, M., Thompson, R.F., Eds.; Elsevier: Amsterdam, The Netherlands, 2010.

40. Wolff, W.; Hirsch, A.; Bieleke, M.; Shenhav, A. Neuroscientific approaches to self-regulatory control in sports. In *Self-Regulation and Motivation in Sport and Exercise Psychology*; Englert, C., Taylor, I., Eds.; Routledge: London, UK, 2020, in press.
41. Rooks, C.R.; Thom, N.J.; McCully, K.K.; Dishman, R.K. Effects of incremental exercise on cerebral oxygenation measured by near-infrared spectroscopy: A systematic review. *Prog. Neurobiol.* **2010**, *92*, 134–150. [CrossRef] [PubMed]
42. Wolff, W.; Bieleke, M.; Hirsch, A.; Wienbruch, C.; Gollwitzer, P.M.; Schüler, J. Increase in prefrontal cortex oxygenation during static muscular endurance performance is modulated by self-regulation strategies. *Sci. Rep.* **2018**, *8*, 15756. [CrossRef]
43. Wolff, W.; Thürmer, J.L.; Stadler, K.-M.; Schüler, J. Ready, set, go: Cortical hemodynamics during self-controlled sprint starts. *Psychol. Sport Exerc.* **2019**, *41*, 21–28. [CrossRef]
44. Fillmore, M.T.; Weafer, J. Alcohol impairment of behavior in men and women. *Addiction* **2004**, *99*, 1237–1246. [CrossRef]
45. Yuan, J.; He, Y.; Qinglin, Z.; Chen, A.; Li, H. Gender differences in behavioral inhibitory control: ERP evidence from a two-choice oddball task. *Psychophysiology* **2008**, *45*, 986–993. [CrossRef]
46. Rubia, K.; Russell, T.; Overmeyer, S.; Brammer, M.J.; Bullmore, E.T.; Sharma, T.; Taylor, E. Mapping motor inhibition: Conjunctive brain activations across different versions of go/no-go and stop tasks. *NeuroImage* **2001**, *13*, 250–261. [CrossRef] [PubMed]
47. Serrien, D.J.; Sovijärvi-Spapé, M.M. Cognitive control of response inhibition and switching: Hemispheric lateralization and hand preference. *Brain Cogn.* **2013**, *82*, 283–290. [CrossRef]
48. Logothetis, N.K. The underpinnings of the BOLD functional magnetic resonance imaging signal. *J. Neurosci.* **2003**, *23*, 3963–3971. [CrossRef] [PubMed]
49. Ekkekakis, P. Illuminating the Black Box: Investigating prefrontal cortical hemodynamics during exercise with near-infrared spectroscopy. *J. Sport Exerc. Psychol.* **2009**, *31*, 505–553. [CrossRef] [PubMed]
50. Lin, P.-Y.; Chen, J.-J.J.; Lin, S.-I. The cortical control of cycling exercise in stroke patients: An fNIRS study. *Hum. Brain Mapp.* **2013**, *34*, 2381–2390. [CrossRef]
51. Perrey, S. Non-invasive NIR spectroscopy of human brain function during exercise. *Methods* **2008**, *45*, 289–299. [CrossRef]
52. Piper, S.K.; Krueger, A.; Koch, S.P.; Mehnert, J.; Habermehl, C.; Steinbrink, J.; Schmitz, C.H. A wearable multi-channel fNIRS system for brain imaging in freely moving subjects. *NeuroImage* **2014**, *85*, 64–71. [CrossRef]
53. Scholkmann, F.; Kleiser, S.; Metz, A.J.; Zimmermann, R.; Mata Pavia, J.; Wolf, U.; Wolf, M. A review on continuous wave functional near-infrared spectroscopy and imaging instrumentation and methodology. *NeuroImage* **2014**, *85*, 6–27. [CrossRef]
54. Oostenveld, R.; Praamstra, P. The five percent electrode system for high-resolution EEG and ERP measurements. *Clin. Neurophysiol.* **2001**, *112*, 713–719. [CrossRef]
55. Huppert, T.J.; Diamond, S.G.; Franceschini, M.A.; Boas, D.A. HomER: A review of time-series analysis methods for near-infrared spectroscopy of the brain. *Appl. Opt.* **2009**, *48*, D280–D298. [CrossRef]
56. Brigadoi, S.; Ceccherini, L.; Cutini, S.; Scarpa, F.; Scatturin, P.; Selb, J.; Gagnon, L.; Boas, D.A.; Cooper, R.J. Motion artifacts in functional near-infrared spectroscopy: A comparison of motion correction techniques applied to real cognitive data. *NeuroImage* **2014**, *85*, 181–191. [CrossRef] [PubMed]
57. Chiarelli, A.M.; Maclin, E.L.; Fabiani, M.; Gratton, G. A kurtosis-based wavelet algorithm for motion artifact correction of fNIRS data. *NeuroImage* **2015**, *112*, 128–137. [CrossRef] [PubMed]
58. Cooper, R.J.; Selb, J.; Gagnon, L.; Phillip, D.; Schytz, H.W.; Iversen, H.K.; Ashina, M.; Boas, D.A. A systematic comparison of motion artifact correction techniques for functional near-infrared spectroscopy. *Front. Neurosci.* **2012**, *6*, 147. [CrossRef] [PubMed]
59. Delpy, D.T.; Cope, M.; van der Zee, P.; Arridge, S.; Wray, S.; Wyatt, J. Estimation of optical pathlength through tissue from direct time of flight measurement. *Phys. Med. Biol.* **1988**, *33*, 1433–1442. [CrossRef]
60. Essenpreis, M.; Cope, M.; Elwell, C.E.; Arridge, S.R.; van der Zee, P.; Delpy, D.T. Wavelength dependence of the differential pathlength factor and the log slope in time-resolved tissue spectroscopy. *Adv. Exp. Med. Biol.* **1993**, *333*, 9–20.
61. Cohen, J.D. *Statistical Power Analysis for the Behavioral Sciences, Revised Edition*; Academic Press: New York, NY, USA, 1977.

62. Koechlin, E.; Ody, C.; Kouneiher, F. The Architecture of cognitive control in the human prefrontal cortex. *Science* **2003**, *302*, 1181–1185. [CrossRef]
63. Li, C.S.; Huang, C.; Constable, R.T.; Sinha, R. Gender differences in the neural correlates of response inhibition during a stop signal task. *NeuroImage* **2006**, *32*, 1918–1929. [CrossRef]
64. Huster, R.J.; Westerhausen, R.; Herrmann, C.S. Sex differences in cognitive control are associated with midcingulate and callosal morphology. *Brain Struct. Funct.* **2011**, *215*, 225–235. [CrossRef]
65. Burton, V.S.; Cullen, F.T.; Evans, T.D.; Alarid, L.F.; Dunaway, R.G. Gender, self-control, and crime. *J. Res. Crime Delinq.* **1998**, *35*, 123–147. [CrossRef]
66. Lipps, D.B.; Galecki, A.T.; Ashton-Miller, J.A. On the implications of a sex difference in the reaction times of sprinters at the Beijing Olympics. *PLoS ONE* **2011**, *6*, e26141. [CrossRef]
67. McEwan, D.; Ginis, K.A.M.; Bray, S.R. The effects of depleted self-control strength on skill-based task performance. *J. Sport Exerc. Psychol.* **2013**, *35*, 239–249. [CrossRef] [PubMed]
68. McNair, P.M.; Lorr, M.; Droppleman, L.F. *POMS Manual*, 2nd ed.; Educational and Industrial Testing Service: San Diego, CA, USA, 1981.
69. Borg, G. *Borg's Perceived Exertion and Pain Scales*; Human Kinetics: Champaign, IL, USA, 1998.

© 2020 by the authors. Licensee MDPI, Basel, Switzerland. This article is an open access article distributed under the terms and conditions of the Creative Commons Attribution (CC BY) license (http://creativecommons.org/licenses/by/4.0/).

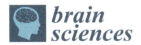

Article

"No Pain No Gain": Evidence from a Parcel-Wise Brain Morphometry Study on the Volitional Quality of Elite Athletes

Gaoxia Wei [1,2,3,*], Ruoguang Si [4], Youfa Li [5], Ying Yao [1,3], Lizhen Chen [1,3], Shu Zhang [1,3], Tao Huang [6], Liye Zou [7], Chunxiao Li [8] and Stephane Perrey [9]

1. CAS Key Laboratory of Mental Health, Institute of Psychology, Chinese Academy of Sciences, Beijing 100101, China; yaoy@psych.ac.cn (Y.Y.); chenlz@psych.ac.cn (L.C.); zhangs@psych.ac.cn (S.Z.)
2. CAS Key Laboratory of Behavioral Science, Institute of Psychology, Chinese Academy of Sciences, Beijing 100101, China
3. Department of Psychology, University of Chinese Academy of Sciences, Beijing 100049, China
4. CUBRIC, Cardiff University, Maindy Road, Wales Cardiff CF24 4HQ, UK; SiR@Cardiff.ac.uk
5. Collaborative Innovation Center of Assessment toward Basic Education Quality, Beijing Normal University, Beijing 100875, China; liyoufa@bnu.edu.cn
6. Department of Physical Education, Shanghai Jiao Tong University, Shanghai 200030, China; taohuang@sjtu.edu.cn
7. Department of Psychology, Shenzhen University, Shenzhen 518061, China; liyezou123@gmail.com
8. School of Physical Education and Sports Science, South China Normal University, Guangzhou 510006, China; chunxiao.li@nie.edu.sg
9. EuroMov Digital Health in Motion, Univ Montpellier, IMT Mines Ales, 34090 Montpellier, France; stephane.perrey@umontpellier.fr
* Correspondence: weigx@psych.ac.cn; Tel.: +86-010-64850898

Received: 7 June 2020; Accepted: 14 July 2020; Published: 17 July 2020

Abstract: Volition is described as a psychological construct with great emphasis on the sense of agency. During volitional behavior, an individual always presents a volitional quality, an intrapersonal trait for dealing with adverse circumstances, which determines the individual's persistence of action toward their intentions or goals. Elite athletes are a group of experts with superior volitional quality and, thereby, could be regarded as the natural subject pool to investigate this mental trait. The purpose of this study was to examine brain morphometric characteristics associated with volitional quality by using magnetic resonance imaging (MRI) and the Scale of Volitional Quality. We recruited 16 national-level athletes engaged in short track speed skating and 18 healthy controls matched with age and gender. A comparison of a parcel-wise brain anatomical characteristics of the healthy controls with those of the elite athletes revealed three regions with significantly increased cortical thickness in the athlete group. These regions included the left precuneus, the left inferior parietal lobe, and the right superior frontal lobe, which are the core brain regions involved in the sense of agency. The mean cortical thickness of the left inferior parietal lobe was significantly correlated with the independence of volitional quality (a mental trait that characterizes one's intendency to control his/her own behavior and make decisions by applying internal standards and/or objective criteria). These findings suggest that sports training is an ideal model for better understanding the neural mechanisms of volitional behavior in the human brain.

Keywords: volition; brain structure; sense of agency; sport; MRI

1. Introduction

Volition or the will is a univocal concept with a long history in philosophy. From a psychological perspective, it has been considered as a psychological construct, being used to describe one's endogenous mental act of forming, maintaining, and implementing an intention or goal [1,2]. This mental process or conscious experience is unique to human beings and associated with a sense of agency [3]. From the developmental perspective, volitional quality is an intrapersonal trait for dealing with adverse circumstances that determines an individual's persistence of action upon intentions or goals [4,5]. This capability is of great significance for individual survival, development, and achievement.

Distinguished from concepts or terms such as grit [6], willpower [7], mental toughness [8,9], and resilience [10], volitional quality has a great emphasis on the sense of agency within four components (self-conscientiousness, independence, determination, and resilience) [5,11–14]. This theoretical model has been widely used in education, physical activity, and sports settings. For instance, junior school students who regularly participated in rock climbing showed greater levels of volitional quality than those without regular participation [15]. A study observed that a four-month outdoor survival training program significantly improved performances in independence, determination, and resilience among college students [16]. Even three-month-long professional sports training was found to enhance an individual's volitional quality [17]; however, the brain structures related to volitional quality are largely unexplored.

With the advance of human brain imaging techniques, a growing body of evidence indicates that the brain structure can be reorganized through learning and life experiences. A magnetic resonance imaging (MRI) study that was performed on experts suggested that the brain volume of the posterior hippocampi in taxi drivers was significantly larger than those of age-matched controls, and the greater brain volume of the posterior hippocampi was positively associated with their driving experiences [18]. Meditators and Tai Chi Chuan masters also showed greater cortical thickness in multiple brain areas related to high-level cognitive processes as compared with the sedentary controls [19,20]. Additionally, some longitudinal studies provide direct evidence on use-dependent brain plasticity. Currently, a growing body of evidence has demonstrated that physical training could induce structural plasticity. Rogge, et al. [21] investigated the effect of a twelve-week whole-body training with minor metabolic demands on the brain structure, which showed that balance training could increase the cortical thickness in the visual and vestibular cortical regions. A recent study indicated that the alteration of the volume and cortical thickness of grey matter could be induced by three-week motor training in adults [22].

Elite athletes are a group of experts with extraordinary physical abilities and mental attributes that are developed over long-term sports training. Professional training may also have a pronounced effect on cortical organization, and some neurocognitive researchers have examined the brain plasticity in elite athletes. For instance, elite short track speed skating (STSS) players exhibited larger volumes in the right cerebellar hemisphere and vermian lobules VI-VII relative to the matched controls [23]. Our previous studies observed that elite diving players showed greater grey matter density in the thalamus and the left precentral gyrus [24] as well as greater cortical thickness in the left superior temporal sulcus, the right orbitofrontal cortex, and the right parahippocampal gyri, as compared to the controls [25]. Similarly, highly practiced golf players showed larger gray matter volumes in the frontoparietal network relative to controls without any golfing practice and less experience [26]. Another study on male adolescent elite footballers showed that increased training volumes improve the cortical area [27]. Overall, these findings suggest that sports training may reorganize cortical and subcortical structures.

Winter sports are sports that have great requirements for physical endurance and independent decision-making capabilities to navigate the snow and ice equipment. Of note, short track speed skate (STSS) athletes who engaged in winter sports often experienced many physical and mental setbacks, limb injuries, and performance slumps, providing a unique opportunity to investigate their volitional quality. A recent behavioral study involving 169 winter sports athletes (alpine skiers) by a retrospective design found that their grit and perfectionistic strivings were closely associated with increased engagements in practice hours, suggesting winter sports athletes might have outstanding volitional qualities [28]. Skaters tend to peak at their late teens and early adulthood, the age at which people also often experienced a dramatic cortical reorganization; therefore, alterations in cortical structures associated with volitional quality are expected in winter sports players. In this study, we aimed to compare elite athletes and control subjects through vertex-wise and parcel-wise analyses to detect multiple morphological differences. Both of two approaches are based on surface-based morphometry. The vertex-wise analysis is a method used to compute local morphological parameters based on each voxel, whereas the parcel-wise method is used to analyze large-scale cortical organization at the level of cortical parcellation [29]. The use of both vertex-wise and parcel-wise analyses can help researchers better understand the gray matter structures from different levels. In order to comprehensively understand mental trait-related anatomical correlates, the combination of two analysis approaches in one study is an ideal approach to completely measure the cortical morphometric changes behind the training-induced mental traits. Using MRI, we aimed to identify the cortical organization associated with volitional quality by comparing their anatomical differences between STSS elite athletes and control subjects. Specifically, we recruited STSS elite athletes from the Chinese national team who are world-class athletes and have experienced many international competitions as an expert group.

2. Methods

2.1. Ethics Statement

This study was approved by the institutional review board of the Institute of Psychology, Chinese Academy of Sciences (Approval date: 20180316). It was performed following the ethical standards laid down in the 1964 Declaration of Helsinki. The written informed consent forms were obtained from all participants and their parents/guardians for those participants aged under 18 years.

2.2. Participants

The participants were 34 right-handed young adults, including 16 STSS athletes from the Chinese national team (age: 18.3 ± 1.5; 7 males) with extensive sports training experiences (8.6 ± 1.9 years) and 18 college students as controls (age: 19.2 ± 1.2; 9 males) matched for sex and age. The participants in the control group were recruited from a local university and had no regular exercise or sports training experiences. All participants were right-handed and healthy. They did not have any history of substance dependence, e.g., alcohol or nicotine. Before the experiment, participants completed a screening form to ensure they did not have a history of hearing or vision problems, physical injury, seizures, metal implants, head trauma with loss of consciousness, or pregnancy.

2.3. Measures

2.3.1. Volitional Quality

Participants' volitional qualities were measured by the 36-item BTL-L-YZ 2.0 Scale of Volitional Quality [11,30]. This scale measures four dimensions of volitional quality, including self-consciousness (12 items), independence (8 items), determination (8 items), and resilience (8 items). The factorial validity, concurrent validity, internal reliability, and test-retest reliability of the scale were supported [11]. A 7-point Likert scale that ranged from 1 (strongly disagree) to 7 (strongly agree) was used for the responses.

2.3.2. Scanning Protocol

An MRI was performed on a 3-tesla scanner (Discovery MR750, GE, USA) with a 12-channel head matrix coil. All high-resolution anatomical images were obtained using the spoiled gradient recalled acquisition in a steady-state (SPGR) sequence with the following scan parameters: echo time (TE) = 2992 ms, repetition time (TR) = 6896 ms, flip angle (FA) = 8°, slice thickness = 1.0 mm, and Field of View (FOV) = 256 mm × 256 mm. The imaging data included 176 sagittal slices. During scanning, all participants reclined in a supine position on the bed of the scanner and were asked to lie still during the imaging procedure. A foam head holder and padding were placed around their head. Moreover, headphones were provided to block background noise.

2.3.3. Image Processing

After the image acquisitions, all images were visually checked for major artifacts, including head motions, brain lesions, and dissection, before further processing. Brain reconstructions from the structural images were conducted with the VolBrain system [31] (http://volbrain.upv.es/) and FreeSurfer (version 6.0), which were integrated into the pipeline of the Connectome Computation System (CCS, [32]). All individual images went through the same pipeline, including the following steps. First, a nonlocal mean-filtering operation was used to remove the spatial noise [33,34]. Second, the MR-inhomogeneity-induced image intensity variance was corrected [35]. Third, the brain images were extracted, and images containing nonbrain tissues were removed using a hybrid approach [36]. Fourth, the brain tissues were segmented into the cerebrospinal fluid (CSF), white matter (WM), and deep gray matter (GM), and the two hemispheres and subcortical structures were disconnected [35]. Fifth, the GM-WM boundary was tessellated with a triangular mesh and smoothed by a mesh deformation [35]. Sixth, the topographical defects were corrected on the surface, and the individual surface mesh was inflated into a sphere [37,38]. Finally, the individual surface (volume) was normalized by estimating the deformation between the individual brain volume and the common spherical coordinate system [39].

2.3.4. Parcel-Wise Cortical Thickness Computation

It was computed by the *recon-all* command implemented in FreeSurfer (version 6.0). The local cortical thickness was measured by averaging the shortest distance from a vertex on the white matter surface to the pial surface and the shortest distance from a point on the pial surface to the white matter surface [40]. There are 163,842 vertices in each hemisphere, and there are 327,684 total vertices in the whole brain. This measurement has a good test-retest reliability across field strengths, scanner upgrade, and scanner manufacturers [41]. Individual cortical thickness maps were registered to the *fsaverage* and smoothed to enhance the interindividual correspondence in the anatomical structure using a Gaussian filter of 10-mm full width at half-maxima (FWHM) [42].

The Desikan-Killiany atlas [43,44] was employed to parcel the cortical surface into 34 regions of interest (ROIs) in each hemisphere to explore the large-scale structures. The mean brain morphometric parameter in cortical thickness in each parcel was then calculated for each participant.

2.4. Statistical Analysis

Vertex-wise group differences in cortical thickness were examined. For each vertex, a general linear model (GLM) was employed with the gender, age, education, and Intracranial Volume (ICV) entered as covariates. Between-group comparisons were then computed, and a cluster-level correction for multiple comparisons was conducted using the random field theory with vertex $p < 0.001$ and cluster $p < 0.05$. These analyses were conducted in FreeSurfer 6.0.

Parcel-wise group differences in cortical thickness were computed using analysis of covariance (ANCOVA). Gender, age, education, and ICV were included as covariates. The adjusted *p*-threshold for the group difference was set to 0.00073 (i.e., 0.05/(2*34)) using Bonferroni correction for a multiple comparison of 68 ROIs in total.

Multivariate analysis of covariance (MANCOVA) was conducted to test the group difference in four dimensions of volitional qualities, with gender, age, and education as covariates. The *p*-value was set to 0.0125 (i.e., 0.05/4) using Bonferroni correction for multiple comparisons of four dimensions in total.

To examine the association between cortical thickness and volitional quality in each group, two separate partial correlation analyses were performed, with gender, age, education, and ICV as covariates. We also performed a partial correlation between the differed cortical thickness in the brain regions and training experiences in the athlete group, with the age and sex as covariates. The p-value was set to $0.05/n$ using Bonferroni correction for multiple comparisons of the brain regions with significant difference. These analyses were conducted with SPSS Statistics 22.0 (IBM Corp., Armonk, NY, USA).

3. Results

3.1. Demographic Data

There was no group difference in age ($t(32) = -1.994$, $p = 0.055$), gender ($\chi^2 = -0.133$, $p = 0.716$), body mass index (BMI) (t = -0.850, $p = 0.401$), and ICV volumes ($t(32) = -0.706$, $p = 0.485$); however, the control group had finished more years of education than the athlete group ($t(32) = -9.962$, $p = 0.000$) (Table 1).

Table 1. Demographic data of athletes and controls.

	Age	Gender	Education (Years)	Body Mass Index (BMI)	Years of Training	Intracranial Volume (ICV) (cm^3)
Athletes ($n = 19$)	18.3 ± 1.5	10 M	9.8 ± 1.8	21.2 ± 1.1	8.6 ± 1.9	1178.06 ± 85.20
Controls ($n = 19$)	19.2 ± 1.2	9 M	13.7 ± 1.0	22.0 ± 3.9	—	1210.68 ± 87.10

3.2. Group Difference in Volitional Qualities

The athlete group showed significantly higher scores in all dimensions, including self-conscientiousness (($F(1,29) = 12.086$, $p = 0.002$), independence ($F(1,29) = 28.386$, $p < 0.001$), determination ($F(1,29) = 7.850$, $p < 0.001$), and resilience ($F(1,29) = 7.842$, $p < 0.001$), relative to the control group (Table 2).

Table 2. Group differences in dimensions of volitional quality.

Dimensions	Athletes (M ± SD)	Controls (M ± SD)	F	p
Self-Conscientiousness	58.38 ± 7.99	45.72 ± 4.35	28.386	0.000
Independence	42.56 ± 7.53	27.50 ± 2.23	12.086	0.002
Determination	35.56 ± 4.75	27.11 ± 3.25	7.850	0.009
Resilience	32.94 ± 4.40	23.11 ± 2.59	7.842	0.009

3.3. Group Difference in Cortical Thickness

The results of the vertex-wise analysis did not show any significant group differences after a multiple comparison correction. The results of the parcel-wise analysis showed that the athlete group had significantly greater cortical thickness in the left precuneus ($F(1,29) = 22.105$, $p = 0.00006$), the left inferior parietal lobe ($F(1,29) = 16.046$, $p = 0.00041$), and the right superior frontal lobe ($F(1,29) = 23.971$, $p = 0.00004$) than the control group (Figures 1 and 2).

Brain Sci. 2020, 10, 459

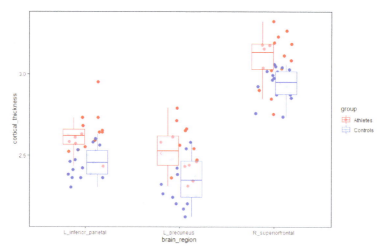

Figure 1. Parcel-wise difference of cortical thickness in the left precuneus, the left inferior parietal lobe, and the right superior frontal lobe between the athlete group and the control group. Data are presented by dot plots, whiskers, and box plots (median and error bars representing the first and third quartiles, respectively).

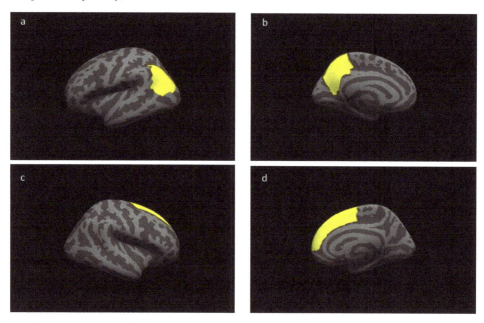

Figure 2. Compared with the control group, the athlete group showed greater cortical thickness in the colored brain regions based on the parcel-wise analysis: (**a**) indicates the left inferior parietal lobe, (**b**) indicates the left precuneus, and (**c**,**d**) the lateral view of the inferior view of the right superior frontal lobe.

3.4. Correlation Analyses

Regarding three brain regions with significant differences of cortical thickness, the adjusted *p*-value was set to 0.05/3 (0.017). As Figure 3 showed, the score of independence was significantly correlated with the cortical thickness in the left inferior parietal lobe ($r = 0.701$, $p = 0.011$). The other three dimensions showed no association with cortical thickness ($r = -0.335$ to 0.609, $ps > 0.017$). However, we did not observe any significant correlation between years of training and the score of any volitional qualities in the athlete group ($r = -0.001$. to 0.372, $ps > 0.05$).

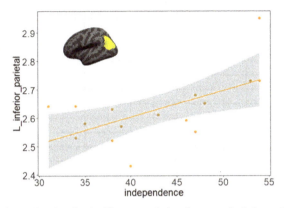

Figure 3. Scatter plots indicating the significant correlations between the independence scores of the volitional qualities and cortical thickness of the left inferior parietal lobule.

4. Discussion

To the best of our knowledge, this is the first brain imaging study to identify cortical architecture associated with volitional qualities. Our study found that STSS athletes showed better volitional qualities than the control group. Regarding the differences in brain morphometry, the athletes group had greater cortical thickness in the left precuneus, the left inferior parietal lobe, and the right superior frontal lobe. The greater cortical thickness in the left inferior parietal lobe was significantly associated with dimension independence of the volitional qualities.

As hypothesized, the behavioral results showed that athletes had better volitional qualities relative to the controls. In addition to the total score of the volitional qualities, all dimensions, including consciousness, independence, determination, and resilience, were significantly higher in the athlete group compared to the control group. This result is consistent with a previous study, which also revealed that STSS athletes scored higher in goal clarity, persistence, determination, and confidence compared to the controls [45]. Similarly, a study on national-level professional basketball players observed that they showed better performances in consciousness and independence than players in other levels [46]. Nonetheless, some studies on other antagonistic sports observed that professional players had significantly better performances in the total scores of volitional qualities but showed different advantages in specific dimensions. For instance, a study on boxers showed a significant correlation between competition scores and resilience in volitional qualities [47]. Moreover, another study comparing the effect of training experience on volitional qualities showed that beach volleyball athletes with above 15 years of training experience had better continence and resilience than those under 15 years of training experience [48]. All these findings indicate that sports training selectively improves the components of volitional qualities. STSS is a sport that requires the adjustment of pacing and tactical positioning [49]. It was found that the optimal pacing strategy varies among STSS projects of different distances. A 500-m race needs a fast start, whereas a 1500-m race has a greater emphasis of physical exertion in the last five laps [50,51]. So, STSS athletes need to make decisions on their own regarding how to distribute the energy and what moment to invest their energy during the race bout [52]. Moreover, they have to keep clear goals during the competition and adhere to a chosen strategy throughout the whole bout. Therefore, in this study, we observed that long-term professional training might improve their mental characteristics of volitional qualities.

The basis of volitional qualities is closely related to the sense of agency [3]. A sense of agency is also called the sense of control, i.e., a subjective awareness of initiating, executing, and controlling one's own volitional actions in the world, as well as the experience of oneself as the agent of one's own motor acts [53]. Therefore, it is accepted that our experiences of volitional behaviors include a vivid sense of agency [3,54,55]. Of note, dimension independence in volitional qualities is a mental construct that is closely associated with a sense of agency, which is a mental trait that characterizes one's tendency to control his/her own behavior and making decisions by applying internal standards and/or objective criteria [56]. An individual having a good sense of agency is capable of controlling their behaviors, which is a prerequisite for volitional qualities and independence. On the other side, impairments in the sense of agency have been reported in neurological and psychiatric disorders [57], indicating that these patients find it difficult to control their own behaviors and present poor volitional qualities. The athletes recruited in this study are professional athletes engaged in their career for at least ten years and have rich experiences in dealing with difficulties in important national and international competitions. It is believed that a sense of agency is strongest when there is a strong motivation to act with a clear goal [58]. Although the mechanism underlying the association of sports training and the sense of agency remains largely unclear, it has been reported that the sense of agency was improved by listening to music in one's daily life [59]. Hence, it is likely that long-term sports training under adverse circumstances likely reshapes elite athletes' sense of agency, which further enhances their volitional qualities.

Intriguingly, all of these brain regions (the precuneus, the inferior parietal lobule, and the superior frontal cortex) are consistently linked to the function of the sense of agency [60]. Precuneus is a posteromedial portion of the parietal lobe responsible for processing self-relevant information. A task-based fMRI study observed that the bilateral anterior precuneus was activated when participants were exposed to psychological trait words describing their own attributes [61]. Apart from the explicit external information, the precuneus is also involved in implicit internal self-related processes, especially in making intentional behaviors [62]. During this process, the precuneus contributes to the sense of agency [53,60]. A recent study investigated the focal lesion areas among 50 patients with a disrupted sense of agency and found a persuasive causal relationship between the intactness of the functional networks related to the precuneus and a sense of agency [55]; therefore, it is speculated that individuals with good performances of independence have a better sense of agency, which is tightly linked to the greater cortical thickness of the precuneus. In addition to the precuneus, the left inferior parietal lobule (IPL) is another anatomical difference related to the sense of agency. A study observed that the IPL was less-activated when the right-handed subjects felt that the behavior was performed by themselves compared to when they felt that the behavior was not performed by themselves [63]. The frontal and prefrontal lobes play a crucial role in the planning and initiation of voluntary action [64]. Notably, parts of the superior frontal gyrus are involved in inhibitory control. For instance, the inhibitory control was slowed in patients with right superior medial frontal damage [65]. Another study also found that the right superior frontal cortical activations to conflict anticipation are related to impulse control in healthy participants [66]. The inhibitory control is a cognitive function also associated with the sense of agency, since a fluency of action selection contributes heavily to the sense of control [67]; therefore, it indicates that the greater cortical thickness in the right superior frontal gyrus might also be associated with an improved sense of agency. Although it is unclear what the underlying mechanism is that causes different cortical thicknesses between the athlete group and the control group, an increased cortical thickness is likely associated with a complex change in the microstructure, e.g., the increases in dendritic arborization, axonal elongation and thickening, synaptogenesis, and glial proliferation [68,69]. Numerous animal models and human studies have consistently reported that training selectively improves neurogenesis and induce changes in the cortical volume [70]. Therefore, our results of greater cortical thicknesses in these brain regions reflect the training-induced changes in the cellular and neuronal levels.

Several limitations should be acknowledged in this study. First, we could not conclude the causal relationship between volitional quality and parcel-wised cortical thickness. Future investigation on a less-skillful amateur group is needed to elucidate whether the difference is induced by training or nurture. Secondly, the relationship between the cortical thicknesses and the years of training was not evident. Instead of years of training, training volume and/or intensity might have a closer association with the changes in the cortical thickness [19,25]; therefore, multiple indices to measure training experiences such as the training load (intensity x volume) should be used in future research to gain a better understanding about the issue. Thirdly, the cross-sectional study design could not completely exclude the confounding effects of nature or nurture on the brain structures in the two groups. These confounding variables include individual differences such as lifestyle, nutrition, and personality. In this study, the difference in education between the two groups might be a potential factor that influences the current results. In future studies, a longitudinal study is needed to rule out the effects of individual differences.

5. Conclusions

Although some limitations existed in this study, it still identified the cortical architecture associated with volitional qualities. Professional athletes exhibited excellent volitional qualities, as well as thicker cortexes in the left precuneus, the left inferior parietal lobule, and the right superior frontal gyrus. Better performance in the dimension independence of the volitional qualities was correlated with a greater cortical thickness in the left inferior parietal lobule. These findings suggest that sports training is an ideal model for better understanding the neural mechanisms of volitional behaviors in the human brain.

Author Contributions: Conceptualization, G.W. and Y.L.; methodology, R.S.; software, R.S.; validation, G.W. and R.S.; formal analysis, R.S. and Y.Y.; investigation, Y.Y., L.C., and S.Z.; resources, G.W.; data curation, G.W.; writing—original draft preparation, G.W., R.S., and Y.Y.; writing—review and editing, G.W., T.H., L.Z., C.L., and S.P.; visualization, R.S.; supervision, G.W.; project administration, G.W.; and funding acquisition, G.W. All authors have read and agreed to the published version of the manuscript.

Funding: This work was supported by the National Natural Science Foundation of China (grant number 31671163) and the CAS Key Laboratory of Mental Health, Institute of Psychology (grant number KLMH2011ZK07), as well as the Open Research Fund of the CAS Key Laboratory of Behavioral Science, Institute of Psychology.

Acknowledgments: We thank the participants from Chinese National Team of Short-track Speeding Skating for their involvement in the study. Our special thanks also goes to Zhi Wang for recruiting participants and Michelle Jiang for editing the manuscript.

Conflicts of Interest: The authors declare no conflicts of interest.

References

1. Searle, J. *Intentionality: An Essay in the Philosophy of Mind*; Cambridge University Press: Cambridge, UK, 1983.
2. Zhu, J. Intention and volition. *Can. J. Philos.* **2004**, *34*, 175–193. [CrossRef]
3. Frith, C. The psychology of volition. *Exp. Brain Res.* **2013**, *229*, 289–299. [CrossRef]
4. Li, Y. A Qualitative Study, Model Constructing and Measuement of Volition. Ph.D. Thesis, Beijing Sport University, Beijing, China, 2007.
5. Liang, C.; Fu, Q.; Cheng, Y.; Yu, J. Development and application of BTL-YZ-1.1 elite athlete volition scale. *J. Wuhan Sports Univ.* **2005**, *2*, 44–47.
6. Duckworth, A.L.; Peterson, C.; Matthews, M.D.; Kelly, D.R. Grit: Perseverance and passion for long-term goals. *J. Personal. Soc. Psychol.* **2007**, *92*, 1087. [CrossRef] [PubMed]
7. Bechara, A. Decision making, impulse control and loss of willpower to resist drugs: A neurocognitive perspective. *Nat. Neurosci.* **2005**, *8*, 1458. [CrossRef]
8. Jones, G. What is this thing called mental toughness? An investigation of elite sport performers. *J. Appl. Sport Psychol.* **2002**, *14*, 205–218. [CrossRef]
9. Jones, G.; Hanton, S.; Connaughton, D. A framework of mental toughness in the world's best performers. *Sport Psychol.* **2007**, *21*, 243–264. [CrossRef]

10. Fletcher, D.; Sarkar, M. Psychological resilience: A review and critique of definitions, concepts, and theory. *Eur. Psychol.* **2013**, *18*, 12. [CrossRef]
11. Li, Y.; Wang, T. Qualitative analyses and model construction of volitional qualities. *J. Beijing Sport Univ.* **2011**, *34*, 4.
12. Li, Y.; Liang, C. BTL—L—YZ2. 0 Development and application of athletes' volitional quality scale. *Sports Sci.* **2008**, *28*, 8.
13. Song, Y.; Li, S. Development of volitional quality scale for Chinese wushu sanda athletes. *J. Beijing Sport Univ.* **2006**, *29*, 1345–1347.
14. Sun, X.; Yang, N. The method for quantitative evaluation of athletes' volitional qualities—Inflection point. *J. Chengdu Inst. Phys. Educ.* **1988**, *3*, 35–37.
15. Zhang, Y. The Effect of Rock Climbing on Volitional Quality of Junior School Students. Master's Thesis, Xi'an Physical Education University, Xi'an, China, 2017.
16. Hu, R. Study on the influence of field living training on college students' volition quality. *Chengdu Inst. Phys. Educ.* **2019**.
17. Wang, X. Study on the influence of sanda on adolescent's volition quality and self-confidence. *Beijing Sport Univ.* **2016**.
18. Maguire, E.A.; Gadian, D.G.; Johnsrude, I.S.; Good, C.D.; Ashburner, J.; Frackowiak, R.S.; Frith, C.D. Navigation-related structural change in the hippocampi of taxi drivers. *Proc. Natl. Acad. Sci. USA* **2000**, *97*, 4398–4403. [CrossRef]
19. Wei, G.-X.; Xu, T.; Fan, F.-M.; Dong, H.-M.; Jiang, L.-L.; Li, H.-J.; Yang, Z.; Luo, J.; Zuo, X.-N. Can Taichi reshape the brain? A brain morphometry study. *PLoS ONE* **2013**, *8*, e61038. [CrossRef] [PubMed]
20. Lazar, S.W.; Kerr, C.E.; Wasserman, R.H.; Gray, J.R.; Greve, D.N.; Treadway, M.T.; McGarvey, M.; Quinn, B.T.; Dusek, J.A.; Benson, H.; et al. Meditation experience is associated with increased cortical thickness. *Neuroreport* **2005**, *16*, 1893–1897. [CrossRef]
21. Rogge, A.K.; Röder, B.; Zech, A.; Hötting, K. Exercise-induced neuroplasticity: Balance training increases cortical thickness in visual and vestibular cortical regions. *Neuroimage* **2018**, *179*, 471–479. [CrossRef]
22. Weber, B.; Koschutnig, K.; Schwerdtfeger, A.; Rominger, C.; Papousek, I.; Weiss, E.M.; Tilp, M.; Fink, A. Learning unicycling evokes manifold changes in gray and white matter networks related to motor and cognitive functions. *Sci. Rep.* **2019**, *9*, 4324. [CrossRef]
23. Park, I.S.; Lee, N.J.; Kim, T.-Y.; Park, J.-H.; Won, Y.-M.; Jung, Y.-J.; Yoon, J.-H. Volumetric analysis of cerebellum in short-track speed skating players. *Cerebellum* **2012**, *11*, 925–930. [CrossRef]
24. Wei, G.; Luo, J.; Li, Y. Brain structure in diving players on MR imaging studied with voxel-based morphometry. *Prog. Nat. Sci.* **2009**, *19*, 1397–1402. [CrossRef]
25. Wei, G.; Zhang, Y.; Jiang, T.; Luo, J. Increased cortical thickness in sports experts: A comparison of diving players with the controls. *PLoS ONE* **2011**, *6*, e17112. [CrossRef] [PubMed]
26. Jäncke, L.; Koeneke, S.; Hoppe, A.; Rominger, C.; Hänggi, J. The Architecture of the Golfer's Brain. *PLoS ONE* **2009**, *4*, e4785. [CrossRef] [PubMed]
27. Varley, I.; Hughes, D.C.; Greeves, J.P.; Fraser, W.D.; Sale, C. Increased training volume improves bone density and cortical area in adolescent football players. *Int. J. Sports Med.* **2017**, *38*, 341–346. [CrossRef]
28. Fawver, B.; Cowan, R.L.; DeCouto, B.S.; Lohse, K.R.; Podlog, L.; Williams, A.M. Psychological characteristics, sport engagement, and performance in alpine skiers. *Psychol. Sport Exerc.* **2020**, *47*, 10. [CrossRef]
29. Schaer, M.; Cuadra, M.B.; Schmansky, N.; Fischl, B.; Thiran, J.P.; Eliez, S. How to measure cortical folding from MR images: A step-by-step tutorial to compute local gyrification index. *J. Vis. Exp.* **2012**, e3417. [CrossRef]
30. Li, Y. *The Qualitative Research of Volitional Qualities*; Beijing Sport University Press: Beijing, China, 2014.
31. Manjón, J.V.; Coupé, P. volBrain: An online MRI brain volumetry system. *Front. Aging Neurosci.* **2016**, *10*, 30. [CrossRef]
32. Xu, T.; Yang, Z.; Jiang, L.; Xing, X.-X.; Zuo, X.-N. A connectome computation system for discovery science of brain. *Sci. Bull.* **2015**, *60*, 86–95. [CrossRef]
33. Xing, X.-X.; Zhou, Y.-L.; Adelstein, J.S.; Zuo, X.-N. PDE-based spatial smoothing: A practical demonstration of impacts on MRI brain extraction, tissue segmentation and registration. *Reson. Imaging* **2011**, *29*, 731–738. [CrossRef]
34. Zuo, X.-N.; Xing, X.-X. Effects of non-local diffusion on structural MRI preprocessing and default network mapping: Statistical comparisons with isotropic/anisotropic diffusion. *PLoS ONE* **2011**, *6*, e26703. [CrossRef]

35. Dale, A.M.; Fischl, B.; Sereno, M.I. Cortical surface-based analysis: I. Segmentation and surface reconstruction. *NeuroImage* **1999**, *9*, 179–194. [CrossRef] [PubMed]
36. Ségonne, F.; Dale, A.M.; Busa, E.; Glessner, M.; Salat, D.; Hahn, H.K.; Fischl, B.J.N. A hybrid approach to the skull stripping problem in MRI. *Neuroimage* **2004**, *22*, 1060–1075. [CrossRef] [PubMed]
37. Fischl, B.; Liu, A.; Dale, A. Automated manifold surgery: Constructing geometrically accurate and topologically correct models of the human cerebral cortex. *IEEE Trans. Med Imaging* **2001**, *20*, 70–80. [CrossRef] [PubMed]
38. Ségonne, F.; Pacheco, J.; Fischl, B. Geometrically accurate topology-correction of cortical surfaces using nonseparating loops. *IEEE Trans. Med Imaging* **2007**, *26*, 518–529. [CrossRef]
39. Fischl, B.; Sereno, M.I.; Tootell, R.B.; Dale, A. High-resolution intersubject averaging and a coordinate system for the cortical surface. *Human brain mapping* **1999**, *8*, 272–284. [CrossRef]
40. Fischl, B.; Dale, A. Measuring the thickness of the human cerebral cortex from magnetic resonance images. *Proc. Natl. Acad. Sci. USA* **2000**, *97*, 11050–11055. [CrossRef]
41. Han, X.; Jovicich, J.; Salat, D.; van der Kouwe, A.; Quinn, B.; Czanner, S.; Busa, E.; Pacheco, J.; Albert, M.; Killiany, R.J.N. Reliability of MRI-derived measurements of human cerebral cortical thickness: The effects of field strength, scanner upgrade and manufacturer. *NeuroImage* **2006**, *32*, 180–194. [CrossRef]
42. Bernal-Rusiel, J.L.; Atienza, M.; Cantero, J.L.J.N. Determining the optimal level of smoothing in cortical thickness analysis: A hierarchical approach based on sequential statistical thresholding. *NeuroImage* **2010**, *52*, 158–171. [CrossRef]
43. Desikan, R.S.; Ségonne, F.; Fischl, B.; Quinn, B.T.; Dickerson, B.C.; Blacker, D.; Buckner, R.L.; Dale, A.M.; Maguire, R.P.; Hyman, B.T.J.N. An automated labeling system for subdividing the human cerebral cortex on MRI scans into gyral based regions of interest. *NeuroImage* **2006**, *31*, 968–980. [CrossRef]
44. Fischl, B.; Van Der Kouwe, A.; Destrieux, C.; Halgren, E.; Ségonne, F.; Salat, D.H.; Busa, E.; Seidman, L.J.; Goldstein, J.; Kennedy, D.; et al. Automatically parcellating the human cerebral cortex. *Cereb. Cortex* **2004**, *14*, 11–22. [CrossRef]
45. Wang, C. Comparison of volitional qualities in short track speed skaters with different gender and athletic levels. *J. Phys. Educ.* **2008**, *15*, 96–99.
46. Wang, Q. Universite High Level Male Basketball Player Will Quality of Research in Wuhan. Master's Thesis, Wuhan Institute of Physical Education, Wuhan, China, 2015.
47. Zhu, D.; Hu, Y.; Yu, Y.; Wang, M.; Gao, P. Relationship between excellent chinese male boxers' personality, volitional quality, psychological tenacity and the performance. *J. Chengdu Sport Univ.* **2013**, *39*, 89–94.
48. Qiao, S.; Wang, Y. Status quo of the will-quality of chinese beach volleyball players. *Sports Sci. Res.* **2011**, *32*, 78–81.
49. Abbiss, C.R.; Laursen, P.B. Describing and understanding pacing strategies during athletic competition. *Sports Med.* **2008**, *38*, 239–252. [CrossRef] [PubMed]
50. Konings, M.J.; Noorbergen, O.S.; Parry, D.; Hettinga, F.J. Pacing behavior and tactical positioning in 1500-m short-track speed skating. *Int. J. Sports Physiol. Perform.* **2016**, *11*, 122–129. [CrossRef] [PubMed]
51. Noorbergen, O.S.; Konings, M.J.; Micklewright, D.; Elferink-Gemser, M.T.; Hettinga, F. Pacing behavior and tactical positioning in 500-and 1000-m short-track speed skating. *Int. J. Sports Physiol. Perform.* **2016**, *11*, 742–748. [CrossRef] [PubMed]
52. Smits, B.L.; Pepping, G.-J.; Hettinga, F. Pacing and decision making in sport and exercise: The roles of perception and action in the regulation of exercise intensity. *Sports Med.* **2014**, *44*, 763–775. [CrossRef]
53. David, N.; Newen, A.; Vogeley, K. The "sense of agency" and its underlying cognitive and neural mechanisms. *Conscious. Cogn.* **2008**, *17*, 523–534. [CrossRef]
54. Roskies, A.L. How does neuroscience affect our conception of volition? *Annu. Rev. Neurosci.* **2010**, *33*, 109–130. [CrossRef]
55. Darby, R.R.; Joutsa, J.; Burke, M.J.; Fox, M.D. Lesion network localization of free will. *Proc. Natl. Acad. Sci. USA* **2018**, *115*, 10792–10797. [CrossRef]
56. Pfabigan, D.M.; Wucherer, A.M.; Wang, X.; Pan, X.; Lamm, C.; Han, S. Cultural influences on the processing of social comparison feedback signals-an ERP study. *Soc. Cogn. Affect Neurosci.* **2018**, *13*, 1317–1326. [CrossRef] [PubMed]
57. Nahab, F.B.; Kundu, P.; Maurer, C.; Shen, Q.; Hallett, M. Impaired sense of agency in functional movement disorders: An fMRI study. *PLoS ONE* **2017**, *12*, e0172502. [CrossRef] [PubMed]

58. Bandura, A. Social cognitive theory: An agentic perspective. *Annu. Rev. Psychol.* **2001**, *52*, 1–26. [CrossRef]
59. Saarikallio, S.H.; Randall, W.M.; Baltazar, M. Music listening for supporting adolescents' sense of agency in daily life. *Front. Psychol.* **2020**, *10*, 2911. [CrossRef] [PubMed]
60. Haggard, P. Sense of agency in the human brain. *Nat. Rev. Neurosci.* **2017**, *18*, 196. [CrossRef]
61. Kircher, T.T.; Senior, C.; Phillips, M.L.; Benson, P.J.; Bullmore, E.T.; Brammer, M.; Simmons, A.; Williams, S.C.; Bartels, M.; David, A.S. Towards a functional neuroanatomy of self processing: Effects of faces and words. *Cogn. Brain Res.* **2000**, *10*, 133–144. [CrossRef]
62. Den Ouden, H.E.; Frith, U.; Frith, C.; Blakemore, S.-J. Thinking about intentions. *NeuroImage* **2005**, *28*, 787–796. [CrossRef]
63. Chaminade, T.; Decety, J.J.N. Leader or follower? Involvement of the inferior parietal lobule in agency. *NeuroReport* **2002**, *13*, 1975–1978. [CrossRef]
64. Marmot, M.G.; Stansfeld, S.; Patel, C.; North, F.; Head, J.; White, I.; Brunner, E.; Feeney, A.; Marmot, M.G.; Smith, G.D. Health inequalities among British civil servants: The Whitehall II study. *Lancet* **1991**, *337*, 1387–1393. [CrossRef]
65. Floden, D.; Stuss, D. Inhibitory control is slowed in patients with right superior medial frontal damage. *J. Cogn. Neurosci.* **2006**, *18*, 1843–1849. [CrossRef]
66. Hu, S.; Ide, J.S.; Zhang, S.; Chiang-shan, R. The right superior frontal gyrus and individual variation in proactive control of impulsive response. *J. Neurosci.* **2016**, *36*, 12688–12696. [CrossRef] [PubMed]
67. Chambon, V.; Haggard, P. Sense of control depends on fluency of action selection, not motor performance. *Cognition* **2012**, *125*, 441–451. [CrossRef]
68. Wang, F.; Lian, C.; Wu, Z.; Zhang, H.; Li, T.; Meng, Y.; Wang, L.; Lin, W.; Shen, D.; Li, G. Developmental topography of cortical thickness during infancy. *Proc. Natl. Acad. Sci. USA* **2019**, *116*, 15855–15860. [CrossRef] [PubMed]
69. Collins, C.E.; Airey, D.C.; Young, N.A.; Leitch, D.B.; Kaas, J.H. Neuron densities vary across and within cortical areas in primates. *Proc. Natl. Acad. Sci. USA* **2010**, *107*, 15927–15932. [CrossRef] [PubMed]
70. Firth, J.; Stubbs, B.; Vancampfort, D.; Schuch, F.; Lagopoulos, J.; Rosenbaum, S.; Ward, P.B. Effect of aerobic exercise on hippocampal volume in humans: A systematic review and meta-analysis. *NeuroImage* **2018**, *166*, 230–238. [CrossRef] [PubMed]

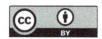

© 2020 by the authors. Licensee MDPI, Basel, Switzerland. This article is an open access article distributed under the terms and conditions of the Creative Commons Attribution (CC BY) license (http://creativecommons.org/licenses/by/4.0/).

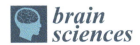

Article

Investigating Performance in a Strenuous Physical Task from the Perspective of Self-Control

Louis-Solal Giboin [1],*, Markus Gruber [1], Julia Schüler [2] and Wanja Wolff [2,3]

1. Sensorimotor Performance Lab, Human Performance Research Centre, University of Konstanz, 78464 Konstanz, Germany; m.gruber@uni-konstanz.de
2. Department of Sport Science, Sport Psychology, University of Konstanz, 78464 Konstanz, Germany; julia.schueler@uni-konstanz.de
3. Department of Educational Psychology, Institute of Educational Science, University of Bern, 3012 Bern, Switzerland; wanja.wolff@uni-konstanz.de
* Correspondence: louis-solal.giboin@uni-konstanz.de

Received: 4 October 2019; Accepted: 7 November 2019; Published: 9 November 2019

Abstract: It has been proposed that one reason physical effort is perceived as costly is because of the self-control demands that are necessary to persist in a physically demanding task. The application of control has been conceptualized as a value-based decision, that hinges on an optimization of the costs of control and available reward. Here, we drew on labor supply theory to investigate the effects of an Income Compensated Wage Decrease (ICWD) on persistence in a strenuous physical task. Research has shown that an ICWD reduced the amount of self-control participants are willing to apply, and we expected this to translate to a performance decrement in a strenuous physical task. Contrary to our expectations, participants in the ICWD group outperformed the control group in terms of persistence, without incurring higher levels of muscle fatigue or ratings of perceived exertion. Improved performance was accompanied by increases in task efficiency and a lesser increase in oxygenation of the prefrontal cortex, an area of relevance for the application of self-control. These results suggest that the relationship between the regulation of physical effort and self-control is less straightforward than initially assumed: less top-down self-control might allow for more efficient execution of motor tasks, thereby allowing for improved performance. Moreover, these findings indicate that psychological manipulations can affect physical performance, not by modulating how much one is willing to deplete limited physical resources, but by altering how tasks are executed.

Keywords: Muscle fatigue; voluntary activation; self-control; performance; motivation

1. Introduction

Many situations require the capability to sustain physical effort for prolonged durations. Most prototypically, this is required in the context of physical exercise (e.g., running, cycling). A large body of research has been targeted towards understanding the limits to human endurance performance. Most of this research centers around the idea that a strenuous physical task is terminated because physiological limits have been reached (e.g., [1–4]). Recently, this assumption has been challenged by the idea that physical performance is limited by the perception of the effort a task induces and not by the limits of the physiological system [5–8]. This implies that psychological factors are also important regulators of how long physical effort can be sustained. More specifically, this ascribes a key role to the psychological concept of self-control in the effective regulation of physical performance. Self-control has been defined as the 'efforts people exert to stimulate desirable responses and inhibit undesirable responses' [9] (p. 77). For example, when a runner has the goal of breaking the two-hour mark in the marathon (given adequate physiological capabilities), self-control is needed to inhibit undesirable responses that might derail goal pursuit (e.g., slowing down because of fatigue) and to facilitate desirable responses that increase the likelihood of goal attainment (e.g., sticking to the target pace). In line with this example, it has been suggested that the decision to continue or persist in a strenuous task largely depends on how much self-control one is willing to apply [10–12].

While self-control conveys substantial societal and personal benefits [13], its exertion also carries intrinsic costs [14,15], and people prefer tasks that pose less self-control demands [16]. This begets an important question: how do individuals decide whether or not to apply control? Although a plethora of different explanations exist, many recent models conceptualize the allocation of control as some form of value-based decision [10,17]. Thus, whether or not (or how much) control is exerted hinges on a continuous cost–benefit analysis and people try to maximize the value of control [18,19]. This means that when the cost of control is expected to be higher than the expected benefits of applying it, it is no longer worth applying. Going back to the marathon example, if, at kilometer 23, one is already considerably fatigued and far behind one's target pace, then the costs of control (i.e., dealing with all the aversive sensations that arise during the race) might outweigh their expected value (i.e., finishing the race, but not in the expected time) and one may stop racing.

The costs of applying self-control could partly explain why people do not always perform up to their physiological limit [5,7]. For example, when performing an incremental cycling exercise to exhaustion, the relevant muscles still contain a large enough functional reserve to produce the required power output. This indicates that the mechanisms inducing task failure may lie closer to central than peripheral levels [7]. These central mechanisms are most likely a mix between psychological processes (like the one hypothesized in the present study) and non-psychological processes directly altering the motor command, e.g., physiological processes inducing central fatigue (for a review, see [20]). There is now a large body of research, showing that previous exertion of self-control (on completely unrelated cognitive tasks) reduces the performance people achieve in physical tasks [12,21], or the duration for which they are able to sustain aversive sensations [22]. In the same vein, imposing demands on executive functions that rely on self-control while subjects complete a strenuous physical task also leads to performance decrements [23]. Taken together, there is now ample empirical evidence showing that performance in strenuous physical tasks depends on the application of self-control.

Research indicates that the cost of applying a given control command is monitored and computed by the dorsal anterior cingulate cortex (dACC), and then further relayed to structures like the lateral pre-frontal cortex (lPFC) that implement the control command in a top-down fashion [18]. Interestingly, during incremental cycling exercises, oxygenation of the prefrontal cortex (PFC), measured with functional near-infrared spectroscopy (fNIRS), increases with effort and decreases when subjects reach exhaustion [24], indicating that central components, possibly at the PFC level, may influence task termination decisions [8] (importantly, this drop in oxygenation is probably not task-specific, as it has also been observed in tasks that pose different physiological demands [25]). In addition, psychological strategies that supposedly automate behavior (i.e., make it less reliant on cognitive control) are associated with a reduced increase in PFC oxygenation during a strenuous physical task [26]. Thus, these findings add preliminary neuroscientific support to the conceptual and empirical evidence that emphasizes that the regulation of physical effort relies on self-control, with the PFC as the prime candidate signaling the application of self-control.

2. The Present Study

In this transdisciplinary study, we use labor supply theory [27,28] as a framework for investigating how changes in rewards translate to changes in psychological (perception of effort), neuronal (oxygenation in the lPFC), and physiological (neuromuscular measures of fatigue) markers of effort and performance. Labor supply theory proposes that when workers determine their preferred hours of work, they choose their subjective point of maximum utility, where labor and leisure are optimally balanced [29]. The point of maximum utility depends on the reward per hour (wage) and the number of hours one can allocate to work (budget constraint). Because it describes decision-making on the base of a balance between work and leisure (which can both be desired), the labor supply theory can allow for a description of more complex behaviors than value-based models, based only on go/no go decisions. Research has shown that the propositions of labor supply theory can be used to explain the allocation of cognitive control to a cognitive task, and that the allocation of cognitive control can be described as a utility function, that weighs the costs of control against its payoff [29]. This indicates that people treat the application of control as labor and choose to invest the amount of control that has the highest subjective utility. Such a combination can be altered by an income manipulation in ways that are predicted by labor supply theory [29]: for example, when wage per unit of time was reduced—but was compensated by an upfront payment (income compensated wage decrease; ICWD)—in a second session, subjects reduced the time spent doing demanding cognitive tasks (Study 1 in [29]). This result indicates that, even with the possibility to earn the same exact income for the same exact amount of cognitive control applied, participants have chosen not to do so (see Figure 1A). Interestingly, these results of cognitive labor/leisure decisions are in agreement with economic labor/leisure decisions, and even animal foraging-related decisions [29]. As hypothesized here and elsewhere [10], the capacity to apply cognitive and physical effort may rely on self-control. Therefore, the labor supply theory seems well suited to model the performance of a strenuous physical task within the paradigm described at the beginning of the introduction. In this paradigm, the performance of the strenuous task would depend on the chosen combination between the reward associated with the task performance and control costs that are required to continue to perform the task.

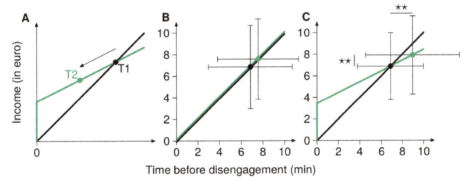

Figure 1. The utility of cognitive control. In this figure, adapted from Kool and Botvinik [29], the black and green dots correspond to the mean combination of income (in euro) and time (in min) before disengagement at t1 and t2, respectively. The black and green lines represent the mean budget constraint at t1 and t2, respectively. The budget constraint line corresponds to all the possible combinations of income and time before disengagement, in the given experimental context. The higher ordinate at the abscissa zero corresponds to the mean upfront payment. The error bars represent SD and the double five-pointed stars correspond to a p-value < 0.01. (**A**) Prediction of the iso–utility curve of the task with an ICWD condition at t2, according to the model of cognitive effort control [29]. (**B**) Results at t1 and t2 of the control group. (**C**) Results at t1 and t2 of the ICWD group.

In the present study, our goal was to assess whether the voluntary termination of a strenuous physical task could be altered by an income manipulation, in the same way as the regulation of cognitive effort applied during cognitive tasks [29]. Importantly, we have chosen a type of physical task (submaximal isometric contraction) for which it has already been shown that manipulation of self-control by ego depletion or mental fatigue experimental paradigms could affect time of disengagement (e.g., [30,31]). Therefore, we predicted that receiving an ICWD in a second session would reduce the amount of self-control participants were willing to apply and, thus, reduce the length of engagement in the strenuous physical task (Figure 1A, t1 vs. t2). Accordingly, we expected the ICWD condition to be accompanied by limited tolerance of perceived effort, less pronounced increases in lPFC oxygenation, and less severe central and peripheral muscle fatigue.

3. Methods

3.1. Participants

The study was approved by the ethics committee of the University of Konstanz and in accordance with the Declaration of Helsinky. All methods used in this study were approved by the ethics committee of the University of Konstanz. Participants gave written informed consent before being enrolled in the study. Participants (N = 34; mean ± SD; age: 25.5 ± 4.7 years, height: 179.6 ± 4.8 cm, weight: 80.9 ± 11.1) took part in two experimental sessions, separated by 1 week. We recruited only male participants, since we performed electrical femoral nerve stimulations with the electrodes fixed over the gluteus muscle and the femoral triangle.

3.2. General Procedure

For each participant, the two experiments were always performed on the same day of the week and at the same time of day. Participants were asked to not consume alcohol or caffeine the day of the experiment and had to prevent any unusual leg exertion 48 h before the experiments. Beside this, participants had to maintain their usual activity. The first 10 participants were allocated randomly in the control or ICWD group. Then, participants were allocated in both groups to match baseline maximal voluntary contraction (MVC) and time before self-disengagement at time 1, during the strenuous physical task (a knee extension fatiguing task). Details of the anthropomorphic characteristics of each group are displayed in Table 1. During the experiment, participants were facing a computer screen that displayed the force information necessary to properly execute the given task. An experimental session proceeds as follows. First, participants were told what would happen during the experiment and gave informed consent. Then, participants were prepared for the neuromuscular and fNIRS measurements and the main task they had to perform. For this, instructions regarding the fatiguing knee extension task and how it was incentivized were given to participants by means of a standardized text, followed by standardized oral instructions (the full instruction sheet for t1 and t2 is uploaded to this manuscript as Supplementary Materials). Before the participant started the task, we measured fNIRS baseline for 1 min. Then, the investigator said "start" and the participant started the task. Participants were kept unaware of both their group attribution and other participant's results.

Table 1. Anthropometric characteristics of each group. Height in cm, weight in kg and age in years. Mean ± standard deviation. For each variable, the difference between groups was assessed with a t-test. ICWD corresponds to income compensated wage decrease.

	Control (N = 17)	ICWD (N = 17)	p-Value
Height	179.1 ± 3.3	180.2 ± 5.9	0.49
Weight	81.5 ± 8.9	80.4 ± 13.2	0.78
Age	25.7 ± 3.8	25.2 ± 5.7	0.78

3.3. Experimental Manipulation and Payment

For the control group (N = 17) at t1 and t2, and for the ICWD group (N = 17) at t1, the wage was 1 Euro per minute spent on the knee extension fatiguing task. Here, the summarized instruction was as follows: "you work on the strength task as long as you want. For each trial you will receive one Euro. Thus, you will receive one Euro per minute. The task lasts until you stop, or until it is terminated because the stopping criterion [i.e., the target force is not produced anymore] has been met". For the ICWD group, at t2, participants received an upfront payment equal to 50% of t1 income and the wage was 0.5 Euros per minute. Therefore, at t2, ICWD participants, although not explicitly made aware of this possibility, could still reach the same income–time combination (Figure 1A, crossing of budget constraint lines). Here, the summarized instruction was as follows: "you work on the strength task as long as you want. For each trial you will receive 50 Cent. Thus, you will receive 50 Cent per minute. Prior to the task you will receive a bonus of X Euro [bonus amount differed as a function of t1 performance]. The task lasts until you stop, or until it is terminated because the stopping criterion [i.e., the target force is not produced anymore] has been met". Participants were paid 5 supplementary Euros for coming into the lab (not considered in the total income calculation).

3.4. Neuromuscular Procedure

Participants started with a warm-up consisting of bodyweight exercises: 2 × 10 squats (30 s rest) followed by 2 × 3 counter movement jumps (30 s rest). Then, we taped electromyography (EMG) sensors (Trigno wireless EMG system, Delsys Inc.) on the skin, which had been previously shaved, abraded and cleaned with alcohol of the vastus lateralis (VL) and biceps femoris (BF) muscles, following SENIAM recommendation. We taped stimulation electrodes (custom made) on the end part of the gluteus maximus muscle (anode; copper, 7 × 5 cm, wrapped in a soaked sponge) and on the femoral triangle (cathode; copper, circular, 2 cm diameter, wrapped in a water-soaked sponge), in order to stimulate the femoral nerve. Participants were then seated in a custom-made chair, with their right knee forming an angle of around 100°. Participants were then tightly fastened with non-compliant straps at the torso, hip and right ankle levels. The strap at the ankle was fixed according to anatomical landmarks (2 cm higher than the line parallel to the floor passing below the lateral malleolus) to ensure an identical placement in the two experimental sessions. The ankle was fixed to a force transducer, to measure isometric knee extension force (Model 9321A, Kistler, Winterthur, Switzerland). Both EMG (high-pass- and low-pass-filtered at 20 Hz ± 10% and 450 Hz ± 10%, respectively) and force signal were sampled with a Power 1401 interface (Cambridge Electronic Design, Cambridge, UK) at 4000 Hz and stored on a computer with the Signal software (Cambridge Electronic Design). Participants had their arms crossed over their chest during the measurement parts of the experiment.

We then stimulated (squared pulse of 1 ms duration, DS7A stimulator, Digitimer) the femoral nerve with incremental stimulation intensities, until reaching the maximal amplitude of the M-wave (Mmax) in the VL muscle and until the twitch of knee extensors muscles when at rest did not increase anymore. Intensity was then set at 150%. Then, participants performed 15–20 incremental voluntary contractions, until reaching around 90% of perceived maximal effort. These contractions had two purposes: to warm-up, specifically to produce an isometric MVC, and to familiarize participants with the control of the cursor. All participants were able to produce a stable 15% MVC contraction and an MVC with a decent force plateau. Then, after 2 min rest, participants performed an MVC for 3 s. For every MVC performed during the experiment, participants were encouraged with standardized shouts. During this MVC, peripheral nerve stimulation (PNS) was delivered during the contraction plateau (to obtain the amplitude of the superimposed twitch) and at rest (to obtain the amplitude of the potentiated twitch at rest, Ptw), 2 s after the end of the contraction. This procedure allows the estimation of voluntary activation (VA) using the interpolated twitch method [32] with the following formula: VA = (1−superimposed twitch amplitude/potentiated twitch amplitude) × 100. This procedure was done a second time after 2 min of rest. If an increase of 5% or more in MVC was observed at baseline, the procedure was repeated.

For the readers not familiar with neuromuscular measurements, a decrease in MVC following the fatigue task indicates the occurrence of neuromuscular fatigue. Roughly, neuromuscular fatigue can stem from events occurring in the nervous system (central fatigue) and events occurring distal to the neuromuscular junction (peripheral fatigue). A decrease in VA indicates a decrease in the capacity to voluntarily recruit muscles and is an estimate of central fatigue. A reduction in Ptw indicates a reduction in muscle excitability and is an estimate of peripheral fatigue. The present measurements can therefore help to quantify the amount of physiological resources spent during the task. For more details, please see [33].

3.5. Knee Extension Task

The knee extension task consisted of keeping a cursor over a threshold line (dashed line in Figure 2) displayed on a screen in front of the participant until self-disengagement (1 m distance). If, at one time point, the cursor stayed below the line for more than 2 s, the task was terminated. The cursor was moved by the isometric knee extension contraction, and the threshold was equal to 15% of their maximal voluntary contraction (MVC). Participants were naïve regarding this calculation. The task was displayed on the screen in 1 min long frames. Before starting the task, standardized oral instructions were given: "You can stop at any time you want. When you stop, say "I stop" and then relax totally your leg and then immediately contract maximally". At the beginning of the frame, an investigator indicated that the participant could initiate the contraction by saying "start". After 4 s, the investigator told the participant how much money he had already earned and how much money he will earn if he completes the 1 min frame (e.g. "you have earned 1 euro, if you finish this frame you will earn 2 euros"). After 30 s, a peripheral nerve stimulation (PNS) of the femoral nerve was triggered to elicit a maximal M-wave. After 48 s, participants were asked to give their rate of perceived exertion (RPE, scale of 1 to 10, with the possibility of going beyond 10 [34]). At 57 s, the participant was told to fully relax their knee extensor muscles ("relax"). This rest had two purposes. First, it allowed us to ensure that there was no drift in the force transducer during the task. Second, this short rest allowed the muscle to recover substantially (as seen with the recovery of the force production variation at the beginning of the next frame [35]), therefore making the task's termination "more psychological". The participant had to say "I stop" when stopping the task, and fully relax their leg. As soon as the cursor reached zero on the y axis and, following the instructions of the investigator ("fully relax the leg, maximal contraction, go!"), the participant had to produce an MVC, and PNS was performed to measure VA and Ptw. Strong verbal encouragements were given. Other than this, there was no interaction between participants and investigators.

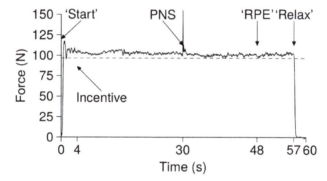

Figure 2. The knee extension task. The task consisted of keeping a cursor over a threshold line (dashed line on the present figure, corresponding to 15% maximal voluntary contraction(MVC)) displayed on a screen in front of the participant, until self-disengagement, by means of an isometric knee extension. If, at one time point, the cursor stayed below the line for more than 2 s, the task was terminated. Participants were told that they could stop the task at any time they wanted. The task was displayed on the screen in 1 min long frames. At the beginning of the frame, an investigator indicated that the participant could initiate the contraction by saying "start". At 4 s, the investigator told the participant how much money he had already earned and how much money he would earn if he completes the 1 min frame. At 30 s, a peripheral nerve stimulation (PNS) of the femoral nerve was triggered to elicit a maximal M-wave. At 48 s, participants were asked to give their rate of perceived exertion. At 57 s, the participant was told to fully relax their knee extensor muscles.

3.6. fNIRS

Changes in cerebral Oxyhemoglobin were continuously measured with an 8 Emitter + 8 Detector multichannel continuous-wave fNIRS imaging system (NIRSport, NIRx Medical Technologies LLC, NY, USA). The NIR wavelengths were 760 nm and 850 nm, and data were collected at a sampling rate of 7.81 Hz. Two 4 emitter + 4 detector arrays were bilaterally positioned over scalp sites that corresponded to the lPFC (see Figure 3A). Emitters and detectors were positioned according to the international 5/10 system: E1 at F1, E2 at AF3, E3 at FC3, E4 at F5, D1 at F3, D2 at AF7, D3 at FC5, D4 at F7, E5 at F6, E6 at AF4, E7 at FC4, E8 at F2, D5 at F8, D6 at AF8, D7 at FC6, and D8 at F4. This montage was designed to measure activity over the dorsal (Emitter–Detector combinations: E1_D1, E2_D1, E3_D1, E6_D8, E7_D8, E8_D8, E2_D2, E3_D3, E6_D6) and ventral (Emitter–Detector combinations: E4_D1, E4_D2, E4_D3, E5_D5, E5_D6, E5_D8) areas of the lPFC. Channels of interest were emitter–detector pairs with 3 mm separation. This resulted in nine channels on the left (channels 1–9) and nine channels on the right (channels 10–18) hemisphere. Channels 9, 12, and 16 had to be excluded from the analyses, due to detector malfunction. The probes were fixated in a NIRScap (EASYCAP GmbH, Herrsching, Germany) with an interoptode distance of 30 mm. The NIRScaps for optode placement were available in three different sizes (head circumferences of 54, 56, and 58 cm) and suitable for all subjects. To ensure better signal quality, a retaining overcap (EASYCAP GmbH, Herrsching, Germany) was placed over the NIRScap.

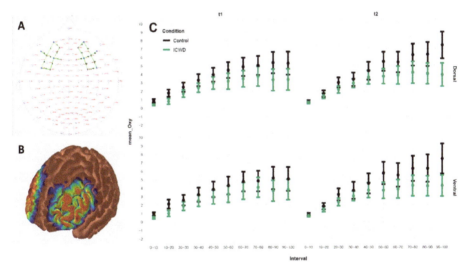

Figure 3. fNIRS measurements. (**A**). The sensitivity profile was created with Atlas Viewer (Aasted, et al., 2015) and it indicates that the chosen optode placements capture the lateral prefrontal cortex (lPFC) reasonably well. It represents Monte Carlo random walks of 1e7 photons (per optode) migrating through a standard atlas (Colin27, **B**). Panel **C** displays the change in oxygenation throughout the fatiguing task [0%–10%] vs. [10%–20%] vs. [90%–100%]) and is displayed separately for experimental conditions, experimental session and regions of interest (ROI; ventral and dorsal lPFC). Error bars represent SEM. ICWD corresponds to income compensated wage decrease.

3.7. Analysis and Statistics

fNIRS data of each subject were preprocessed using HOMER2 (MathWorks Inc., 2016) [36]. The enPruneChannels function was used to remove channels when the signal was too weak or too strong and then optical intensity was converted to optical density using the Intensity_to_OD function. Then, a discrete wavelet transform was performed to identify and correct motion artifacts [37]. Finally, data were low-pass filtered (0.5 Hz) and converted to Oxy- and Deoxyhemoglobin with the modified Beer–Lambert law [38], using the default differential path length factor of 6.0 for both wavelengths. Finally, fNIRS data were time-normalized, to allow for comparison between groups and sessions across the whole duration of the task.

We measured the peak-to-peak amplitude of MVC and Ptw, and calculated VA with the amplitude of the superimposed twitch and Ptw. The baseline values were taken from the biggest MVC performed before the fatiguing task. For the EMG, we used root mean square over the whole frame (from 3 s to 28 s and from 32 s to 57 s, to avoid analyzing the contraction initiation and termination, as well as the Mmax potential) and normalized it to the amplitude of the Mmax measured during the same frame. The RPE and EMG were time-normalized, in order to make comparisons between sessions and groups across the duration of the task. For the mean force produced during the task, we averaged the force for the whole duration of the task (without the final MVC). Statistics were performed with JASP (for the two-way ANOVAs) and with R (for the linear mixed-effects analyses). We used two-way ANOVAs with group (control vs. ICWD, between subject) and session (t1 vs. t2, within subject) as a factor in the time before self-disengagement in the knee extension task, income, and mean force during the task. These ANOVAs were followed by paired t-tests at the time factor level. Three-way ANOVAs were used to test whether groups, session, or time within sessions (pre fatigue task vs. post fatigue task, within subject) had an effect on MVC, VA and Ptw. We estimated linear mixed-effects models (LMM) with LME4, and used the Satterthwaite approximation for degrees of freedom implemented in LMERTEST to establish the significance of fixed-effects. All LMM were estimated with random effects for participants. We tested whether there was an interaction between groups and time within sessions separately for the RPE and EMG at t1 and t2. In the model estimate for fNIRS data, we tested the interaction between groups and session and added a fixed effect of the time within a session.

4. Results

4.1. Behavioral Results

ANOVAs showed an effect of the sessions ($F_{1,32}=13.6$, $p < 0.001$; $F_{1,32} = 9.3$, $p = 0.005$) but no clear sessions × group interaction ($F_{1,32} = 3.23$, $p = 0.08$; $F_{1,32} = 0.31$, $p = 0.57$) between the time before self-disengagement and income, respectively, during the knee extension task. In the control group, no change in time before self-disengagement and the reward obtained from t1 to t2 was observed (Figure 1B; $t_{16} = -1.4$, $p = 0.17$ for both performance and income), indicating the robustness of the initially determined point of maximum utility. In the ICWD group, income and time before self-disengagement increased at t2 (Figure 1C; $t_{16} = -3.7$, $p = 0.002$ for both).

4.2. Perceived and Physiological Effort

LMM showed no difference in the time-normalized rate of perceived exertion (RPE), measured every minute during the task, between groups for each experimental session (see Figure 4). The Three way ANOVAs showed no difference between groups or sessions in maximal voluntary contractions (MVC), voluntary activation (VA) or the potentiated twitch at rest (Ptw). Only an effect within sessions (pre vs. post strenuous task) was observed for each dependent variable (p-values all < 0.001; see Table 2 for numerical values). With LMM, we observed no difference between groups and across the task for each experimental session in vastus lateralis (VL) electromyogram (EMG), normalized to Mmax (see Figure 5). Finally, LMM revealed a significant increase of oxygenation over the course of the time-normalized fatiguing task ($F_{9,1116.2} = 72.91$, $p < 2.2e-16$). In addition, there was an interaction between experimental session and group ($F_{1,67.69} = 10.99$, $p = 0.0014$), indicating higher oxygenation in the control group in the second experimental session (see Figure 3).

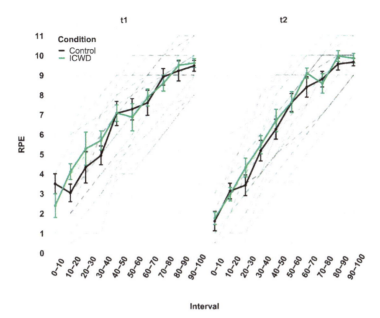

Figure 4. Rate of perceived effort. Mean rate of perceived exertion (RPE) are displayed throughout the time normalized task (Interval) during the first (t1) and second (t2) experimental session for the control (black) and ICWD (green) groups. The dashed lines correspond to individual data. Error bars correspond to SEM.

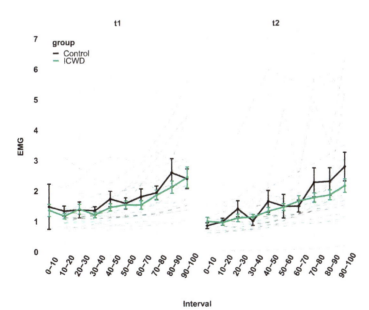

Figure 5. EMG. Mean rms EMG, normalized to Mmax (%), are displayed throughout the time normalized task (Interval) during the first (t1) and second (t2) experimental session for the control (black) and ICWD (green) groups. The dashed lines correspond to individual data. Error bars correspond to SEM.

Table 2. Neuromuscular results. Mean ± SD of maximal voluntary contraction (MVC) in N), voluntary activation (VA in %) and potentiated twitch at rest (Ptw in N) of both groups (Control vs. ICWD) at T1 and T2 sessions and pre- and post-knee extension task.

Group	Control				ICWD			
Session	T1		T2		T1		T2	
Within Session	Pre	Post	Pre	Post	Pre	Post	Pre	Post
MVC (N)	651 ± 131	354 ± 115	660 ± 141	367 ± 123	637 ± 121	360 ± 179	628 ± 123	376 ± 163
VA (%)	93.1 ± 5.3	81.8 ± 15	92.6 ± 6.3	84.5 ± 17.3	94.4 ± 5.5	84.1 ± 11.1	93.7 ± 3.9	86.6 ± 13
Ptw (N)	153 ± 29	74 ± 27	154 ± 34	72 ± 3	150 ± 21	76 ± 41	146 ± 24	81 ± 35

4.3. Task Efficiency

A two-way ANOVA showed the session × group interaction effect of the total mean force produced during the knee extension task ($F_{1,32}$ = 4.95, p = 0.033; see Figure 6), indicating a lower mean force produced during the task at t2 for the ICWD group.

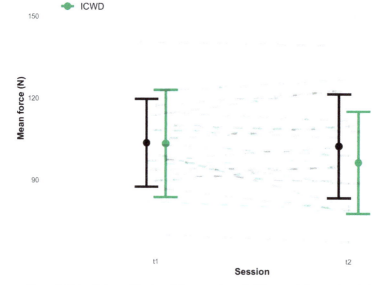

Figure 6. Task efficiency. Display of the mean force (in N) exerted during the whole task duration at t1 and t2 for both groups. The dashed lines represent individual data and the error bars represent SD. The black horizontal bar crowned by a star represents a time × group interaction with a p-value = 0.03.

5. Discussion

This is the first study to use labor supply theory to explain self-controlled persistence in a physically demanding task. We found that receiving an ICWD in a second session resulted in longer time before disengagement in a strenuous physical task, and not the expected decrease in performance. This is a puzzling result: from a utility maximization perspective this increase appears to be irrational, because, compared to t1, each unit of income increase requires two units of effort. Thus, the ICWD manipulation apparently triggered a shift in the subjective point of maximum utility, leading subjects to apply more self-control, allowing them to tolerate greater physical exertion, in order to increase income. However, if heightened motivation is the reason for the improved performance, then this should have been accompanied by a greater depletion of psychological (RPE), neuronal (lPFC oxygenation), and physiological (neuromuscular measures of fatigue) markers of effort and performance. To test this, we estimated the task-induced physiological costs by measuring muscle fatigue and it's central and peripheral components. Further, we estimated the psychological costs by assessing RPE throughout the task, and we indirectly estimated the application of self-control by continuously monitoring blood oxygenation in the lPFC throughout the task [15,39,40]. Interestingly, for none of the physiological measures did we observe greater levels of fatigue in the ICWD group, indicating that the longer time before disengagement was not achieved via a greater depletion of physiological resources. This finding was mirrored by the observation that participants in the ICWD group did not report higher ratings of perceived exertion. Thus, the longer time before disengagement was not achieved by a greater tolerance to the sensation of effort. This result is important, since previous research indicates that perceived effort (as measured with RPE) is "the cardinal exercise stopper" [41], thereby making tolerance of effort a crucial determinant of time before disengagement. Our results are in line with this reasoning, as participants apparently did not go over a certain threshold of RPE, irrespective of incentivization. Finally, compared to the control group, participants in the ICWD group displayed a less pronounced increase in lPFC oxygenation over the course of the task, indicating comparatively less activation in an area that is relevant for the application of control. Taken together, the longer time before disengagement was achieved without greater depletion of psychological and physiological resources and even with reduced involvement of self-control relevant brain areas. As no differences in the amount of resource depletion could be measured, the longer time before disengagement likely stems from a change in the utilization of available resources. Indeed, post-hoc analyses revealed that the mean force produced during the task was reduced in the ICWD condition. This means that subjects were able to produce force curves that were closer to the target force of t2. This equates to a more efficient use of resources while performing the task, allowing for a longer time before self-disengagement without a change in physiological and psychological costs.

6. Implications

Our findings are surprising in at least two ways: first, in contrast with our hypotheses, participants in the ICWD condition increased their task duration at t2. Second, this increase was not achieved by a greater depletion of physiological and psychological resources but by a more efficient use of available resources and a less pronounced engagement of a cerebral correlate of self-control application. While we did not expect to find this pattern of results, we believe that research on the effects of rewards on movement efficiency and the predictions of labor supply theory might allow for a tentative explanation of these findings: the increase in physiological movement efficiency that was observed in the ICWD condition falls in line with research demonstrating that the noise or metabolic costs of low-demand physical tasks can be influenced by rewards [42,43]. Thus, performing a low-demand physical task with greater accuracy (i.e., with less noise in the movement) requires the allocation of more self-control [42]. However, the control–noise relationship is likely reversed in strenuous physical tasks: if a task is performed more efficiently (i.e., with less noise), less self-control is needed to fight against the urge to disengage from the task. In other words, if a physically demanding task can be performed more efficiently, the amount and magnitude of aversive signals (e.g., muscle receptor feedback [44], corollary discharge [45]) that have to be integrated by areas relevant for self-controlled task continuation should be reduced. In line with this, a steeper increase in lPFC activation was observed in the control group from time 1 to 2, but no such change occurred in the ICWD group. Thus, if the ICWD manipulation lowered the amount of self-control participants were willing to allocate to the task (as measured by lPFC oxygenation), then—ironically—this might have, in fact, increased the time before disengagement, by allowing for a more efficient task execution. To summarize, looking solely at performance, our results seem to suggest that the predictions derived from labor supply theory do not hold in the case of regulation of physical effort. However, it is important to note that lPFC oxygenation, which was used to operationalize the allocation of self-control, changed in a way that was consistent with the expected effect of the

ICWD manipulation. Thus, our results suggest that the amount of self-control one applies is not linearly—and is possibly even counterintuitively—related to the to-be regulated physical performance. In our data, this is exemplified by a counterintuitive increase in performance, despite a less pronounced involvement of the lPFC. Thus, further research should focus on disentangling the relationship between self-control and physical performance, and specifically investigate instances where less control leads to a more efficient use of resources and, hence, improved performance.

According to research on the neuronal mechanisms that govern control [18,19], the shift in movement and cognitive control is monitored and specified by the dACC. One possible explanation for our findings is that the dACC diverted the control-signal from a mainly top-down regulated control signal (i.e. lPFC activity) to striatal areas that play a role in movement control. Indeed, these latter networks are sensitive to reward and could modulate movement efficiency [46]. This falls in line with the dopaminergic-dependent, reward-induced reduction in noise demonstrated in low-demand physical tasks [19,42]. Supporting this, compared to healthy controls, neurological patients who suffer from disease-induced decrements in motor performance experience steeper increases in RPE [47] and higher activity in the cortico-striatal network, which has been implicated in fatigue [48]. This has been interpreted as a compensatory activation to account for the inordinate amount of resources (i.e., cognitive effort) that patients are required to spend to reach an intended outcome (physical task).

7. Limitations

It must be noted that the task structure used in the present study differs in important ways from the only other study we know of that used labor supply to predict the allocation of self-control controls [29]. In our study, subjects performed a physical task, whereas, in the study by Kool and Botvinick [29], subjects performed a cognitive task. Thus, the latter is a more direct measure of control allocation, whereas, in our study, self-control allocation represents a mediator between subjects' capacity to perform the task and actual task performance [10]. The tasks also differed on a structural level: instead of a task with the possibility of allocating time spent doing a difficult or an easy contraction, according to participant preference (which would mirror Kool and Botvinick's approach [29]), participants had to perform a continuous contraction until self-disengagement. We opted for this setup for two reasons. First, physiological processes leading to neuromuscular fatigue are dependent on the way contractions are performed and the resting time between hard efforts (for example, see [49]). If using a paradigm with choices of physical effort allocation, we would not be able to control whether a different combination of the total time spent doing a hard contraction and subsequent income was induced by a better strategy, limiting the accumulation of neuromuscular fatigue (e.g., a more optimal effort/rest sequence) or due to the psychological manipulation. A scripted set of contractions, or a continuous contraction, like in the present study, reduces this bias and allows the quantification of the effect from the psychological manipulation on physical effort. Second, many real life decisions are about whether or not to further invest effort into one, ongoing task and researchers have explicitly called for the investigation of such scenarios within the framework of labor supply theory [29]. Thus, we chose to respond to this call and use a single continuous task.

It should also be noted that, in the lPFC activity results, while we expected to see a lower slope in activation increase in the ICWD group compared to the control group, it is surprising that this difference is driven by an altered oxygenation pattern in the control group and not in the ICWD group.

Finally, evidence indicates that manipulation of self-control by the means of ego depletion or a mental fatigue experimental paradigm affects whole-body and isolation tasks differently [21]. Therefore, the present results may not generalize to all kinds of strenuous physical effort.

8. Conclusions

We tested the hypothesis that a manipulation intended to reduce the amount of self-control participants were willing to apply to a strenuous physical task would also reduce performance of an isometric knee extension task. While such an ICWD has been shown to reduce the amount of effort participants were willing to invest into a cognitive task [29], on a phenomenological level a reversed effect was observed in regards to a physical task: surprisingly, reducing the rewards participants could obtain per unit of time led to better performance in the strenuous physical task. This increase was not achieved with an increase in psychological (RPE), neuronal (lPFC oxygenation), or physiological costs (neuromuscular measures of fatigue) but, rather, with an increase in movement efficiency. Thus, on the neuronal level, our results appear to be in line with labor supply theory, but the mechanisms by which control affects net outcome in a strenuous physical task (where subjects have to make do with limited resources) might be less straightforward and actually cause a behavioral outcome that is in contrast to the theoretical predictions. This finding highlights the intriguing possibility that, in some situations, higher persistence in demanding physical tasks may not necessarily require more self-control. In such a situation, a shift in motivation may not lead to a more excessive use of resources, but to more efficient resource utilization. This result may have important implications for the effects of reward structures in sport, economic, psychological and motor control domains.

Supplementary Materials: The following are available online at http://www.mdpi.com/2076-3425/9/11/317/s1, File S1: Study Materials.

Author Contributions: Conceptualization, L.-S.G. and W.W.; Methodology, L.-S.G. and W.W.; Formal Analysis, L.-S.G. and W.W.; Investigation, L.-S.G. and W.W.; Resources, J.S. and M.G.; Data Curation, L.-S.G. and W.W.; Writing-Original Draft Preparation, L.-S.G. and W.W.; Writing-Review & Editing, L.-S-G., W.W., J.S. and M.G.; Visualization, L.-S.G. and W.W.

Funding: This research received no external funding.

Conflicts of Interest: The authors declare no conflict of interest.

References

1. Allen, D.G.; Lamb, G.D.; Westerblad, H. Skeletal muscle fatigue: Cellular mechanisms. *Physiol. Rev.* **2008**, *88*, 287–332. [CrossRef] [PubMed]
2. Amann, M.; Calbet, J.A.L. Convective oxygen transport and fatigue. *J. Appl. Physiol.* **2008**, *104*, 861–870. [CrossRef] [PubMed]
3. Burnley, M.; Jones, A.M. Oxygen uptake kinetics as a determinant of sports performance. *Eur. J. Sport Sci.* **2007**, *7*, 63–79. [CrossRef]
4. Secher, N.H.; Seifert, T.; Lieshout, J.J.V. Cerebral blood flow and metabolism during exercise: Implications for fatigue. *J. Appl. Physiol.* **2008**, *104*, 306–314. [CrossRef] [PubMed]
5. Marcora, S.M.; Staiano, W. The limit to exercise tolerance in humans: Mind over muscle? *Eur. J. Appl. Physiol.* **2010**, *109*, 763–770. [CrossRef] [PubMed]
6. Walsh, V. Is sport the brain's biggest challenge? *Curr. Biol.* **2014**, *24*, R859–R860. [CrossRef] [PubMed]
7. Morales-Alamo, D.; Losa-Reyna, J.; Torres-Peralta, R.; Martin-Rincon, M.; Perez-Valera, M.; Curtelin, D.; Ponce-Gonzalez, J.G.; Santana, A.; Calbet, J.A. What limits performance during whole-body incremental exercise to exhaustion in humans? *J. Physiol.* **2015**, *593*, 4631–4648. [CrossRef]
8. Robertson, C.V.; Marino, F.E. A role for the prefrontal cortex in exercise tolerance and termination. *J. Appl. Physiol.* **2016**, *120*, 464–466. [CrossRef]
9. De Ridder, D.T.D.; Lensvelt-Mulders, G.; Finkenauer, C.; Stok, F.M.; Baumeister, R.F. Taking stock of self-control: A meta-analysis of how trait self-control relates to a wide range of behaviors. *Personal. Soc. Psychol. Rev.* **2012**, *16*, 76–99. [CrossRef]
10. Shenhav, A.; Musslick, S.; Lieder, F.; Kool, W.; Griffiths, T.L.; Cohen, J.D.; Botvinick, M.M. Toward a rational and mechanistic account of mental effort. *Annu. Rev. Neurosci.* **2017**, *40*, 99–124. [CrossRef]
11. Meeusen, R.; Pires, F.O.; Pinheiro, F.A.; Lutz, K.; Cheung, S.S.; Perrey, S.; Radel, R.; Brisswalter, J.; Rauch, H.G.; Micklewright, D.; et al. Commentaries on viewpoint: A role for the prefrontal cortex in exercise tolerance and termination. *J. Appl. Physiol.* **2016**, *120*, 467–469. [PubMed]
12. Van Cutsem, J.; Marcora, S.; De Pauw, K.; Bailey, S.; Meeusen, R.; Roelands, B. The effects of mental fatigue on physical performance: A systematic review. *Sports Med.* **2017**, *47*, 1569–1588. [CrossRef] [PubMed]
13. Duckworth, A.L. The significance of self-control. *Proc. Natl Acad. Sci. USA* **2011**, *108*, 2639–2640. [CrossRef] [PubMed]

14. Kool, W.; McGuire, J.T.; Wang, G.J.; Botvinick, M.M. Neural and behavioral evidence for an intrinsic cost of self-control. *PLoS ONE* **2013**, *8*, e72626. [CrossRef]
15. McGuire, J.T.; Botvinick, M.M. Prefrontal cortex, cognitive control, and the registration of decision costs. *Proc. Natl. Acad. Sci. USA* **2010**, *107*, 7922–7926. [CrossRef]
16. Inzlicht, M.; Shenhav, A.; Olivola, C.Y. The effort paradox: Effort is both costly and valued. *Trends Cogn. Sci.* **2018**, *22*, 337–349. [CrossRef]
17. Berkman, E.T.; Hutcherson, C.A.; Livingston, J.L.; Kahn, L.E.; Inzlicht, M. Self-control as value-based choice. *Curr. Dir. Psychol. Sci.* **2017**, *26*, 422–428. [CrossRef]
18. Shenhav, A.; Botvinick, M.M.; Cohen, J.D. The expected value of control: An integrative theory of anterior cingulate cortex function. *Neuron* **2013**, *79*, 217–240. [CrossRef]
19. Shenhav, A.; Cohen, J.D.; Botvinick, M.M. Dorsal anterior cingulate cortex and the value of control. *Nat. Neurosci.* **2016**, *19*, 1286–1291. [CrossRef]
20. Taylor, J.L.; Amann, M.; Duchateau, J.; Meeusen, R.; Rice, C.L. Neural contributions to muscle fatigue: From the brain to the muscle and back again. *Med. Sci. Sports Exerc.* **2016**, *48*, 2294–2306. [CrossRef]
21. Giboin, L.S.; Wolff, W. The effect of ego depletion or mental fatigue on subsequent physical endurance performance: A meta-analysis. *PsyArXiv* **2019**. [CrossRef]
22. Boat, R.; Taylor, I.M. Prior self-control exertion and perceptions of pain during a physically demanding task. *Psychol. Sport Exerc.* **2017**, *33*, 1–6. [CrossRef]
23. Leone, C.; Feys, P.; Moumdjian, L.; D'Amico, E.; Zappia, M.; Patti, F. Cognitive-motor dual-task interference: A systematic review of neural correlates. *Neurosci. Biobehav. Rev.* **2017**, *75*, 348–360. [CrossRef] [PubMed]
24. Rupp, T.; Perrey, S. Prefrontal cortex oxygenation and neuromuscular responses to exhaustive exercise. *Eur. J. Appl. Physiol.* **2008**, *102*, 153–163. [CrossRef]
25. Rooks, C.R.; Thom, N.J.; McCully, K.K.; Dishman, R.K. Effects of incremental exercise on cerebral oxygenation measured by near-infrared spectroscopy: A systematic review. *Prog. Neurobiol.* **2010**, *92*, 134–150. [CrossRef]
26. Wolff, W.; Bieleke, M.; Hirsch, A.; Wienbruch, C.; Gollwitzer, P.M.; Schüler, J. Increase in prefrontal cortex oxygenation during static muscular endurance performance is modulated by self-regulation strategies. *Sci. Rep.* **2018**, *8*, 15756. [CrossRef]
27. Kool, W.; Botvinick, M. Mental labour. *Nat. Hum. Behav.* **2018**, *2*, 899–908. [CrossRef]
28. Kagel, J.H.; Battalio, R.C.; Green, L. *Economic Choice Theory: An Experimental Analysis of Animal Behavior*; Cambridge University Press: Cambridge, UK, 1995.
29. Kool, W.; Botvinick, M. A labor/leisure tradeoff in cognitive control. *J. Exp. Psychol. Gen.* **2014**, *143*, 131–141. [CrossRef]
30. Bray, S.R.; Martin Ginis, K.A.; Hicks, A.L.; Woodgate, J. Effects of self-regulatory strength depletion on muscular performance and EMG activation. *Psychophysiology* **2008**, *45*, 337–343. [CrossRef]
31. Pageaux, B.; Marcora, S.M.; Lepers, R. Prolonged mental exertion does not alter neuromuscular function of the knee extensors. *Med. Sci. Sports Exerc.* **2013**, *45*, 2254–2264. [CrossRef]
32. Merton, P.A. Voluntary strength and fatigue. *J. Physiol.* **1954**, *123*, 553–564. [CrossRef] [PubMed]
33. Millet, G.Y.; Martin, V.; Martin, A.; Vergès, S. Electrical stimulation for testing neuromuscular function: From sport to pathology. *Eur. J. Appl. Physiol.* **2011**, *111*, 2489–2500. [CrossRef] [PubMed]
34. Pageaux, B. Perception of effort in exercise science: Definition, measurement and perspectives. *Eur. J. Sport Sci.* **2016**, *16*, 885–894. [CrossRef] [PubMed]
35. Hunter, S.K.; Enoka, R.M. Changes in muscle activation can prolong the endurance time of a submaximal isometric contraction in humans. *J. Appl. Physiol.* **2003**, *94*, 108–118. [CrossRef] [PubMed]
36. Huppert, T.J.; Diamond, S.G.; Franceschini, M.A.; Boas, D.A. Homer: A review of time-series analysis methods for near-infrared spectroscopy of the brain. *Appl. Opt.* **2009**, *48*, D280–D298. [CrossRef] [PubMed]
37. Molavi, B.; Dumont, G.A. Wavelet-based motion artifact removal for functional near-infrared spectroscopy. *Physiol. Meas.* **2012**, *33*, 259–270. [CrossRef]
38. Delpy, D.T.; Cope, M.; van der Zee, P.; Arridge, S.; Wray, S.; Wyatt, J. Estimation of optical pathlength through tissue from direct time of flight measurement. *Phys. Med. Biol.* **1988**, *33*, 1433–1442. [CrossRef]
39. Hare, T.A.; Camerer, C.F.; Rangel, A. Self-control in decision-making involves modulation of the vmPFC valuation system. *Science* **2009**, *324*, 646–648. [CrossRef]
40. Duverne, S.; Koechlin, E. Rewards and cognitive control in the human prefrontal cortex. *Cereb. Cortex* **2017**, *27*, 5024–5039. [CrossRef]

41. Staiano, W.; Bosio, A.; Morree, H.M.d.; Rampinini, E.; Marcora, S. The cardinal exercise stopper: Muscle fatigue, muscle pain or perception of effort. In *Sport and the Brain: The Science of Preparing, Enduring and Winning, Part C*; Marcora, S., Sarkar, M., Eds.; Progress in Brain Research; Elsevier: Amsterdam, The Netherlands, 2018.
42. Manohar, S.G.; Chong, T.T.; Apps, M.A.; Batla, A.; Stamelou, M.; Jarman, P.R.; Bhatia, K.P.; Husain, M. Reward pays the cost of noise reduction in motor and cognitive control. *Curr. Biol.* **2015**, *25*, 1707–1716. [CrossRef]
43. Shadmehr, R.; Huang, H.J.; Ahmed, A.A. A representation of effort in decision-making and motor control. *Curr. Biol.* **2016**, *26*, 1929–1934. [CrossRef] [PubMed]
44. Hureau, T.J.; Romer, L.M.; Amann, M. The 'sensory tolerance limit': A hypothetical construct determining exercise performance? *Eur. J. Sport Sci.* **2016**, *18*, 1–12. [CrossRef] [PubMed]
45. Marcora, S. Perception of effort during exercise is independent of afferent feedback from skeletal muscles, heart, and lungs. *J. Appl. Physiol.* **2009**, *106*, 2060–2062. [CrossRef] [PubMed]
46. Turner, R.S.; Desmurget, M. Basal ganglia contributions to motor control: A vigorous tutor. *Curr. Opin. Neurobiol.* **2010**, *20*, 704–716. [CrossRef] [PubMed]
47. Thickbroom, G.W.; Sacco, P.; Kermode, A.G.; Archer, S.A.; Byrnes, M.L.; Guilfoyle, A.; Mastaglia, F.L. Central motor drive and perception of effort during fatigue in multiple sclerosis. *J. Neurol.* **2006**, *253*, 1048–1053. [CrossRef] [PubMed]
48. DeLuca, J.; Genova, H.M.; Hillary, F.G.; Wylie, G. Neural correlates of cognitive fatigue in multiple sclerosis using functional mri. *J. Neurol. Sci.* **2008**, *270*, 28–39. [CrossRef] [PubMed]
49. Carroll, T.J.; Taylor, J.L.; Gandevia, S.C. Recovery of central and peripheral neuromuscular fatigue after exercise. *J. Appl. Physiol.* **2016**, *122*, 1068–1076. [CrossRef]

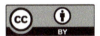

© 2019 by the authors. Licensee MDPI, Basel, Switzerland. This article is an open access article distributed under the terms and conditions of the Creative Commons Attribution (CC BY) license (http://creativecommons.org/licenses/by/4.0/).

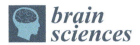

Article

Cerebellar Transcranial Direct Current Stimulation Improves Maximum Isometric Force Production during Isometric Barbell Squats

Rouven Kenville [1,2,*], Tom Maudrich [1,2], Dennis Maudrich [2], Arno Villringer [2,3,4] and Patrick Ragert [1,2]

1. Institute for General Kinesiology and Exercise Science, Faculty of Sport Science, University of Leipzig, D-04109 Leipzig, Germany; maudrich@cbs.mpg.de (T.M.); patrick.ragert@uni-leipzig.de (P.R.)
2. Department of Neurology, Max Planck Institute for Human Cognitive and Brain Sciences, D-04103 Leipzig, Germany; dmaudrich@cbs.mpg.de (D.M.); villringer@cbs.mpg.de (A.V.)
3. Clinic for Cognitive Neurology, University of Leipzig, 04103 Leipzig, Germany
4. MindBrainBody Institute at Berlin School of Mind and Brain, Charité-Universitätsmedizin Berlin and Humboldt-Universität zu Berlin, 10099 Berlin, Germany
* Correspondence: kenville@cbs.mpg.de; Tel.: +49-341-9940-2407

Received: 20 March 2020; Accepted: 11 April 2020; Published: 14 April 2020

Abstract: Maximum voluntary contraction force (MVC) is an important predictor of athletic performance as well as physical fitness throughout life. Many everyday life activities involve multi-joint or whole-body movements that are determined in part through optimized muscle strength. Transcranial direct current stimulation (tDCS) has been reported to enhance muscle strength parameters in single-joint movements after its application to motor cortical areas, although tDCS effects on maximum isometric voluntary contraction force (MIVC) in compound movements remain to be investigated. Here, we tested whether anodal tDCS and/or sham stimulation over primary motor cortex (M1) and cerebellum (CB) improves MIVC during isometric barbell squats (iBS). Our results provide novel evidence that CB stimulation enhances MIVC during iBS. Although this indicates that parameters relating to muscle strength can be modulated through anodal tDCS of the cerebellum, our results serve as an initial reference point and need to be extended. Therefore, further studies are necessary to expand knowledge in this area of research through the inclusion of different tDCS paradigms, for example investigating dynamic barbell squats, as well as testing other whole-body movements.

Keywords: transcranial direct current stimulation (tDCS); whole-body movement; motor system; muscle strength

1. Introduction

Muscle strength not only predicts athletic performance and/or efficacy but also contributes to the accomplishment of various tasks throughout everyday life, for example, walking, climbing stairs, and running [1–3]. Core features of muscle strength, such as maximum isometric voluntary contraction force (MIVC), depend on central nervous control of the number of active motor units and their firing rate. To date, central mechanisms of muscle strength remain insufficiently explored, especially regarding potential differentiations of the neuronal sites responsible for muscle strength regulation between single-joint (e.g., finger-pinch) and whole-body movements (e.g., squats).

Previous neuroimaging studies showed both primary motor cortex (M1) and cerebellum (CB) to change their activity with different force requirements in single-joint movements [4–7], although it remains to be fully understood which cortical/subcortical structures concur to enable muscle strength and control in whole-body movements, i.e., movements that require orchestrated interplay between multiple joints and muscles. Since most neuroimaging methods are not ideally suited to investigating whole-body movements, neuromodulatory approaches have been employed to uncover strength related brain-muscle associations [8].

Transcranial direct current stimulation (tDCS) is a non-invasive procedure, which stimulates brain regions applying weak direct currents through the skull. Depending on the polarity, stimulated regions either show enhanced or decreased excitability. tDCS has been used to uncover neural links between muscle strength and related brain areas through modulating their excitability. Accordingly, numerous studies have demonstrated tDCS related increases in muscle strength endurance [9–11] and MIVC [12–14], particularly for upper extremities. Lower extremity muscle strength modulation has also been assessed through tDCS application, although results are rather inconclusive. For example, some results showed tDCS to be effective in modulating isometric muscle strength [10,14,15], whereas other studies provide evidence to the contrary [16–18]. It is of note that, among others stimulation sites, current density (mA/cm^2), as well as strength training background of participants all differ between studies, making interpretations difficult. Nevertheless, a common ground regarding applicable tDCS protocols can be isolated. As such, most studies examining tDCS–MIVC modulations have stimulated M1, used a current intensity of 2 mA and stimulated for 20 min [8]. Additionally, enhancing effects of tDCS on MIVC have solely been reported for anodal tDCS, although cathodal effects have been examined [9,14], which may be rooted in increased cortical excitability and cross-activation, as well as reduced short-interval intracortical inhibition (SICI) [8,19,20].

TDCS induced modulations of MIVC remain to be investigated in whole-body tasks. During such tasks, potential target areas expand beyond motor cortical regions, as it is known that, apart from M1, SMA, and PMC, the cerebellum plays an essential part in motor control of whole-body movements, especially in movements that require appropriate and continuous postural control, e.g., squats and walking [21]. Here, the cerebellum has been shown to support postural control responses by adapting motor actions concerning specific task requirements [22,23]. Patients suffering from cerebellar pathologies (e.g., dysmetria and cerebellar ataxia) exhibit severe restrictions relating to control of kinematic and dynamic movement parameters during whole-body movement execution [24–26]. Selective studies even report of individual participants being able to jump on one leg, yet unable to coordinate both legs simultaneously after splitting of the cerebellar vermis [27]. Interestingly, in animal studies it could be shown that cerebellar discharge precedes cortical discharge during whole-body movement execution [28], hinting at a temporal hierarchy between both structures favoring the cerebellum. Further, in monkeys, the ability to execute unconstrained movements was greatly impaired during partial cerebellar inactivation when compared to constrained movement execution [29]. Accordingly, different aspects of whole-body movements have been modulated through cerebellar tDCS (CB-tDCS), which relies on the same principles as conventional tDCS. Few studies have examined CB-tDCS effects in compound or whole-body movements. For example, adaptations during a split-belt treadmill walking task were greatest for anodal CB-tDCS in healthy subjects when compared to cathodal and sham conditions [30]. CB-tDCS seems to be most effective (compared to M1-tDCS and sham stimulation (SH-tDCS)) regarding improvements in visuomotor tasks. Additionally, it was demonstrated that CB-tDCS elicits improvements in postural control, both in healthy participants [31] as well as chronic stroke patients [32]. Nevertheless, some studies show no effects of CB-tDCS on balance control in healthy participants [32,33]. To date, no study has tested the effects of CB-tDCS on core features of muscle strength, such as MIVC.

In summary, although the physiological effects of both M1- and CB-tDCS remain to be fully understood, both stimulation sites have been shown to affect motor function. Specifically, M1-tDCS was able to increase muscle strength parameters such as MIVC in some instances, while CB-tDCS proved to be behaviorally beneficial regarding whole-body movement components such as postural control. Based on the aforementioned findings, we here hypothesized that tDCS over M1 and CB is capable of evoking increases in MIVC during isometric barbell squats (iBS) as compared to sham stimulation.

2. Materials and Methods

2.1. Participants

The study was approved by the local ethics committee of the Medical Faculty at the University of Leipzig (ref.-nr. 034/17-ek) and all participants gave their written informed consent to participate in the experiments per the Declaration of Helsinki. Participants were excluded from the present study if the following exclusion criteria were present: neurological/psychological disease, intake of centrally acting drugs, caffeine or alcohol intake 24 h before the experiment, acute, chronic, and/or inadequately regenerated pathologies of the knee joint, the ankle joints, and/or the spine to minimize the risk of injury. Also, participants with regular practice of musical instruments and sports (>3 $^{hrs}/_{week}$) were excluded from participation in this study. This was motivated by the fact that recent studies have shown that musical training induces functional and structural plasticity in the brain [34,35]. Furthermore, we intended to test participants without any background in organized strength training to omit results related to athletic expertise.

Initially, we performed a sample size estimation (G*Power 3.1) [36,37] based on previous results of tDCS induced modulation of MIVC in lower extremities [13,14] using the following parameters: for test family = F-test and statistical test = analysis of variance (ANOVA), a power value (probability of correctly rejecting a false null hypothesis) of 0.8 was chosen given a type I error rate of α= 5%. Additionally, the effect size (f) was set to 0.4, as previous related studies reported values in this range [13,14,18]. The estimated minimum sample size to obtain sufficient test power was $n = 10$. A total number of 25 healthy male ($n = 13$) and female ($n = 12$) participants (age: 23.29 ± 3.66 years (mean ± SD)) were enrolled in the present study. All participants were right-handed, as assessed by the Edinburgh Handedness Inventory with a laterality quotient (LQ) score of 91.98 ± 10.32. Due to incorrect measurements, 4 participants were excluded from further analyses. Additionally, one participant was excluded due to a neck injury during testing. All analyses were performed with the remaining 20 participants (age: 24.00 ± 3.65 years; LQ score: 91.34 ± 10.76).

2.2. Procedure

The experiment consisted of a randomized, counter-balanced, sham-controlled, double-blinded cross-over design where each participant performed during 3 experimental sessions, separated by at least 5 d, to prevent task-related impacts of cognitive and/or muscular fatigue. One researcher randomly assigned participants to CB-tDCS, M1-tDCS, or SH-tDCS using consecutive randomization. This researcher was uninvolved during subsequent data recording. All researchers conducting the experiment were unaware of the stimulation type. All participants performed a behavioral task of the lower extremities on three separate days using a different stimulation type (CB-tDCS, M1-tDCS, or SH-tDCS) for each session. A different tDCS-arrangement was randomly applied for each session to stimulate different brain regions during task performance for 20 min (for details see Figure 1). All participants were naïve in the iBS.

2.3. Behavioral Task (iBS)

At the beginning of each experimental session, instructions were given, focusing on the correct execution of the iBS. Participants were instructed to plant their feet and exert force without raising their heels during the performance of iBS. Additionally, each participant was instructed to keep a slight lumbar lordosis during iBS. Initial instructions were followed by a brief (3 min) warm-up program comprising of supervised executions of dynamic squats without additional weight and focusing on the aforementioned key aspects of correct movement execution (A, planting of the feet, B, slight lumbar lordosis). Before the first experimental session, the barbell position, corresponding to a 95° knee angle, was determined for each participant by using a digital protractor. Before baseline MIVC measurements were carried out, participants practiced the task for familiarization.

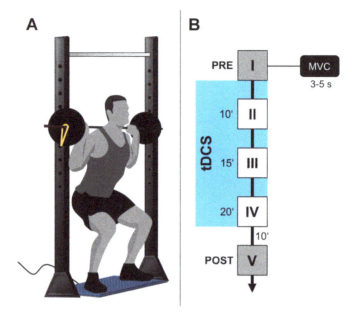

Figure 1. Study design. (**A**) Schematic representation of default positioning during isometric barbell squats (iBS) measurements. (**B**) Overview, regarding study procedures. Illustrated are all five maximum isometric voluntary contraction (MIVC) measurement blocks (I–V) alongside an exemplary depiction of a MIVC measurement conducted per one block for block I. MIVC blocks during stimulation are framed by a blue rectangle.

Each session consisted of five blocks of iBS (before, 10, 15, and 20 min after stimulation onset and 10 min after stimulation termination (POST)). The duration to complete one block of iBS was approximately 30 s. The stimulation was started right after the last MIVC-measurement of the first block (before).

Maximum iBS-force (Newton (N)) was assessed using a multi-component force plate (Kistler type 9286AA, Kistler AG, Winterthur, Switzerland). Data were recorded with a sampling rate of 500 Hz. The force plate was placed in a straight vertical line below a fixed barbell mounted on a squat half rack (Barbarian-Line®Profi Half Rack, IFS GmbH, Wassenberg, Germany). For iBS, participants were instructed to step onto the force plate and under the standard barbell. The feet were placed and aligned along two marked lines on the surface of the force plate to standardize the position of the feet on the force plate. Lastly, shoulders were pressed against the fixed barbell and both hands grabbed the barbell while shoulders were slightly adducted. This position was assumed for all measurements. For MIVC measurements during the performance of iBS, all participants were told to push against the immovable barbell as hard as possible for 3–5 s. Peak force values of each MIVC-measurement were taken for the MIVC value of the respective block. Subjects rested in a seated position on a stool in between MIVC measurements. During rest phases, movements of the lower limbs were prohibited to avoid differences in excitability between participants. No feedback regarding iBS-MIVC-performance was given.

2.4. Transcranial Direct Current Stimulation

A tDCS current of 2 mA was delivered for 20 min (excluding 2 × 30 s of up- and down-ramping before and after stimulation respectively) using a battery-driven stimulator (neuroConn direct current (NC-DC)-stimulator; neuroConn GmbH, Ilmenau, Germany) and a pair of surface-soaked sponge electrodes. All tDCS conditions (M1-tDCS, CB-tDCS, SH-tDCS) were randomly assigned within and counter-balanced across participants. The anode (35 cm^2, current density: 0.057 mA/cm^2) was placed either over the bilateral M1 leg area or the bilateral cerebellum, with the cathode (reference; 100 cm^2, current density 0.020 mA/cm^2) placed on the medial part of the supraorbital bone (tDCS of bilateral M1 leg area) or the right musculus buccinator (tDCS of bilateral cerebellum) [38] respectively. A large cathode was used to maintain the current density of the reference electrode at a low level, as such a reference electrode was demonstrated to be functionally ineffective without compromising the effectiveness of tDCS regarding the stimulation electrode [39,40]. The anatomical landmark for bilateral M1 (leg area) was determined according to previous studies which based their peak coordinates on Transcranial magnetic stimulation (TMS)-measurements [41–43]. For anodal tDCS of M1, we placed the anode 1 cm behind the vertex (Cz) on the mid-sagittal line to cover both leg motor cortices. For anodal cerebellar stimulation, the anode was placed 2 cm below the inion [38,44]. During SH-tDCS, a 2 mA current was maintained for 30 s before being ramped down and terminated. To improve the blinding procedure, M1-tDCS or CB-tDCS montages were randomly used as SH-tDCS montages. Before and after tDCS, participants rated their level of perceived sensation in relation to the stimulation (0 = no sensation, 10 = unbearable sensation) on a visual analog scale (VAS).

2.5. tDCS Current Flow Simulation

We simulated electric field distributions based on a finite element model of a representative head inside the open-source SimNIBS software (www.simnibs.org) to approximate current flow based on our tDCS configurations. For both M1-tDCS and CB-tDCS conditions, anodes, and cathodes were defined according to the above-mentioned positions. For both simulations, a current of 2 mA was selected. For anodal tDCS of M1 (leg area), the maximum electrical field strength (0.53 V/m) was determined below the anode, corresponding to the leg area of M1 with a posterior–anterior current flow direction towards premotor areas (Figure 2A). Anodal cerebellar tDCS electrical field strength was highest in the left cerebellar hemisphere (0.56 V/m) with posterior–anterior current flow direction towards brain stem areas (Figure 2B).

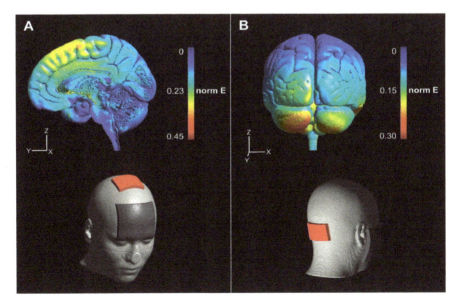

Figure 2. Transcranial direct current stimulation (tDCS) current flow simulation. Simulated current flow is illustrated for primary motor cortex (M1)-tDCS (**A**) as well as cerebellar (CB)-tDCS (**B**). Anodes are depicted as red rectangles and cathodes as gray rectangles projected on a standard head model in the lower half of (**A**) and (**B**), respectively. Normalized electrical field strength (V/m) is indicated through colormaps with blue representing lowest and red representing highest field strengths, respectively.

2.6. Data Analysis

Analyses were performed using customized MATLAB® (v. R2019b, The MathWorks Inc., Natick, MA, USA) scripts. For each subject, data were evaluated thoroughly with incorrect measurements being excluded. Peak force values (N) were extracted out of each measurement and used for further analyses (cf., Figure 1B). Data were then normalized to individual baseline performances on each different session (M1-tDCS, CB-tDCS, SH-tDCS). For an exemplary depiction of MIVC determination, please see Figure 3. Normal distribution was assessed through Lilliefors-testing ($\alpha = 0.05$). All data were subjected to repeated-measures analyses of variance ($_{rm}$ANOVA) with stimulation (STIM) (M1-tDCS, CB-tDCS, and SH-tDCS) and measurement times (TIME) (before stimulation, 10, 15, and 20 during stimulation and 10 min after stimulation termination) as within-subject factors for the dependent variable MIVC to compare tDCS induced MIVC effects. Additionally, we compared online (during tDCS stimulation) and offline (after tDCS stimulation) effects of tDCS. For this purpose, we compared averaged MIVC values across timepoints during stimulation (10, 15, and 20) with MIVC values during POST. Potential sphericity violations were adjusted according to Greenhouse–Geisser (epsilon < 0.75) or Huynh–Feldt correction (epsilon > 0.75). Statistical thresholds were set at $p < 0.05$. Post hoc analyses were conducted by way of Bonferroni–Holm correction for multiple comparisons. To examine the effect of potential outliers, we used a common procedure to detect and remove outliers. First, we computed the mean and standard deviation (SD) of all MIVCs per participant and condition. Then, we excluded datasets, which fell more than 2.5 SD from the mean [45–47] and reconducted analyses to uncover potential differences in the obtained results.

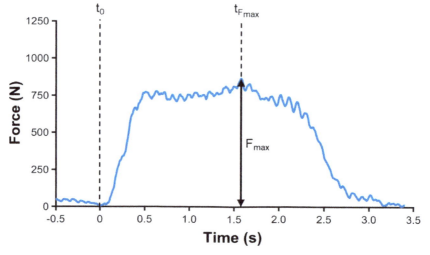

Figure 3. Determination of MIVC. Exemplary MIVC determination is illustrated on a single force–time curve. Force–time onset (t_0), peak force value (F_{max}), as well as time to peak force value (t_{Fmax}) are highlighted.

3. Results

We did not find significant differences regarding perceived stimulation sensation between sessions ($F(2,38) = 0.222$, $p = 0.802$, $\eta p^2 = 0.001$). None of our participants reported any tDCS related side effects and no participant reported discomfort during stimulation.

MIVC During iBS

For an overview of all individual MIVC results per stimulation please see Figure 4.

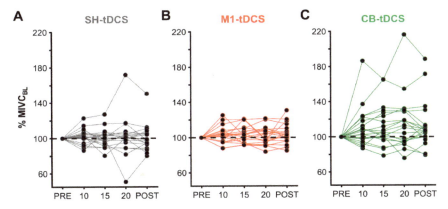

Figure 4. MIVC results I. Individual MIVC results illustrated as percentage-wise increase respective to baseline MIVC values (% MIVC$_{BL}$), per sham (SH)-TDCS (**A**), M1-tDCS (**B**), and CB-tDCS (**C**) for all participants.

Here, we found a significant main effect for STIM (F(2,38) = 4.369, p = 0.027, ηp^2 = 0.187), with post-hoc Bonferroni-Holm tests revealing MIVC values to be higher for CB-tDCS when compared to SH-tDCS (p = 0.028) (Figure 5B), with no significant effects for CB-tDCS vs. M1-tDCS (p = 0.076), as well as M1-tDCS vs. SH-tDCS (p = 0.681). When averaging MIVC values across TIME per stimulation we found MIVC to increase by 1.16% for SH-tDCS and 2.91% for M1-tDCS as compared to 12.70% for CB-tDCS (Figure 5B). We did not find significant main effects for TIME (F(3,57) = 0.099, p = 0.005, ηp^2 = 0.146) (Figure 5A), or a STIM*TIME interaction (F(6,114) = 0.608, p = 0.633, ηp^2 = 0.031). Following the outlier detection, one dataset was removed, and all analyses were reconducted. However, the results did not change as we still observed an effect for STIM (F(2,36) = 4.101, p = 0.033, ηp^2 = 0.186), with post-hoc Bonferroni–Holm tests revealing MIVC values to be higher for CB-tDCS when compared to SH-tDCS (p = 0.022), with no significant effects for CB-tDCS vs. M1-tDCS (p = 0.255), as well as M1-tDCS vs. SH-tDCS (p = 0.833). Accordingly, the outlier had no effect on our results and we therefore elected to display the results with all original data.

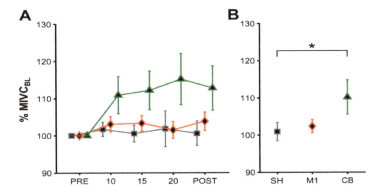

Figure 5. MIVC results II. Mean MIVC and standard error of the mean (SEM) values illustrated as percentage-wise increase respective to baseline MIVC values (% MIVC$_{BL}$), per SH-TDCS (grey squares), M1-tDCS (red diamonds), and CB-tDCS (green triangles) for all participants. (**A**) Depicts mean MIVC results averaged across participants, while (**B**) illustrates mean MIVC results averaged across participants and time to highlight general tDCS effects. Asterisks indicate significant differences between tDCS stimulations. Respective p values are reported in the Results section.

Lastly, we assessed differences in MIVC values averaged across timepoints during stimulation (10, 15, and 20) with MIVC values during POST to compare online and offline tDCS effects. We found a significant main effect for STIM (F(2,38) = 4.049, p = 0.025, ηp^2 = 0.176), with post-hoc Bonferroni–Holm tests revealing MIVC values to be higher for CB-tDCS when compared to SH-tDCS (p = 0.033) with no significant effects for CB-tDCS vs. M1-tDCS (p = 0.109), as well as M1-tDCS vs. SH-tDCS (p = 0.613). We did not find significant main effects for online vs. offline tDCS effects on MIVC (F(1,19) = 0.011, p = 0.918, ηp^2 = 0.001) or an interaction between both factors (F(2,38) = 0.367, p = 0.695, ηp^2 = 0.019).

4. Discussion

In the present study, we evaluated the effects of anodal tDCS (M1-tDCS and CB-tDCS) on MIVC during iBS. We observed a significant increase in MIVC during iBS for CB-tDCS compared to SH-tDCS. To the best of our knowledge, the present study is the first to examine tDCS effects on muscle strength parameters during a whole-body movement. Additionally, we provide the first description of force enhancing effects during non-invasive cerebellar stimulation. Lastly, we did not find differences between online and offline MIVC enhancement. We believe that these results are of importance for several research fields as we provide an initial reference point and highlight potential challenges for future studies.

The main result of this study is an increase in MIVC for CB-tDCS stimulation but no significant increase for M1-tDCS or SH-tDCS. On one hand, an increase in muscular force after tDCS administration is in line with previous studies [12–15], albeit excluding CB-tDCS, yet in contrast to other results that failed to find such effects on muscle strength parameters [16–18]. Several factors may account for this.

First, it seems important to discuss our paradigm within the context of previous related research. Concerning this matter, we believe our tDCS paradigm to be consistent with most studies examining tDCS-induced muscle strength modulations [8]. Stimulation sites of both M1-tDCS, as well as CB-tDCS, were chosen based on common directives from recent literature [8,38,44]. We selected a current of 2 mA, as it has been reported that a current of 2 mA penetrates deeper through the skull when compared to 1.5 mA or 1 mA [48] and is commonly employed when administering tDCS over CB or M1. This might be a critical point considering an absent effect of M1-tDCS on MIVC, as M1 (leg area) is located deep inside the longitudinal cerebral fissure [49]. On the contrary, higher current intensity does not necessarily increase cortical excitability [50,51]. It has been suggested, that lower current intensities (<2 mA) are potentially more beneficial regarding tDCS effects, meaning that even if currents of higher intensity generally penetrate deeper through tissue, they do not always reflect optimal intensities to modulate local excitability [52]. Still, current flow simulations based on both tDCS configurations employed in our study show target areas (M1 and CB) to be extensively covered by the administered current (see Figure 2A,B). It is, therefore, conceivable that M1 plays a subordinate role in the force modulation of iBS. While both target areas are covered, current additionally spread broadly across other areas of the brain. This issue of low spatial focality is well known in tDCS research [8,13,52], although many studies show tDCS modulations of single muscle activity [48] and single muscle performance [12,14,53]. Additionally, concerning the effects of CB-tDCS on MIVC, it could be argued that due to our montage current is spreading beyond the cerebellum, specifically to regions of the brain stem and therefore, our results cannot be attributed to cerebellar modulations exclusively. However, a previous study assessed changes in brainstem excitability using the same CB-tDCS montage we employed in this study [54]. The authors did not find changes in brainstem excitability, which is why we assume such a confound to be unlikely regarding the present study.

Considering the positive effect of CB-tDCS on iBS, it is important to contextualize the results with our task. The iBS task, as performed in the present study, represented a novel challenge to all participants as they were not skilled in iBS with a short familiarization serving as each individual's only experience before testing. In this sense optimized coordination between muscles involved in force transmission during iBS is conceivable. Several studies show such adjustments as a result of CB-tDCS, e.g., during locomotor adaptation tasks [30] and complex overhand throwing tasks [55].

In particular, it should be mentioned that these studies that show such effects used protocols of anodal CB-tDCS in accordance with our results [30,55–57]. Another adaptation relating to coordination that could be induced by CB-tDCS is an optimized antagonist contraction behavior. Several studies have shown that increases in strength and improved force progression, following adaptation to strength training, are associated with reduced antagonist co-contraction [58,59]. It is also known that the cerebellum plays a crucial role in the coordination between agonist–antagonist contractions during exercise. For example, people suffering from cerebellar pathologies may experience increased co-contractions at the start of movement [60], inaccurate timing of antagonist muscles during agonistic contractions [60,61], and delayed onset of agonistic contractions [62]. Furthermore, studies show that the cerebellum contributes to the temporal coordination of movement patterns [61]. Interestingly, anodal stimulation of the cerebellum, combined with subsequent cerebral stimulation has been shown to improve the onset latency of antagonistic movements in patients with cerebellar ataxia [63]. Future studies should investigate the precise mode of action of CB-tDCS on antagonistic contractions and its relationship to improved strength performance in compound whole-body movements. In addition, adaptive motor control and the role of both areas of stimulation (M1-tDCS and CB-tDCS) during adaptive motor control potentially explain our results. In brief, adaptive motor control describes error reduction during motor adaptation [64]. Although both cerebellum and M1 are involved in motor control, their roles during adaptive motor control differ. Here, cerebellar processing is thought to affect online learning, evidenced through reductions in movement-related errors after CB-stimulation during motor tasks using tDCS [30,64,65] and TMS [66] stimulation. Further, cerebellar lesions lead to impaired abilities regarding successful changes in visuomotor positioning which further suggests that error reduction during motor tasks is a process connected to cerebellar activity [24,67]. On the other hand, M1-stimulation yields an offline response concerning adaptive motor control. This is reflected in previous research showing decreased retention time with no effects on error reduction after M1-stimulation [64,65]. These differences could help explain our finding that CB-tDCS increases MIVC during iBS. As CB-tDCS modifies cerebellar output, mainly that of Purkinje cells [54], it is possible that such a stimulation modulates cerebellar responses to sensory prediction error-related input and therefore leads to an increase in cerebellar response to task-related kinematic and dynamic errors [54,64]. Although this remains speculative, our results might, therefore, reflect an increase in the range of operating Purkinje cells as a response to CB-tDCS stimulation, leading to more rapid adaptations following each trial. This potentially results in greater force output, as timely coordination between segments (limbs and constrained body parts) in all joints is enhanced due to these rapid adaptational processes concerning the internal model of iBS. Therefore, we think that our results do not reflect greater force production capacity, but rather a quicker realization of force production due to improved coordination between muscles involved in iBS, possibly as a result of optimized internal models of iBS following CB-tDCS compared to M1-tDCS and SH-tDCS.

Lastly, M1 is not likely involved in online motor control and force production during iBS. Still, previous studies showed force modulations of M1-tDCS [12–14], which is why the absence of such an effect in this study has to be addressed. An initial problem lies in the interindividual heterogeneity of M1 representations [68], inferring that current which sufficiently covers a targeted area and thus enhances local excitability in one participant might fail to do so entirely in another. This issue is closely related to overall variability in tDCS responsiveness. Generally, many participants fail to respond to tDCS stimulation expectedly [69,70]. In particular cases, nearly half of all stimulated participants do not respond to stimulation as anticipated [71]. Inter-individual variability in tDCS responsiveness has been observed for hand [69–71] and leg area of M1 [72,73]. TMS can be used as a countermeasure to ensure consideration of individualities concerning cortical representations. Interestingly, combining TMS-localization with tDCS stimulation does not guarantee responsiveness. Out of two studies that examined tDCS related muscle strength modulations in lower extremities and used TMS to localize and stimulate individual target areas, one reports high responsiveness and behavioral enhancement [14], whilst the second does not [18]. Still, future studies should consider using TMS, as it would have allowed for a definite control measure regarding the effectiveness of tDCS stimulations. High-definition tDCS (HD-tDCS) is another approach to increase the focality of non-invasively administered current. It was shown that HD-tDCS current is generally more spatially focal and able to increase the duration of tDCS induced after-effects compared to conventional tDCS [74]. Two studies have applied HD-tDCS to examine its effects on muscle strength parameters but were unable to find positive results [75,76]. Finally, a limitation of this study is the number of MIVC tests performed per measurement point. We have decided on one MIVC measurement per measurement point since the risk of injury to the participants is increased with each additional measurement per measurement point. We were recommended to do so by biomechanical experts during the evaluation of our test set-up. Since the squat, as a whole-body movement, demands the entire muscle apparatus, we wanted to avoid additional risks due to accumulated fatigue. In addition, the resting periods between several MIVCs, especially during whole-body movements, should be at least 3–5 min apart to ensure maximum force generation in each trial [77].

5. Conclusions

In conclusion, we provide novel evidence that anodal CB-tDCS can enhance MIVC in iBS serving as a whole-body movement. This is the first study to observe force enhancing effects of tDCS on whole-body movements as well as the first study to show force enhancing effects of CB-tDCS. As such, we present an initial framework of references concerning tDCS effects on muscle strength parameters in whole-body movements. A multitude of everyday life activities is comprised of whole-body movements. TDCS induced improvements of movement parameters, such as MIVC, in whole-body movements could prove beneficial to enable improved physical functioning, as well as prevent age-related decline in motor function. Perspectively, it seems important to test dynamic movements as whole-body movements commonly include both dynamic (eccentric and concentric) and static (isometric) movement periods. Therefore, it is necessary to extend our findings by including different protocols as well as examining other whole-body movements in future studies.

Author Contributions: R.K., T.M., P.R., and A.V. were responsible for the conception and design of the study. R.K., T.M., and D.M. were responsible for the acquisition, analysis, and interpretation of data for the work. R.K. drafted the manuscript; R.K., T.M., D.M., A.V., and P.R. provided critical revision. All authors approved the final version of the manuscript and agree to be accountable for all aspects of the work in ensuring that questions related to the accuracy or integrity of any part of the work are appropriately investigated and resolved. All persons designated as authors qualify for authorship, and all those who qualify for authorship are listed. All authors have read and agreed to the published version of the manuscript.

Funding: This study was supported by the Max-Planck Society.

Acknowledgments: We would like to thank Martina Clauß, Lisa Schubert, Ramona Menger, and Hartmut Domröse for organizational and technical support.

Conflicts of Interest: The authors declare no conflict of interest.

References

1. Beckham, G.; Mizuguchi, S.; Carter, C.; Sato, K.; Ramsey, M.; Lamont, H.; Hornsby, G.; Haff, G.; Stone, M. Relationships of isometric mid-thigh pull variables to weightlifting performance. *J. Sports Med. Phys. Fit.* **2013**, *53*, 573–581.
2. Izquierdo, M.; Aguado, X.; Gonzalez, R.; Lopez, J.; Häkkinen, K. Maximal and explosive force production capacity and balance performance in men of different ages. *Eur. J. Appl. Physiol. Occup. Physiol.* **1999**, *79*, 260–267. [CrossRef] [PubMed]
3. Häkkinen, K.; Alen, M.; Kraemer, W.; Gorostiaga, E.; Izquierdo, M.; Rusko, H.; Mikkola, J.; Häkkinen, A.; Valkeinen, H.; Kaarakainen, E. Neuromuscular adaptations during concurrent strength and endurance training versus strength training. *Eur. J. Appl. Physiol.* **2003**, *89*, 42–52. [CrossRef] [PubMed]
4. Grodd, W.; Hulsmann, E.; Lotze, M.; Wildgruber, D.; Erb, M. Sensorimotor mapping of the human cerebellum: fMRI evidence of somatotopic organization. *Hum. Brain Mapp.* **2001**, *13*, 55–73. [CrossRef]

5. Wiestler, T.; McGonigle, D.J.; Diedrichsen, J. Integration of sensory and motor representations of single fingers in the human cerebellum. *J. Neurophysiol.* **2011**, *105*, 3042–3053. [CrossRef]
6. Spraker, M.B.; Corcos, D.M.; Kurani, A.S.; Prodoehl, J.; Swinnen, S.P.; Vaillancourt, D.E. Specific cerebellar regions are related to force amplitude and rate of force development. *Neuroimage* **2012**, *59*, 1647–1656. [CrossRef]
7. Dettmers, C.; Fink, G.R.; Lemon, R.N.; Stephan, K.M.; Passingham, R.E.; Silbersweig, D.; Holmes, A.; Ridding, M.C.; Brooks, D.J.; Frackowiak, R.S. Relation between cerebral activity and force in the motor areas of the human brain. *J. Neurophysiol.* **1995**, *74*, 802–815. [CrossRef]
8. Lattari, E.; Oliveira, B.R.R.; Monteiro Junior, R.S.; Marques Neto, S.R.; Oliveira, A.J.; Maranhao Neto, G.A.; Machado, S.; Budde, H. Acute effects of single dose transcranial direct current stimulation on muscle strength: A systematic review and meta-analysis. *PLoS ONE* **2018**, *13*, e0209513. [CrossRef]
9. Cogiamanian, F.; Marceglia, S.; Ardolino, G.; Barbieri, S.; Priori, A. Improved isometric force endurance after transcranial direct current stimulation over the human motor cortical areas. *Eur. J. Neurosci.* **2007**, *26*, 242–249. [CrossRef]
10. Lattari, E.; Rosa Filho, B.J.; Fonseca Junior, S.J.; Murillo-Rodriguez, E.; Rocha, N.; Machado, S.; Maranhao Neto, G.A. Effects on Volume Load and Ratings of Perceived Exertion in Individuals Advanced Weight-Training After Transcranial Direct Current Stimulation. *J. Strength Cond. Res.* **2018**, *34*, 89–96. [CrossRef]
11. Lattari, E.; Andrade, M.L.; Filho, A.S.; Moura, A.M.; Neto, G.M.; Silva, J.G.; Rocha, N.B.; Yuan, T.F.; Arias-Carrion, O.; Machado, S. Can Transcranial Direct Current Stimulation Improve the Resistance Strength and Decrease the Rating Perceived Scale in Recreational Weight-Training Experience? *J. Strength Cond. Res.* **2016**, *30*, 3381–3387. [CrossRef] [PubMed]
12. Abdelmoula, A.; Baudry, S.; Duchateau, J. Anodal transcranial direct current stimulation enhances time to task failure of a submaximal contraction of elbow flexors without changing corticospinal excitability. *Neuroscience* **2016**, *322*, 94–103. [CrossRef] [PubMed]
13. Vargas, V.Z.; Baptista, A.F.; Pereira, G.O.C.; Pochini, A.C.; Ejnisman, B.; Santos, M.B.; Joao, S.M.A.; Hazime, F.A. Modulation of Isometric Quadriceps Strength in Soccer Players With Transcranial Direct Current Stimulation: A Crossover Study. *J. Strength Cond. Res.* **2018**, *32*, 1336–1341. [CrossRef]
14. Tanaka, S.; Hanakawa, T.; Honda, M.; Watanabe, K. Enhancement of pinch force in the lower leg by anodal transcranial direct current stimulation. *Exp. Brain Res.* **2009**, *196*, 459–465. [CrossRef]
15. Angius, L.; Pageaux, B.; Hopker, J.; Marcora, S.M.; Mauger, A.R. Transcranial direct current stimulation improves isometric time to exhaustion of the knee extensors. *Neuroscience* **2016**, *339*, 363–375. [CrossRef]
16. Lattari, E.; Campos, C.; Lamego, M.K.; Passos de Souza, S.L.; Neto, G.M.; Rocha, N.B.; Jose de Oliveira, A.; Carpenter, S.; Machado, S. Can transcranial direct current stimulation improve muscle power in individuals with advanced resistance training experience? *J. Strength Cond. Res.* **2017**. [CrossRef]
17. Ciccone, A.B.; Deckert, J.A.; Schlabs, C.R.; Tilden, M.J.; Herda, T.J.; Gallagher, P.M.; Weir, J.P. Transcranial Direct Current Stimulation of the Temporal Lobe Does Not Affect High Intensity Work Capacity. *J. Strength Cond. Res.* **2018**. [CrossRef]
18. Maeda, K.; Yamaguchi, T.; Tatemoto, T.; Kondo, K.; Otaka, Y.; Tanaka, S. Transcranial Direct Current Stimulation Does Not Affect Lower Extremity Muscle Strength Training in Healthy Individuals: A Triple-Blind, Sham-Controlled Study. *Front. Neurosci.* **2017**, *11*, 179. [CrossRef]
19. Nitsche, M.A.; Paulus, W. Excitability changes induced in the human motor cortex by weak transcranial direct current stimulation. *J. Physiol.* **2000**, *527 Pt 3*, 633–639. [CrossRef]
20. Hendy, A.M.; Kidgell, D.J. Anodal-tDCS applied during unilateral strength training increases strength and corticospinal excitability in the untrained homologous muscle. *Exp. Brain Res.* **2014**, *232*, 3243–3252. [CrossRef]
21. Jacobs, J.V.; Horak, F.B. Cortical control of postural responses. *J. Neural Transm. (Vienna)* **2007**, *114*, 1339–1348. [CrossRef] [PubMed]
22. Ito, M. Historical review of the significance of the cerebellum and the role of Purkinje cells in motor learning. *Ann. N. Y. Acad. Sci.* **2002**, *978*, 273–288. [CrossRef] [PubMed]
23. Ioffe, M.E.; Chernikova, L.A.; Ustinova, K.I. Role of cerebellum in learning postural tasks. *Cerebellum* **2007**, *6*, 87–94. [CrossRef] [PubMed]

24. Martin, T.A.; Keating, J.G.; Goodkin, H.P.; Bastian, A.J.; Thach, W.T. Throwing while looking through prisms. I. Focal olivocerebellar lesions impair adaptation. *Brain* **1996**, *119 Pt 4*, 1183–1198. [CrossRef]
25. Timmann, D.; Brandauer, B.; Hermsdorfer, J.; Ilg, W.; Konczak, J.; Gerwig, M.; Gizewski, E.R.; Schoch, B. Lesion-symptom mapping of the human cerebellum. *Cerebellum* **2008**, *7*, 602–606. [CrossRef]
26. Topka, H.; Konczak, J.; Schneider, K.; Boose, A.; Dichgans, J. Multijoint arm movements in cerebellar ataxia: Abnormal control of movement dynamics. *Exp. Brain Res.* **1998**, *119*, 493–503. [CrossRef]
27. Bastian, A.J.; Mink, J.W.; Kaufman, B.A.; Thach, W.T. Posterior vermal split syndrome. *Ann. Neurol.* **1998**, *44*, 601–610. [CrossRef]
28. Thach, W.T. Timing of activity in cerebellar dentate nucleus and cerebral motor cortex during prompt volitional movement. *Brain Res.* **1975**, *88*, 233–241. [CrossRef]
29. Goodkin, H.P.; Thach, W.T. Cerebellar control of constrained and unconstrained movements. I. Nuclear inactivation. *J. Neurophysiol.* **2003**, *89*, 884–895. [CrossRef]
30. Jayaram, G.; Tang, B.; Pallegadda, R.; Vasudevan, E.V.; Celnik, P.; Bastian, A. Modulating locomotor adaptation with cerebellar stimulation. *J. Neurophysiol.* **2012**, *107*, 2950–2957. [CrossRef]
31. Poortvliet, P.; Hsieh, B.; Cresswell, A.; Au, J.; Meinzer, M. Cerebellar transcranial direct current stimulation improves adaptive postural control. *Clin. Neurophysiol.* **2018**, *129*, 33–41. [CrossRef] [PubMed]
32. Zandvliet, S.B.; Meskers, C.G.M.; Kwakkel, G.; van Wegen, E.E.H. Short-Term Effects of Cerebellar tDCS on Standing Balance Performance in Patients with Chronic Stroke and Healthy Age-Matched Elderly. *Cerebellum* **2018**, *17*, 575–589. [CrossRef] [PubMed]
33. Steiner, K.M.; Enders, A.; Thier, W.; Batsikadze, G.; Ludolph, N.; Ilg, W.; Timmann, D. Cerebellar tDCS does not improve learning in a complex whole body dynamic balance task in young healthy subjects. *PLoS ONE* **2016**, *11*, e0163598. [CrossRef] [PubMed]
34. Steele, C.J.; Bailey, J.A.; Zatorre, R.J.; Penhune, V.B. Early musical training and white-matter plasticity in the corpus callosum: Evidence for a sensitive period. *J. Neurosci.* **2013**, *33*, 1282–1290. [CrossRef] [PubMed]
35. Vollmann, H.; Ragert, P.; Conde, V.; Villringer, A.; Classen, J.; Witte, O.W.; Steele, C.J. Instrument specific use-dependent plasticity shapes the anatomical properties of the corpus callosum: A comparison between musicians and non-musicians. *Front. Behav. Neurosci.* **2014**, *8*, 245. [CrossRef] [PubMed]
36. Chow, S.; Shao, J.; Wang, H. *Sample Size Calculations in Clinical Research, Chapman & Hall*; CRC: Boca Raton, FL, USA, 2008.
37. Rosner, B. *Fundamentals of Biostatistics. Cengage Learning*; Inc., Kentucky: Boston, MA, USA, 2010.
38. Ferrucci, R.; Cortese, F.; Priori, A. Cerebellar tDCS: How to do it. *Cerebellum* **2015**, *14*, 27–30. [CrossRef]
39. Knoch, D.; Nitsche, M.A.; Fischbacher, U.; Eisenegger, C.; Pascual-Leone, A.; Fehr, E. Studying the neurobiology of social interaction with transcranial direct current stimulation—The example of punishing unfairness. *Cereb. Cortex* **2008**, *18*, 1987–1990. [CrossRef]
40. Nitsche, M.A.; Doemkes, S.; Karakose, T.; Antal, A.; Liebetanz, D.; Lang, N.; Tergau, F.; Paulus, W. Shaping the effects of transcranial direct current stimulation of the human motor cortex. *J. Neurophysiol.* **2007**, *97*, 3109–3117. [CrossRef]
41. Madhavan, S.; Stinear, J.W. Focal and bi-directional modulation of lower limb motor cortex using anodal transcranial direct current stimulation. *Brain Stimul.* **2010**, *3*, 42. [CrossRef]
42. Laczo, B.; Antal, A.; Rothkegel, H.; Paulus, W. Increasing human leg motor cortex excitability by transcranial high frequency random noise stimulation. *Restor. Neurol. Neurosci.* **2014**, *32*, 403–410. [CrossRef]
43. Kaminski, E.; Steele, C.J.; Hoff, M.; Gundlach, C.; Rjosk, V.; Sehm, B.; Villringer, A.; Ragert, P. Transcranial direct current stimulation (tDCS) over primary motor cortex leg area promotes dynamic balance task performance. *Clin. Neurophysiol.* **2016**, *127*, 2455–2462. [CrossRef] [PubMed]
44. Taubert, M.; Stein, T.; Kreutzberg, T.; Stockinger, C.; Hecker, L.; Focke, A.; Ragert, P.; Villringer, A.; Pleger, B. Remote Effects of Non-Invasive Cerebellar Stimulation on Error Processing in Motor Re-Learning. *Brain Stimul.* **2016**, *9*, 692–699. [CrossRef] [PubMed]
45. Van Selst, M.; Jolicoeur, P. A solution to the effect of sample size on outlier elimination. *Q. J. Exp. Psychol. Sect. A* **1994**, *47*, 631–650. [CrossRef]
46. Miller, J. Reaction time analysis with outlier exclusion: Bias varies with sample size. *Q. J. Exp. Psychol.* **1991**, *43*, 907–912. [CrossRef]
47. Pollet, T.V.; van der Meij, L. To Remove or not to Remove: The Impact of Outlier Handling on Significance Testing in Testosterone Data. *Adapt. Hum. Behav. Physiol.* **2017**, *3*, 43–60. [CrossRef]

48. Jeffery, D.T.; Norton, J.A.; Roy, F.D.; Gorassini, M.A. Effects of transcranial direct current stimulation on the excitability of the leg motor cortex. *Exp. Brain Res.* **2007**, *182*, 281–287. [CrossRef]
49. Sasaki, N.; Abo, M.; Hara, T.; Yamada, N.; Niimi, M.; Kakuda, W. High-frequency rTMS on leg motor area in the early phase of stroke. *Acta Neurol. Belg.* **2017**, *117*, 189–194. [CrossRef]
50. Jamil, A.; Batsikadze, G.; Kuo, H.I.; Labruna, L.; Hasan, A.; Paulus, W.; Nitsche, M.A. Systematic evaluation of the impact of stimulation intensity on neuroplastic after-effects induced by transcranial direct current stimulation. *J. Physiol.* **2017**, *595*, 1273–1288. [CrossRef]
51. Kan, B.; Dundas, J.E.; Nosaka, K. Effect of transcranial direct current stimulation on elbow flexor maximal voluntary isometric strength and endurance. *Appl. Physiol. Nutr. Metab.* **2013**, *38*, 734–739. [CrossRef]
52. Neuling, T.; Wagner, S.; Wolters, C.H.; Zaehle, T.; Herrmann, C.S. Finite-Element Model Predicts Current Density Distribution for Clinical Applications of tDCS and tACS. *Front. Psychiatry* **2012**, *3*, 83. [CrossRef]
53. Krishnan, C.; Ranganathan, R.; Kantak, S.S.; Dhaher, Y.Y.; Rymer, W.Z. Anodal transcranial direct current stimulation alters elbow flexor muscle recruitment strategies. *Brain Stimul.* **2014**, *7*, 443–450. [CrossRef] [PubMed]
54. Galea, J.M.; Jayaram, G.; Ajagbe, L.; Celnik, P. Modulation of cerebellar excitability by polarity-specific noninvasive direct current stimulation. *J. Neurosci.* **2009**, *29*, 9115–9122. [CrossRef] [PubMed]
55. Jackson, A.K.; de Albuquerque, L.L.; Pantovic, M.; Fischer, K.M.; Guadagnoli, M.A.; Riley, Z.A.; Poston, B. Cerebellar Transcranial Direct Current Stimulation Enhances Motor Learning in a Complex Overhand Throwing Task. *Cerebellum* **2019**, *18*, 813–816. [CrossRef] [PubMed]
56. Cantarero, G.; Spampinato, D.; Reis, J.; Ajagbe, L.; Thompson, T.; Kulkarni, K.; Celnik, P. Cerebellar direct current stimulation enhances on-line motor skill acquisition through an effect on accuracy. *J. Neurosci.* **2015**, *35*, 3285–3290. [CrossRef] [PubMed]
57. Jongkees, B.J.; Immink, M.A.; Boer, O.D.; Yavari, F.; Nitsche, M.A.; Colzato, L.S. The Effect of Cerebellar tDCS on Sequential Motor Response Selection. *Cerebellum* **2019**, *18*, 738–749. [CrossRef] [PubMed]
58. Carolan, B.; Cafarelli, E. Adaptations in coactivation after isometric resistance training. *J. Appl. Physiol.* **1992**, *73*, 911–917. [CrossRef] [PubMed]
59. Rutherford, O.M.; Jones, D.A. The role of learning and coordination in strength training. *Eur. J. Appl. Physiol. Occup. Physiol.* **1986**, *55*, 100–105. [CrossRef]
60. Hallett, M.; Shahani, B.T.; Young, R.R. EMG analysis of patients with cerebellar deficits. *J. Neurol. Neurosurg. Psychiatry* **1975**, *38*, 1163–1169. [CrossRef]
61. Hore, J.; Flament, D. Changes in motor cortex neural discharge associated with the development of cerebellar limb ataxia. *J. Neurophysiol.* **1988**, *60*, 1285–1302. [CrossRef]
62. Diener, H.C.; Dichgans, J. Pathophysiology of cerebellar ataxia. *Mov. Disord.* **1992**, *7*, 95–109. [CrossRef]
63. Grimaldi, G.; Oulad Ben Taib, N.; Manto, M.; Bodranghien, F. Marked reduction of cerebellar deficits in upper limbs following transcranial cerebello-cerebral DC stimulation: Tremor reduction and re-programming of the timing of antagonist commands. *Front. Syst. Neurosci.* **2014**, *8*, 9. [CrossRef] [PubMed]
64. Galea, J.M.; Vazquez, A.; Pasricha, N.; de Xivry, J.J.; Celnik, P. Dissociating the roles of the cerebellum and motor cortex during adaptive learning: The motor cortex retains what the cerebellum learns. *Cereb. Cortex* **2011**, *21*, 1761–1770. [CrossRef] [PubMed]
65. Ehsani, F.; Bakhtiary, A.H.; Jaberzadeh, S.; Talimkhani, A.; Hajihasani, A. Differential effects of primary motor cortex and cerebellar transcranial direct current stimulation on motor learning in healthy individuals: A randomized double-blind sham-controlled study. *Neurosci. Res.* **2016**, *112*, 10–19. [CrossRef]
66. Jayaram, G.; Galea, J.M.; Bastian, A.J.; Celnik, P. Human locomotor adaptive learning is proportional to depression of cerebellar excitability. *Cereb. Cortex* **2011**, *21*, 1901–1909. [CrossRef] [PubMed]
67. Rabe, K.; Livne, O.; Gizewski, E.R.; Aurich, V.; Beck, A.; Timmann, D.; Donchin, O. Adaptation to visuomotor rotation and force field perturbation is correlated to different brain areas in patients with cerebellar degeneration. *J. Neurophysiol.* **2009**, *101*, 1961–1971. [CrossRef]
68. Hazime, F.A.; da Cunha, R.A.; Soliaman, R.R.; Romancini, A.C.B.; Pochini, A.C.; Ejnisman, B.; Baptista, A.F. Anodal Transcranial Direct Current Stimulation (Tdcs) Increases Isometric Strength of Shoulder Rotators Muscles in Handball Players. *Int. J. Sports Phys. Ther.* **2017**, *12*, 402–407.
69. Laakso, I.; Tanaka, S.; Koyama, S.; De Santis, V.; Hirata, A. Inter-subject Variability in Electric Fields of Motor Cortical tDCS. *Brain Stimul.* **2015**, *8*, 906–913. [CrossRef]

70. Laakso, I.; Tanaka, S.; Mikkonen, M.; Koyama, S.; Sadato, N.; Hirata, A. Electric fields of motor and frontal tDCS in a standard brain space: A computer simulation study. *Neuroimage* **2016**, *137*, 140–151. [CrossRef]
71. Wiethoff, S.; Hamada, M.; Rothwell, J.C. Variability in response to transcranial direct current stimulation of the motor cortex. *Brain Stimul.* **2014**, *7*, 468–475. [CrossRef]
72. Madhavan, S.; Sriraman, A.; Freels, S. Reliability and Variability of tDCS Induced Changes in the Lower Limb Motor Cortex. *Brain Sci.* **2016**, *6*, 26. [CrossRef]
73. Van Asseldonk, E.H.; Boonstra, T.A. Transcranial Direct Current Stimulation of the Leg Motor Cortex Enhances Coordinated Motor Output During Walking With a Large Inter-Individual Variability. *Brain Stimul.* **2016**, *9*, 182–190. [CrossRef] [PubMed]
74. Kuo, H.-I.; Bikson, M.; Datta, A.; Minhas, P.; Paulus, W.; Kuo, M.-F.; Nitsche, M.A. Comparing cortical plasticity induced by conventional and high-definition 4 × 1 ring tDCS: A neurophysiological study. *Brain Stimul.* **2013**, *6*, 644–648. [CrossRef] [PubMed]
75. Flood, A.; Waddington, G.; Keegan, R.J.; Thompson, K.G.; Cathcart, S. The effects of elevated pain inhibition on endurance exercise performance. *PeerJ* **2017**, *5*, e3028. [CrossRef] [PubMed]
76. Radel, R.; Tempest, G.; Denis, G.; Besson, P.; Zory, R. Extending the limits of force endurance: Stimulation of the motor or the frontal cortex? *Cortex* **2017**, *97*, 96–108. [CrossRef] [PubMed]
77. Rahimi, R. Effect of different rest intervals on the exercise volume completed during squat bouts. *J. Sports Sci. Med.* **2005**, *4*, 361–366. [PubMed]

© 2020 by the authors. Licensee MDPI, Basel, Switzerland. This article is an open access article distributed under the terms and conditions of the Creative Commons Attribution (CC BY) license (http://creativecommons.org/licenses/by/4.0/).

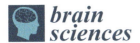

Article

Acute Effects of High-Definition Transcranial Direct Current Stimulation on Foot Muscle Strength, Passive Ankle Kinesthesia, and Static Balance: A Pilot Study

Songlin Xiao [1], Baofeng Wang [1], Xini Zhang [1], Junhong Zhou [2,3,*] and Weijie Fu [1,4,*]

1. School of Kinesiology, Shanghai University of Sport, Shanghai 200438, China; xiao_songlin@126.com (S.X.); wangbaofeng1911@163.com (B.W.); zhangxini1129@163.com (X.Z.)
2. The Hinda and Arthur Marcus Institute for Aging Research, Hebrew SeniorLife, Boston, MA 02131, USA
3. Harvard Medical School, Boston, MA 02131, USA
4. Key Laboratory of Exercise and Health Sciences of Ministry of Education, Shanghai University of Sport, Shanghai 200438, China
* Correspondence: junhongzhou@hsl.harvard.edu (J.Z.); fuweijie@sus.edu.cn or fuweijie315@163.com (W.F.)

Received: 20 March 2020; Accepted: 19 April 2020; Published: 21 April 2020

Abstract: This study aimed to examine the effects of single-session anodal high-definition transcranial direct current stimulation (HD-tDCS) on the strength of intrinsic foot muscles, passive ankle kinesthesia, and static balance. Methods: In this double-blinded self-controlled study, 14 healthy younger adults were asked to complete assessments of foot muscle strength, passive ankle kinesthesia, and static balance before and after a 20-minute session of either HD-tDCS or sham stimulation (i.e., control) at two visits separated by one week. Two-way repeated-measures analysis of variance was used to examine the effects of HD-tDCS on metatarsophalangeal joint flexor strength, toe flexor strength, the passive kinesthesia threshold of ankle joint, and the average sway velocity of the center of gravity. Results: All participants completed all study procedures and no side effects nor risk events were reported. Blinding was shown to be successful, with an overall accuracy of 35.7% in the guess of stimulation type ($p = 0.347$). No main effects of intervention, time, or their interaction were observed for foot muscle strength ($p > 0.05$). The average percent change in first-toe flexor strength following anodal HD-tDCS was 12.8 ± 24.2%, with 11 out of 14 participants showing an increase in strength, while the change following sham stimulation was 0.7 ± 17.3%, with 8 out of 14 participants showing an increase in strength. A main effect of time on the passive kinesthesia threshold of ankle inversion, dorsiflexion, and anteroposterior and medial–lateral average sway velocity of the center of gravity in one-leg standing with eyes closed was observed; these outcomes were reduced from pre to post stimulation ($p < 0.05$). No significant differences were observed for other variables between the two stimulation types. Conclusion: The results of this pilot study suggested that single-session HD-tDCS may improve the flexor strength of the first toe, although no statistically significant differences were observed between the anodal HD-tDCS and sham procedure groups. Additionally, passive ankle kinesthesia and static standing balance performance were improved from pre to post stimulation, but no significant differences were observed between the HD-tDCS and sham procedure groups. This may be potentially due to ceiling effects in this healthy cohort of a small sample size. Nevertheless, these preliminary findings may provide critical knowledge of optimal stimulation parameters, effect size, and power estimation of HD-tDCS for future trials aiming to confirm and expand the findings of this pilot study.

Keywords: high-definition transcranial direct current stimulation (HD-tDCS); foot muscle strength; passive ankle kinesthesia; static balance

1. Introduction

A new paradigm has redefined the complex human foot structure as the foot core system, which includes the active, passive, and neural subsystems [1]. The active subsystem is composed of intrinsic and extrinsic foot muscles that can control foot movement and provide propulsive power, while the neural subsystem comprises sensory receptors that provide accurate motion sensory messages regarding ankle posture [2]. The active and neural subsystems are important in maintaining standing balance and controlling body posture [3]. Impaired movement sense and reduced foot muscle strength increase walking variability, fall risk [4,5], and even sports-related injuries such as plantar fasciitis and chronic ankle instability (CAI) [6,7]. Therefore, many studies have focused on strengthening the foot core system to prevent foot injuries. To our knowledge, previous studies have mainly focused on enhancing foot function and preventing foot injuries by strengthening intrinsic foot muscles and peripheral nervous systems [1,2]. However, the central nervous system plays a critical role in altering motor planning and generating movement patterns, and changes within the central nervous system predispose individuals to re-injury [8]. Decreased excitability of the primary motor cortex (M1) and reduced activation of the somatosensory cortex (S1) have been reported in individuals with foot injuries, e.g., CAI [8]. Therefore, strategies designed to target the cortical sensorimotor regions of the brain hold great promise for improving functional performance pertaining to the foot, and may thus help prevent foot-related injuries in sports.

Transcranial direct current stimulation (tDCS) is a safe method for modulating the excitability of brain regions noninvasively by inducing a low-amplitude current flow between two or more electrodes placed on the scalp [9]. Several systematic reviews and meta-analyses have demonstrated that anodal tDCS applied over M1 can improve balance control, promote muscle strength and muscular endurance, and enhance exercise performance in cycling [10–12]. Studies have also shown that anodal tDCS designed to target the sensorimotor regions of the brain improves physical performance, including muscle strength and sensory function [13]. Specifically, researchers observed that one session of tDCS targeting M1 enhanced the isometric strength of quadricep femoris [14] and the toe pinch force [15]. Zhou et al. [16] recently observed that single-session tDCS over S1 induced the improvement of vibrotactile sensation of the foot sole of older adults under weight-bearing conditions. These studies suggested that anodal tDCS can improve muscle strength and foot sole somatosensation by increasing the cortical excitability of the sensorimotor regions of the brain.

However, these studies used conventional tDCS with large sponge electrodes. This may cause a tingling sensation over the scalp. Moreover, the results indicated large interpersonal variance, which may be due to the current delivered by conventional tDCS diffusing in the cortical regions [17]. Fortunately, novel high-definition tDCS (HD-tDCS) has been developed by employing advanced neuro-modeling techniques; small electrodes enable the navigation of current flow in cortical regions and thus induce a "focal" electric field on targets [18]. The effects of this HD-tDCS technique on human motion function and performance, however, have not been explored. We here anticipate that anodal HD-tDCS can be used as an effective approach to improve foot muscle strength, ankle kinesthesia, and balance performance pertaining to these functions.

This study aimed to examine the effects of single-session anodal HD-tDCS on the strength of foot plantar muscles, passive ankle kinesthesia, and static balance ability. We hypothesized that compared to sham stimulation (i.e., control), single-session anodal HD-tDCS could enhance metatarsophalangeal joint (MPJ) flexor and toe flexor strength, decrease the passive kinesthesia threshold of the ankle joint, and improve static balance ability in healthy younger adults.

2. Methods

2.1. Participants

Fourteen healthy young male adults (age: 22.8 ± 1.2 years; height: 174.6 ± 6.6 cm; body mass: 72.2 ± 8.8 kg; dominant leg: right, as defined by the preferred kicking leg [19]) were recruited. The sample size was calculated using a power analysis with a statistical power of 0.80, a probability level of 0.05, and an effect size f of 0.38 [20] via G*Power 3.1.9.2 software [21,22]. The analysis gave a sample of 11 participants. Considering a 20% drop-out rate, 14 participants were recruited in this study. Participants were recruited from a university community through the distribution of flyers and email announcements of the study. The inclusion criteria were as follows: (1) good health of participants in terms of normal muscle strength and sensory function and (2) no history of lower extremity injuries in the past 6 months. Those who had skin allergies, were using neuropsychiatric medication, had a major neurological disease, or had any contraindications with respect to the use of tDCS (e.g., metal-implanted devices in the brain) were excluded. The participants were asked not to engage in strenuous exercises within 24 h prior to testing and not to drink any beverages containing stimulants such as caffeine within 4 h prior to testing to limit the potential influence of heavy-load physical activity or caffeine on their performance. All participants provided a written informed consent as approved by the Institutional Review Board of the Shanghai University of Sport (2019RT020).

2.2. Experimental Protocol

In this randomized double-blinded, self-controlled study, each participant completed two visits consisting of functional tests (i.e., passive ankle kinesthesia, foot muscle strength, and static balance) immediately before and after a 20-minute session of either HD-tDCS or sham stimulation in a randomized order. The tests started at the same time of a day on each visit, and the two visits were separated by one week to largely eliminate the after-effects of stimulation and to diminish repetition effects. All participants completed the tests in the same order: passive ankle kinesthesia first, then foot muscle strength, and finally static balance. Between different types of tests, a 5-min break was provided to eliminate the effects of fatigue on task performance.

2.3. High-Definition Transcranial Direct Current Stimulation Intervention

The DC-STIMULATOR PLUS (neuroConn, Ilmenau, Germany) device was used to connect to a 4 × 1 multichannel stimulation adapter. The tDCS montage was designed to increase the lower limb area of the sensorimotor regions, i.e., M1 and S1. Five silver chloride-sintered circular electrodes with size of 1 cm^2 were used. The anodal electrode was placed over the Cz electrode of a 10/20 electroencephalogram (EEG) system and was surrounded by four cathodal electrodes (each at a ring center-to-ring center distance of 3.5 cm from the anodal electrode, i.e., C3, C4, Fz, and Pz) (Figure 1A–C) [23]. HD-tDCS was administered for 20 min continuously at a target current intensity of 2.0 mA. This dose of HD-tDCS could exert prominent, long-lasting excitatory following stimulation. Moreover, this intensity has been proven to be safe and well-tolerated by participants [24,25]. Anodal HD-tDCS was applied with an electric current intensity of 2 mA for 20 min. In the anodal HD-tDCS, the current was ramped up to 2 mA over 30 s at 0.1-mA intervals. After 20 min of stimulation, the current was then ramped down to 0 mA over 30 s. In the sham stimulation, the parameters were the same as those in HD-tDCS, but the current was ramped up to 2 mA over 30 s and then immediately ramped down to 0 mA. According to previous studies, this provided enough time to identify the presence of the current with no effective brain stimulation [26,27]. The type of stimulation (i.e., HD-tDCS or sham) was programmed using a code only known by personnel uninvolved in any study procedure before the stimulation. Thus, neither the participants nor the study personnel knew the stimulation type (double-blinded method). The participants were asked to complete a questionnaire at the end of each stimulation to evaluate the potential side effects. They were also asked to "guess" whether they had received HD-tDCS or sham stimulation to assess the blinding efficacy.

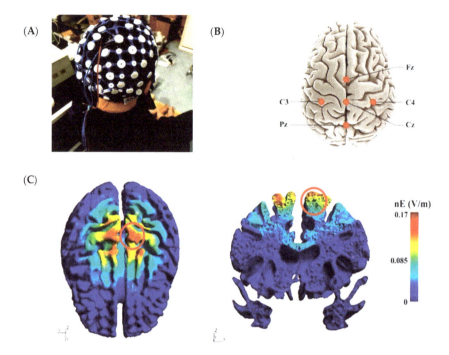

Figure 1. High-definition transcranial direct current stimulation (HD-tDCS) electrode placement and electrical current flow model. (**A**) The experimental setup for HD-tDCS. (**B**) Placement of 4 × 1 HD-tDCS electrodes. The anodal electrode was placed over the Cz electrode of a 10/20 electroencephalogram (EEG) system and surrounded by four cathodal electrodes i.e., C3, C4, Fz, and Pz. (**C**) Electrical current flow model of the cortical surface (left), and the cortical cross-section (right). The electrical field influenced the lower limb area of the sensorimotor regions (red circle).

2.4. Data Collection

2.4.1. Passive Ankle Kinesthesia

The passive kinesthesia threshold of the ankle joint was assessed by using an ankle proprioception tester (KP-11, Toshimi, Shandong, China). The test–retest reliability of this instrument was verified with an intraclass correlation coefficient in range of 0.737–0.935 [28]. Each participant sat on an adjustable seat, and their hip, knee, and ankle joints were fixed at 90°. They each wore an eye mask and noise reduction earphones during the test. The dominant foot was bare, and the sole was wrapped with an air cushion to remove any tactile sense. The dominant foot was then relaxed and placed on the bottom of the foot pedal. Only half the weight of the lower extremity was loaded onto the platform. The platform was randomly activated to drive the participant's ankle in plantarflexion (PF), dorsiflexion (DF), inversion (INV), and eversion (EV). Each participant was then instructed to complete at least three familiarity tests in each direction of ankle motion (i.e., PF, DF, INV, and EV). After confirming the trigger and the direction of foot movement, the participant was asked to press the stop button. The experimenter then recorded the angular displacement and movement direction. The participant lifted his foot from the platform, and the experimenter reset the instrument. After the familiarization test, the participant completed three trials of the test in each movement direction (i.e., PF, DF, INV, and EV) in a randomized order. A rest period of 1 min was given between trials.

2.4.2. Metatarsophalangeal Joint Flexor Strength

MPJ flexor strength was measured using an MPJ flexor strength testing system customized by our team. The validity and reliability were reported previously [29,30]. Each participant was seated in the system with bare feet and legs. The position and height of the seat were adjusted to make the thighs parallel to the ground and the knee joint was fixed at 90°. The heels, ankles, and knees were fixed (Figure 2). When the test started, the participant was asked to flex the MPJ and press the pedal for 10 s with maximum force. The measurement was repeated thrice with a rest period of 1 min. The peak MPJ flexor strength was then obtained and normalized according to the body weight of each participant.

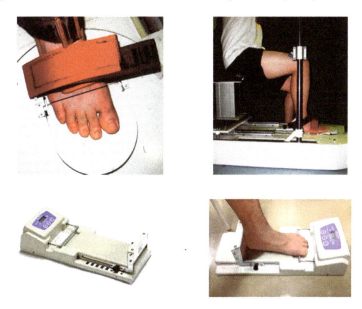

Figure 2. Metatarsophalangeal joint flexor strength tester (upper panels) and toe grip dynamometer and toe flexor strength measurement (lower panels).

2.4.3. Toe Flexor Strength

Toe flexor strength was measured in the sitting position using a toe grip dynamometer (T.K.K.3361, Takei Scientific Instruments Co., Niigata, Japan). Details of the tester, testing process, and its reliability are available in the literature [31,32]. Each participant was asked to sit on an adjustable seat, with the hip, knee, and ankle joints fixed at 90°. The dominant foot was placed on the dynamometer and fixed with the heel stopper, and the other foot was positioned next to the testing instrument. During the measurements, the toes were flexed vigorously for at least 3 s, and the trunk was kept upright while keeping the hands on the chest (Figure 2). The peak flexor strengths of the first toe, the other four toes, and all toes were recorded and normalized by body weight of each participant. The measurement was repeated thrice with an interval of 1 min.

2.4.4. Static Balance Ability

In the standing balance test, each participant stood on the balance testing system (Super Balance, Acmeway, Beijing, China) while wearing a sports uniform (i.e., vest, shorts, and socks). While looking straight ahead, the participants stood in a position in which the width of their bare feet was the same as that of their shoulders. Each participant completed three trials in each of the following conditions: two-leg standing with eyes open (TL_EO) and eyes closed (TL_EC) and one-leg standing with eyes open (OL_EO) and eyes closed (OL_EC). Two-leg trials lasted 30 s, and one-leg trials lasted 10 s.

A break of 30 s was provided between trials. The system recorded the sway velocity of the center of gravity (CoG) in the medial–lateral (ML) and anteroposterior (AP) directions.

2.5. Statistics

SPSS 22.0 (SPSS Inc., Chicago, IL, USA.) was used to complete the statistical analysis, and all data were expressed by mean ± standard deviation. The Shapiro–Wilk test was used to examine the normal distribution of the outcomes. Fisher's exact test was used to test the blinding efficacy of HD-tDCS. Two-way repeated measures analysis of variance (ANOVA) was used to examine the main effects (intervention and time) and their interaction on functional performance. Post-hoc analysis was used if a significance in the interaction was observed. The significance level was set as $p < 0.05$. Effect size values (η_p^2) were reported for ANOVA.

3. Results

Fourteen participants received 2 mA of stimulation and completed all study procedures. No side effects or risk events were reported. For blinding efficacy, Fisher's exact test showed a successful blinding procedure with an overall accuracy of 35.7% ($p = 0.347$).

The two-way repeated measures ANOVA revealed no significant intervention by time interaction effects for flexor strengths of the MPJ ($F_{(1, 26)} = 0.472$, $p = 0.50$, $\eta_p^2 = 0.018$), the first toe ($F_{(1, 26)} = 3.124$, $p = 0.09$, $\eta_p^2 = 0.107$), the other four toes ($F_{(1, 26)} = 0.001$, $p = 0.97$, $\eta_p^2 < 0.001$), and all five toes ($F_{(1, 26)} = 0.547$, $p = 0.47$, $\eta_p^2 = 0.021$). Further, no significant main effects of time and intervention were observed for any of these variables ($p > 0.05$). Specifically, the average percent change of the first-toe flexor strength following anodal HD-tDCS was 12.8 ± 24.2%, with 11 out of 14 participants showing an increase in strength, while the change following sham stimulation was 0.7 ± 17.3%, with 8 out of 14 participants showing an increase in strength.

No significant intervention by time interaction effects were observed for the passive kinesthesia thresholds of PF ($F_{(1, 26)} = 0.329$, $p = 0.57$, $\eta_p^2 = 0.012$), DF ($F_{(1, 26)} = 0.158$, $p = 0.69$, $\eta_p^2 = 0.006$), INV ($F_{(1, 26)} = 0.072$, $p = 0.79$, $\eta_p^2 = 0.003$), and EV ($F_{(1, 26)} = 0.237$, $p = 0.63$, $\eta_p^2 = 0.009$). A significant main effect of time was observed for the INV kinesthesia threshold ($F_{(1, 26)} = 9.606$, $p = 0.005$, $\eta_p^2 = 0.270$) and the DF kinesthesia threshold ($F_{(1, 26)} = 5.409$, $p = 0.03$, $\eta_p^2 = 0.172$), whereas no significance was observed in the main effects of the intervention. The INV and DF kinesthesia thresholds were significantly decreased after the stimulation as compared to pre-stimulation regardless of the two stimulation types ($p < 0.05$). Moreover, the INV kinesthesia threshold in 13 out of the 14 participants specifically decreased after anodal HD-tDCS, while this occurred in 8 out of the 14 participants after sham stimulation. The average percent decrease in the INV and DF kinesthesia thresholds following anodal HD-tDCS was 13.1 ± 17.6% (0.4 ± 0.4°) and 3.3 ± 17.1% (0.1 ± 0.3°), respectively, while the average percent change following sham stimulation was 9.4 ± 22.1% (0.3 ± 0.8°) and 7.4 ± 18.0% (0.2 ± 0.3°), respectively (Table 1).

Table 1. Effects of HD-tDCS on passive ankle kinesthesia and foot muscle strength.

Variables	HD-tDCS Pre	HD-tDCS Post	Sham Pre	Sham Post
PF (°)	1.29 ± 0.46	1.19 ± 0.45	1.38 ± 0.52	1.35 ± 0.39
DF (°)	1.48 ± 0.65	1.36 ± 0.42	1.44 ± 0.53	1.28 ± 0.32
INV (°)	2.73 ± 1.31	2.33 ± 1.15	2.77 ± 1.23	2.44 ± 1.22
EV (°)	2.43 ± 0.61	2.17 ± 0.95	2.37 ± 0.82	2.22 ± 0.79
MPJ flexor strength (N/kg)	1.56 ± 0.53	1.64 ± 0.38	1.43 ± 0.50	1.57 ± 0.49
Flexor strength of the first toe (N/kg)	1.45 ± 0.58	1.61 ± 0.67	1.46 ± 0.58	1.43 ± 0.49
Flexor strength of the other four toes (N/kg)	1.25 ± 0.41	1.30 ± 0.39	1.19 ± 0.41	1.24 ± 0.44
Flexor strength of the all five toes (N/kg)	2.84 ± 0.57	2.80 ± 0.63	2.62 ± 0.54	2.74 ± 0.56

Notes: PF: plantarflexion; DF: dorsiflexion; INV: inversion; EV: eversion; MPJ: metatarsophalangeal joint; HD-tDCS: high-definition transcranial direct current stimulation.

The two-way repeated measures ANOVA revealed no significant intervention by time interaction effects for the ML average CoG sway velocity in TL_EO ($F_{(1, 26)} = 0.250$, $p = 0.62$, $\eta_p^2 = 0.010$), AP average CoG sway velocity in TL_EO ($F_{(1, 26)} = 1.063$, $p = 0.312$, $\eta_p^2 = 0.039$), ML average CoG sway velocity in TL_EC ($F_{(1, 26)} = 1.056$, $p = 0.314$, $\eta_p^2 = 0.039$), AP average CoG sway velocity in TL_EC ($F_{(1, 26)} = 0.020$, $p = 0.89$, $\eta_p^2 = 0.001$), ML average CoG sway velocity in OL_EO ($F_{(1, 26)} = 0.615$, $p = 0.44$, $\eta_p^2 = 0.023$), AP average CoG sway velocity in OL_EO ($F_{(1, 26)} = 4.202$, $p = 0.051$, $\eta_p^2 = 0.139$), ML average CoG sway velocity in OL_EC ($F_{(1, 26)} = 0.029$, $p = 0.87$, $\eta_p^2 = 0.001$), and AP average CoG sway velocity in OL_EC ($F_{(1, 26)} = 1.755$, $p = 0.20$, $\eta_p^2 = 0.063$). A significant main effect of time was observed for the AP average CoG sway velocity in OL_EO ($F_{(1, 26)} = 5.473$, $p = 0.03$, $\eta_p^2 = 0.174$), ML average CoG sway velocity in OL_EC ($F_{(1, 26)} = 14.103$, $p = 0.001$, $\eta_p^2 = 0.352$), and AP average CoG sway velocity in OL_EC ($F_{(1, 26)} = 24.281$, $p < 0.001$, $\eta_p^2 = 0.483$), but no main effect of intervention. It was found that the AP average CoG sway velocity in OL_EO, ML average CoG sway velocity in OL_EC, and AP average CoG sway velocity in OL_EC were significantly decreased after the stimulation as compared to pre-stimulation regardless of the two stimulation types ($p < 0.05$). Specifically, the average percent decreases in the AP average CoG sway velocity in OL_EO, ML average CoG sway velocity in OL_EC, and AP average CoG sway velocity in OL_EC following anodal HD-tDCS were 0.8 ± 11.5%, 8.5 ± 11.4%, and 10.7 ± 9.5%, respectively, while the average percent changes following sham stimulation were 9.7 ± 15.2%, 11.0 ± 13.1%, and 17.0 ± 16.5%, respectively (Table 2).

Table 2. Effects of HD-tDCS on static balance.

Posture Conditions	Variables	HD-tDCS Pre	HD-tDCS Post	Sham Pre	Sham Post
TL_EO	ML average CoG sway velocity (mm/s)	6.53 ± 1.12	6.60 ± 1.03	6.40 ± 1.06	6.60 ± 1.09
	AP average CoG sway velocity (mm/s)	8.48 ± 1.45	8.41 ± 1.23	8.43 ± 1.40	8.72 ± 1.76
TL_EC	ML average CoG sway velocity (mm/s)	6.64 ± 0.82	7.03 ± 0.97	6.40 ± 1.17	6.46 ± 1.36
	AP average CoG sway velocity (mm/s)	9.40 ± 1.54	9.28 ± 1.43	9.19 ± 2.02	9.01 ± 1.75
OL_EO	ML average CoG sway velocity (mm/s)	31.63 ± 7.28	30.89 ± 7.80	33.42 ± 12.31	31.38 ± 10.52
	AP average CoG sway velocity (mm/s)	29.04 ± 4.65	28.75 ± 5.28	33.63 ± 11.35	29.34 ± 6.55
OL_EC	ML average CoG sway velocity (mm/s)	65.43 ± 15.80	59.56 ± 14.70	65.94 ± 17.23	59.52 ± 18.56
	AP average CoG sway velocity (mm/s)	67.73 ± 14.45	60.20 ± 13.39	71.79 ± 17.05	58.73 ± 13.64

Notes: TL_EO: two-leg standing with eyes open; TL_EC: two-leg standing with eyes closed; OL_EO: one-leg standing with eyes open; OL_EC: one-leg standing with eyes closed; ML: medial–lateral; AP: anteroposterior; HD-tDCS: high-definition transcranial direct current stimulation; CoG: the center of gravity.

4. Discussion

The tDCS procedure has been applied to the treatment and rehabilitation of multiple mental and neurological diseases [33]. However, its effectiveness has not been fully assessed in the field of human movement science, including in the rehabilitation and improvement of foot-related physical performance. In this pilot study, the direction of effects suggested that single-session HD-tDCS may improve the flexor strength of the first toe, although this increase in strength did not significantly differ from sham stimulation. Moreover, participants also showed improvements in the passive ankle kinesthesia threshold and static standing balance performance from pre to post stimulation, while no significant differences were observed between anodal HD-tDCS and sham stimulation. To our knowledge, this is the first study designed to examine the effects of HD-tDCS on foot-related physical performance, demonstrating that tDCS may be a promising method to improve the foot muscle strength and potentially sensation, and could provide novel insights into the potential role of brain cortical regions in the regulation of foot function.

For both athletes and those with diminished foot function, improving foot muscle strength, kinesthesia, and static balance is related to better sports performance and can help the prevention and rehabilitation of injuries and risk events in daily life [34]. Previous studies have provided preliminary evidence that anodal tDCS can improve muscle strength, foot sensory function, and static balance. Tanaka et al. [15] reported that tDCS significantly increased the toe pinch force by stimulating M1, with the observed effect remaining for at least 30 min. Zhou et al. [16] observed that anodal tDCS lowered foot sole vibratory thresholds of the elderly when standing. Studies have also demonstrated that tDCS can improve the postural stability of young adults when standing quietly with TL_EC [35] and enhance the adjustment ability to respond to complex postures [36], indicating that tDCS may be considered as a novel approach to improve foot-related function. However, several other studies showed the opposite results, reporting that tDCS may not significantly improve these functions. Maeda et al. [37], for example, observed that anodal tDCS failed to enhance the lower extremity muscle strength in healthy participants. Similarly, studies also showed that anodal tDCS did not significantly elevate the maximal force production of knee extensors [38] nor enhance static balance ability [39]. In this pilot study, we observed that a significant improvement in passive ankle kinesthesia and static standing balance performance from pre to post intervention was induced by HD-tDCS, which was in line with results from previous studies showing tDCS-induced benefits on physical performance. On the other hand, no statistically significant differences were observed in foot muscle strength, passive kinesthesia threshold, and static balance between the two stimulation types, consistent with the studies showing no significant improvement induced by tDCS.

Several reasons may account for the interesting findings in this study. One is related to potential ceiling effects. In this study, only healthy younger adults were enrolled, and they had excellent physical performance, including high-level muscle strength, great capacity to perceive the trivial changes in ankle motion, and thus great ability to maintain standing balance. Thus, it was possible that the benefit induced by HD-tDCS in physical performance was limited by a "ceiling effect" [16]. Besides, it should also be noted that in addition to sensory-motor regions, other brain regions are also involved in the regulation of the foot strength, sensation, and standing postural sway, such as the prefrontal cognitive regions, insular cortex, and the supplementary motor area. Targeting only one region in this healthy cohort may not be able to induce significant functional improvement.

Meanwhile, though HD-tDCS was used in this study, we know that the brain structure varies across individuals even in healthy younger cohorts, and such inter-subject variance in brain structure may increase the diffusion of the current in the targeted brain regions. Studies have shown that "on-target" current intensity was associated with an increase in functional performance [40]. Therefore, a "personalized" HD-tDCS montage design by using the brain structure MRI data of each individual in combination with advanced neuro-modelling techniques may boost the effects of tDCS interventions on these functional improvements.

Interestingly, although our study had a good blinding effect (35.7%), the INV and DF kinesthesia threshold and the AP and ML average CoG sway velocity in OL_EC were decreased from pre- to post-stimulation both the HD-tDCS and sham groups, and sham stimulation induced similar percent changes in these outcomes compared to HD-tDCS. In this conventional sham control protocol, it was believed only feelings on the scalp similar to those in anodal stimulation would be sensed, but not those of induced cortical activation [41]. However, it was unavoidable that the 30-second stimulation at the beginning of sham would potentially induce certain neurobiological effects on the targeting cortex and lead to improvements in functional performance [42]. A previous study, for example, revealed that event-related electroencephalogram components (P3) related to response time and accuracy were significantly lowered in sham stimulation, and changes in P3 amplitude were moderately correlated with changes in work memory accuracy. This suggested that sham stimulation may have biological effects and alter neuronal function [43]. This may partially explain the effects of sham stimulation we observed here. Novel active sham stimulation has been found to more effectively blind participants and operators to the stimulation condition without affecting functional outcomes [44]. Implementing this new approach in future studies would be worthwhile to help better examine the effects of HD-tDCS on functional performance pertaining to the foot.

To date, the mechanisms by which tDCS might improve physical performance remain largely unclear and the effects of tDCS on physical performance have been found to be inconsistent. The high inter-individual variability, the different electrode montages, and various stimulation protocols (i.e., stimulation types, electrode size and position, intensity, duration) may be contributors to the variable results [13]. Thus, this pilot study may provide some implications for selecting optimal stimulation parameters for future study. Besides, several studies have reported that tDCS applied over the M1 had a positive effect on motor imagery [36], providing some implications in order to explore the beneficial effects of imagery conditions on physical performance during tDCS in future studies [45,46].

There are some limitations in this study. In this pilot study, only a small sample of male participants was enrolled; future studies with a larger sample size of participants with similar numbers of men and women are thus needed. This study focused on only a healthy cohort, and the exploration of the effects of tDCS on the foot function and balance in those with diminished or impaired functionality, such as those with foot injuries, would be worthwhile. It is also necessary to examine the effects of both anodal and cathodal tDCS on cortical activation of the brain and functional performance. This may help to better understand the causal role of brain activity in the regulation of behavior.

5. Conclusions

This pilot study was the first to examine the effects of single-session anodal HD-tDCS designed to target the sensory-motor regions of the brain with respect to foot muscle strength, passive ankle kinesthesia, and static balance. The results suggested that single-session HD-tDCS may improve the flexor strength of the first toe, passive ankle kinesthesia, and static standing balance performance, although no significant differences were observed with regard to such effects between anodal HD-tDCS and sham stimulation. This may be potentially due to ceiling effects and the small sample size in this study. Nevertheless, these preliminary findings may inform future studies with larger sample sizes aimed at confirming and expanding the findings of this pilot study by providing knowledge on optimal stimulation parameters, effect size, and power estimation of the tDCS intervention.

Author Contributions: Conceptualization, W.F.; methodology, J.Z. and S.X.; formal analysis, S.X., B.W., and X.Z.; investigation, S.X., B.W., X.Z., J.Z., and W.F.; resources, W.F.; data curation, S.X.; writing—original draft preparation, S.X.; writing—review and editing, J.Z. and W.F.; project administration, W.F.; funding acquisition, W.F. All authors have read and agreed to the published version of the manuscript.

Funding: This research was funded by the National Natural Science Foundation of China (11772201, 11932013), the National Key Technology Research and Development Program of the Ministry of Science and Technology of China (2019YFF0302100), the "Dawn" Program of Shanghai Education Commission (19SG47), and the Talent Development Fund of Shanghai Municipal (2018107).

Conflicts of Interest: The authors declare no conflict of interest. The funders had no role in the design of the study; in the collection, analyses, or interpretation of data; in the writing of the manuscript, or in the decision to publish the results.

References

1. McKeon, P.O.; Hertel, J.; Bramble, D.; Davis, I. The foot core system: A new paradigm for understanding intrinsic foot muscle function. *Br. J. Sports Med.* **2015**, *49*, 290. [CrossRef]
2. McKeon, P.O.; Fourchet, F. Freeing the foot: Integrating the foot core system into rehabilitation for lower extremity injuries. *Clin. Sports Med.* **2015**, *34*, 347–361. [CrossRef] [PubMed]
3. Lephart, S.M.; Pincivero, D.M.; Giraldo, J.L.; Fu, F.H. The role of proprioception in the management and rehabilitation of athletic injuries. *Am. J. Sports Med.* **1997**, *25*, 130–137. [CrossRef] [PubMed]
4. Li, Y.; Ko, J.; Zhang, S.; Brown, C.N.; Simpson, K.J. Biomechanics of ankle giving way: A case report of accidental ankle giving way during the drop landing test. *J. Sport Health Sci.* **2019**, *8*, 494–502. [CrossRef] [PubMed]
5. Lowrey, C.R.; Strzalkowski, N.D.J.; Bent, L.R. Skin sensory information from the dorsum of the foot and ankle is necessary for kinesthesia at the ankle joint. *Neurosci. Lett.* **2010**, *485*, 6–10. [CrossRef] [PubMed]
6. Cheung, R.T.H.; Sze, L.K.Y.; Mok, N.W.; Ng, G.Y.F. Intrinsic foot muscle volume in experienced runners with and without chronic plantar fasciitis. *J. Sci. Med. Sport.* **2016**, *19*, 713–715. [CrossRef]
7. Lee, E.; Cho, J.; Lee, S. Short-foot exercise promotes quantitative somatosensory function in ankle instability: A randomized controlled trial. *Med. Sci. Monit.* **2019**, *25*, 618–626. [CrossRef]

8. Needle, A.R.; Lepley, A.S.; Grooms, D.R. Central nervous system adaptation after ligamentous injury: A summary of theories, evidence, and clinical interpretation. *Sports Med.* **2017**, *47*, 1271–1288. [CrossRef]
9. Nitsche, M.A.; Paulus, W. Excitability changes induced in the human motor cortex by weak transcranial direct current stimulation. *J. Physiol.* **2000**, *527*, 633–639. [CrossRef]
10. De Moura, M.C.D.S.; Hazime, F.A.; Marotti Aparicio, L.V.; Grecco, L.A.C.; Brunoni, A.R.; Hasue, R.H. Effects of transcranial direct current stimulation (tDCS) on balance improvement: A systematic review and meta-analysis. *Somatosens. Mot. Res.* **2019**, *36*, 122–135. [CrossRef]
11. Lattari, E.; Oliveira, B.R.R.; Monteiro Júnior, R.S.; Marques Neto, S.R.; Oliveira, A.J.; Maranhão Neto, G.A.; Machado, S.; Budde, H. Acute effects of single dose transcranial direct current stimulation on muscle strength: A systematic review and meta-analysis. *PLoS ONE* **2018**, *13*, e0209513. [CrossRef] [PubMed]
12. Machado, D.; Unal, G.; Andrade, S.M.; Moreira, A.; Altimari, L.R.; Brunoni, A.R.; Perrey, S.; Mauger, A.R.; Bikson, M.; Okano, A.H. Effect of transcranial direct current stimulation on exercise performance: A systematic review and meta-analysis. *Brain Stimul.* **2019**, *12*, 593–605. [CrossRef] [PubMed]
13. Angius, L.; Pascual-Leone, A.; Santarnecchi, E. Brain stimulation and physical performance. *Prog. Brain Res.* **2018**, *240*, 317–339. [PubMed]
14. Vargas, V.Z.; Baptista, A.F.; Pereira, G.; Pochini, A.C.; Ejnisman, B.; Santos, M.B.; João, S.; Hazime, F.A. Modulation of isometric quadriceps strength in soccer players with transcranial direct current stimulation: A crossover study. *J. Strength Cond. Res.* **2018**, *32*, 1336–1341. [CrossRef]
15. Tanaka, S.; Hanakawa, T.; Honda, M.; Watanabe, K. Enhancement of pinch force in the lower leg by anodal transcranial direct current stimulation. *Exp. Brain Res.* **2009**, *196*, 459–465. [CrossRef]
16. Zhou, J.; Lo, O.-Y.; Lipsitz, L.A.; Zhang, J.; Fang, J.; Manor, B. Transcranial direct current stimulation enhances foot sole somatosensation when standing in older adults. *Exp. Brain Res.* **2018**, *236*, 795–802. [CrossRef]
17. Datta, A.; Bansal, V.; Diaz, J.; Patel, J.; Reato, D.; Bikson, M. Gyri-precise head model of transcranial direct current stimulation: Improved spatial focality using a ring electrode versus conventional rectangular pad. *Brain Stimul.* **2009**, *2*, 201–207. [CrossRef]
18. Reckow, J.; Rahman-Filipiak, A.; Garcia, S.; Schlaefflin, S.; Calhoun, O.; DaSilva, A.F.; Bikson, M.; Hampstead, B.M. Tolerability and blinding of 4x1 high-definition transcranial direct current stimulation (HD-tDCS) at two and three milliamps. *Brain Stimul.* **2018**, *11*, 991–997. [CrossRef]
19. Fu, W.; Fang, Y.; Gu, Y.; Huang, L.; Li, L.; Liu, Y. Shoe cushioning reduces impact and muscle activation during landings from unexpected, but not self-initiated, drops. *J. Sci. Med. Sport* **2017**, *20*, 915–920. [CrossRef]
20. Yamamoto, S.; Ishii, D.; Ichiba, N.; Yozu, A.; Kohno, Y. Cathodal tDCS on the motor area decreases the tactile threshold of the distal pulp of the hallux. *Neurosci. Lett.* **2020**, *719*, 133887. [CrossRef]
21. Faul, F.; Erdfelder, E.; Buchner, A.; Lang, A.G. Statistical power analyses using G*Power 3.1: Tests for correlation and regression analyses. *Behav. Res. Methods* **2009**, *41*, 1149–1160. [CrossRef] [PubMed]
22. Faul, F.; Erdfelder, E.; Lang, A.G.; Buchner, A. G*Power 3: A flexible statistical power analysis program for the social, behavioral, and biomedical sciences. *Behav. Res. Methods* **2007**, *39*, 175–191. [CrossRef] [PubMed]
23. DaSilva, A.F.; Truong, D.Q.; DosSantos, M.F.; Toback, R.L.; Datta, A.; Bikson, M. State-of-art neuroanatomical target analysis of high-definition and conventional tDCS montages used for migraine and pain control. *Front. Neuroanat.* **2015**, *9*, 89. [CrossRef] [PubMed]
24. Borckardt, J.J.; Bikson, M.; Frohman, H.; Reeves, S.T.; Datta, A.; Bansal, V.; Madan, A.; Barth, K.; George, M.S. A pilot study of the tolerability and effects of high-definition transcranial direct current stimulation (HD-tDCS) on pain perception. *J. Pain* **2012**, *13*, 112–120. [CrossRef]
25. Villamar, M.F.; Volz, M.S.; Bikson, M.; Datta, A.; Dasilva, A.F.; Fregni, F. Technique and considerations in the use of 4x1 ring high-definition transcranial direct current stimulation (HD-tDCS). *J. Vis. Exp.* **2013**, *77*, e50309. [CrossRef]
26. Cole, L.; Giuffre, A.; Ciechanski, P.; Carlson, H.L.; Zewdie, E.; Kuo, H.-C.; Kirton, A. Effects of high-definition and conventional transcranial direct-current stimulation on motor learning in children. *Front. Neurosci.* **2018**, *12*, 787. [CrossRef]
27. Gandiga, P.C.; Hummel, F.C.; Cohen, L.G. Transcranial DC stimulation (tDCS): A tool for double-blind sham-controlled clinical studies in brain stimulation. *Clin. Neurophysiol.* **2006**, *117*, 845–850. [CrossRef]
28. Sun, W.; Song, Q.; Yu, B.; Zhang, C.; Mao, D. Test-retest reliability of a new device for assessing ankle joint threshold to detect passive movement in healthy adults. *J. Sports Sci.* **2015**, *33*, 1667–1674. [CrossRef]

29. Xiao, S.; Zhang, X.; Deng, L.; Zhang, S.; Cui, K.; Fu, W. Relationships between foot morphology and foot muscle strength in healthy adults. *Int. J. Environ. Res. Public Health* **2020**, *17*, 1274. [CrossRef]
30. Zhang, S.; Fu, W.; Liu, Y. Does habitual rear-foot strike pattern with modern running shoes affect the muscle strength of the longitudinal arch? *Isoki. Exer. Sci.* **2019**, *27*, 213–218. [CrossRef]
31. Kurihara, T.; Yamauchi, J.; Otsuka, M.; Tottori, N.; Hashimoto, T.; Isaka, T. Maximum toe flexor muscle strength and quantitative analysis of human plantar intrinsic and extrinsic muscles by a magnetic resonance imaging technique. *J. Foot Ankle Res.* **2014**, *7*, 26. [CrossRef] [PubMed]
32. Yamauchi, J.; Koyama, K. Influence of ankle braces on the maximum strength of plantar and toe flexor muscles. *Int. J. Sports Med.* **2015**, *36*, 592–595. [CrossRef] [PubMed]
33. Lefaucheur, J.P.; Antal, A.; Ayache, S.S.; Benninger, D.H.; Brunelin, J.; Cogiamanian, F.; Cotelli, M.; De Ridder, D.; Ferrucci, R.; Langguth, B.; et al. Evidence-based guidelines on the therapeutic use of transcranial direct current stimulation (tDCS). *Clin. Neurophysiol.* **2017**, *128*, 56–92. [CrossRef]
34. Luan, X.; Tian, X.; Zhang, H.; Huang, R.; Li, N.; Chen, P.; Wang, R. Exercise as a prescription for patients with various diseases. *J. Sport Health Sci.* **2019**, *8*, 422–441. [CrossRef] [PubMed]
35. Dutta, A.; Chugh, S. Effect of transcranial direct current stimulation on cortico-muscular coherence and standing postural steadiness. In *Proceedings of the 2nd IASTED International Conference on Assistive Technologies*; ACTA Press: Innsbruck, Austria, 2012.
36. Saruco, E.; Di Rienzo, F.; Nunez-Nagy, S.; Rubio-Gonzalez, M.A.; Jackson, P.L.; Collet, C.; Saimpont, A.; Guillot, A. Anodal tDCS over the primary motor cortex improves motor imagery benefits on postural control: A pilot study. *Sci. Rep.* **2017**, *7*, 480. [CrossRef] [PubMed]
37. Maeda, K.; Yamaguchi, T.; Tatemoto, T.; Kondo, K.; Otaka, Y.; Tanaka, S. Transcranial Direct Current Stimulation Does Not Affect Lower Extremity Muscle Strength Training in Healthy Individuals: A Triple-Blind, Sham-Controlled Study. *Front. Neurosci.* **2017**, *11*, 179. [CrossRef]
38. Flood, A.; Waddington, G.; Keegan, R.J.; Thompson, K.G.; Cathcart, S. The effects of elevated pain inhibition on endurance exercise performance. *PeerJ* **2017**, *5*, e3028. [CrossRef]
39. Grimaldi, G.; Manto, M. Anodal transcranial direct current stimulation (tDCS) decreases the amplitudes of long-latency stretch reflexes in cerebellar ataxia. *Ann. Biomed. Eng.* **2013**, *41*, 2437–2447. [CrossRef]
40. Kim, J.H.; Kim, D.W.; Chang, W.H.; Kim, Y.H.; Kim, K.; Im, C.H. Inconsistent outcomes of transcranial direct current stimulation may originate from anatomical differences among individuals: Electric field simulation using individual MRI data. *Neurosci. Lett.* **2014**, *564*, 6–10. [CrossRef]
41. Fertonani, A.; Ferrari, C.; Miniussi, C. What do you feel if I apply transcranial electric stimulation? Safety, sensations and secondary induced effects. *Clin. Neurophysiol.* **2015**, *126*, 2181–2188. [CrossRef]
42. Fonteneau, C.; Mondino, M.; Arns, M.; Baeken, C.; Bikson, M.; Brunoni, A.R.; Burke, M.J.; Neuvonen, T.; Padberg, F.; Pascual-Leone, A.; et al. Sham tDCS: A hidden source of variability? Reflections for further blinded, controlled trials. *Brain Stimul.* **2019**, *12*, 668–673. [CrossRef] [PubMed]
43. Nikolin, S.; Martin, D.; Loo, C.K.; Boonstra, T.W. Effects of TDCS dosage on working memory in healthy participants. *Brain Stimul.* **2018**, *11*, 518–527. [CrossRef] [PubMed]
44. Dagan, M.; Herman, T.; Harrison, R.; Zhou, J.; Giladi, N.; Ruffini, G.; Manor, B.; Hausdorff, J.M. Multitarget transcranial direct current stimulation for freezing of gait in Parkinson's disease. *Mov. Disord.* **2018**, *33*, 642–646. [CrossRef] [PubMed]
45. O'Shea, H.; Moran, A. Does motor simulation theory explain the cognitive mechanisms underlying motor imagery? A critical review. *Front. Hum. Neurosci.* **2017**, *11*, 72. [CrossRef] [PubMed]
46. Palmiero, M.; Piccardi, L.; Giancola, M.; Nori, R.; D'Amico, S.; Olivetti Belardinelli, M. The format of mental imagery: From a critical review to an integrated embodied representation approach. *Cogn. Process.* **2019**, *20*, 277–289. [CrossRef] [PubMed]

© 2020 by the authors. Licensee MDPI, Basel, Switzerland. This article is an open access article distributed under the terms and conditions of the Creative Commons Attribution (CC BY) license (http://creativecommons.org/licenses/by/4.0/).

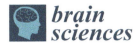

Article

Effects of Multiple Sessions of Cathodal Priming and Anodal HD-tDCS on Visuo Motor Task Plateau Learning and Retention

Pierre Besson [1,†], Makii Muthalib [1,2,†], Christophe De Vassoigne [1], Jonh Rothwell [3] and Stephane Perrey [1,*]

[1] EuroMov Digital Health in Motion, Univ Montpellier, IMT Mines Ales, 34090 Montpellier, France; pierre.besson@umontpellier.fr (P.B.); makii.muthalib@gmail.com (M.M.); ch.de.vassoigne@gmail.com (C.D.V.)
[2] SilverLine Research, 4127 Brisbane, Australia
[3] Institute of Neurology, University College London, London WC1N 3BG, UK; j.rothwell@ucl.ac.uk
* Correspondence: stephane.perrey@umontpellier.fr; Tel.: +33-(0)434-432-623
† Both authors contributed equally to this work.

Received: 30 September 2020; Accepted: 18 November 2020; Published: 19 November 2020

Abstract: A single session of priming cathodal transcranial direct current stimulation (tDCS) prior to anodal tDCS (c-a-tDCS) allows cumulative effects on motor learning and retention. However, the impact of multiple sessions of c-a-tDCS priming on learning and retention remains unclear. Here, we tested whether multiple sessions of c-a-tDCS (over 3 consecutive days) applied over the left sensorimotor cortex can further enhance motor learning and retention of an already learned visuo-motor task as compared to anodal tDCS (a-tDCS) or sham. In a between group and randomized double-blind sham-controlled study design, 25 participants separated in 3 independent groups underwent 2 days of baseline training without tDCS followed by 3-days of training with both online and offline tDCS, and two retention tests (1 and 14 days later). Each training block consisted of five trials of a 60 s circular-tracing task intersected by 60 s rest, and performance was assessed in terms of speed–accuracy trade-off represented notably by an index of performance (IP). The main findings of this exploratory study were that multiple sessions of c-a-tDCS significantly further enhanced IP above baseline training levels over the 3 training days that were maintained over the 2 retention days, but these learning and retention performance changes were not significantly different from the sham group. Subtle differences in the changes in speed–accuracy trade-off (components of IP) between c-a-tDCS (maintenance of accuracy over increasing speed) and a-tDCS (increasing speed over maintenance of accuracy) provide preliminary insights to a mechanistic modulation of motor performance with priming and polarity of tDCS.

Keywords: transcranial direct current stimulation (tDCS); motor performance; priming tDCS; cathodal; multiple sessions; motor learning; neuroplasticity

1. Introduction

Transcranial direct current stimulation (tDCS) is a noninvasive neuromodulation technique that can increase or decrease cortical excitability depending on the polarity of the induced electric field [1]. Anodal tDCS (a-tDCS) of the primary motor cortex (M1) has generally been shown to enhance motor performance and learning, but this depends on the specific motor task utilized [2], as well as tDCS parameters (electrode position [3]; current intensity/density [4]) and the timing of application [5,6]. However, even with strict control of these considerations, intra- and inter-individual variability of responses to tDCS have been reported in several studies [7,8]. Although anatomical differences between subjects will always be a major factor influencing tDCS responses, one way to enhance tDCS responses is to design new tDCS protocols where personalization of stimulation parameters is the ultimate goal [9]. Regarding the tDCS setup, high-definition (HD)-tDCS montage can be one solution to improve optimization of the technique due to the expected focality of the induced-current [10,11] and the persistence of the after-effects on cortical excitability [12,13].

For either motor or cognitive tasks, concurrent (online) application of a-tDCS and task training is a potential way to enhance the performance and learning [14,15]. Motor learning [16] is typically defined as practice- or experience-induced acquisition of either fine motor skills from increased accuracy and reduced performance variability (speed–accuracy trade-off phenomenon) or gross skilled motor performance permitting functions as jumping, walking, maintaining a body balance, etc. Most studies (e.g., [4,5]) have tested the efficacy of tDCS coupled with learning of fine motor skills. The greater facilitative effect of concurrent a-tDCS on motor performance/learning is thought to be due to enhanced synaptic efficacy in the simultaneously engaged neural network through a "gating" mechanism [17]. The seminal work of Antal et al. [18] has shown that the excitability enhancement of M1 induced by a-tDCS improved performance in the early phase of learning in a visuo-motor coordination task compared to sham. Offline a-tDCS (i.e., tDCS before the task) has been suggested to limit motor performance/learning compared to online a-tDCS due to homeostatic metaplastic mechanisms based on the Bienenstock–Cooper–Munro theory claiming a "sliding threshold" for bidirectional synaptic plasticity [17]. Accordingly, a-tDCS, which increases the likelihood of long-term potentiation (LTP)-like plasticity, would increase the modification threshold for LTP during the subsequent motor task and thus adversely affect motor performance/learning [14]. Simultaneous application of tDCS and training appears a requirement to promote offline gains in favour of retention process [5]. Our recent functional near infrared spectroscopy neuroimaging study [6] observed that although online a-HD-tDCS showed reduced sensorimotor cortex activation to offline a-HD-tDCS relative to when the motor task is performed. However, after a 30 min delay in motor task performance, sensorimotor cortex activation was similarly increased for both online and offline compared to sham. Altogether, in healthy adults, a meta-analysis [19] concluded that multiple sessions of a-tDCS are more efficacious than a single session for enhancing both motor learning and retention, due to combined incremental online and offline skill gains.

The sequence and timing of the tDCS polarity are two factors that can also be manipulated to enhance motor performance and learning with regard to the homeostatic metaplasticity phenomenon [20]. Sub-threshold neuronal membrane depolarization induced by a-tDCS has an intensity- and time-dependent effect to strengthen synaptic efficacy [21]. Reducing corticospinal excitability with priming cathodal tDCS (c-tDCS) before a-tDCS (c-a-tDCS) and motor task training can influence homeostatic metaplastic mechanisms as well [22,23]. Applying priming c-tDCS followed 10-min later by concurrent a-tDCS and motor task training appears promising to induce significantly greater enhancement in acquisition [23] and retention of motor skills two weeks later [22] as compared to sham and training with concurrent a-tDCS. However, to the best of our knowledge, no study has compared multiple sessions of c-tDCS priming and a-tDCS (c-a-tDCS) to further enhance plateau learning and retention of an already learned motor skill. Herein we aimed to investigate the beneficial effect of a new tDCS protocol exploiting c-tDCS priming on online gains, offline gains and long-term retention after multiple days of motor practice. For that purpose, 3–5 training days are regularly used [2,5,24,25]. We adopted a 3-day training phase as carried out in the studies of Saucedo Marquez et al. [2] regarding fine motor skills, or Kumari et al. [24] regarding gross motor skills.

Therefore, the aim of this exploratory study was to determine if multiple sessions (over 3 consecutive days) of c-a-tDCS can further enhance motor learning and retention of an already learned visuo-motor task. Based on the aforementioned studies, we hypothesized that c-a-tDCS would induce a greater improvement in learning and retention compared to a-tDCS or sham.

2. Materials and Methods

2.1. Participants

Twenty-five healthy adults (9 females, 19–45 years old, mean age ± SD: 31.0 ± 9.9) volunteered to participate in the study. All participants gave written informed consent prior to participation in the study according to the Declaration of Helsinki. All procedures were approved by the local Ethics Committee (IRB-EM 17-01B, EuroMov-Montpellier). The laterality index for right handers (n = 21 with a-tDCS = 6, c-a-tDCS = 8 and sham = 7) and left handers (n = 4 with a-tDCS = 3 and c-a-tDCS = 1) assessed with the Edinburg handedness inventory [26] was 75 ± 23 and −70 ± 33, respectively. All participants had no history of neurology or physical disorders or any upper extremity muscle or joint injuries. The respect of safety recommendations (e.g., current duration, current density, charge density) associated with the use of tDCS was strictly followed [27].

2.2. Study Design and Protocol

This study is a part of Dr. Pierre Besson's PhD thesis. In a double-blind sham-controlled study [28], the 25 participants were randomly distributed into 3 groups: anodal anodal-task (a-tDCS, n = 9, 3 females, age 31.0 ± 8.9); cathodal priming/anodal-task (c-a-tDCS, n = 9, 4 females, age 31.7 ± 12.0); sham (n = 7, 3 females, age 30.1 ± 8.9). For sham, 3 participants underwent a-tDCS and 4 underwent c-a-tDCS. All participants were required to undertake 6 testing days (5 successive days and one day 2 weeks later). For the baseline (day 0) and the 2 retention testing days (day 4 and day 18), no tDCS was applied and only the tracing-motor task consisting of 1 block (B) of 5 trials (1 min task interspersed by 1-min rest, total 10 min duration) was performed. Days 1, 2 and 3 were training days and included either sham or real tDCS. Figure 1 presents the schematic of the experimental design for a training day. Each training day was comprised of 3 blocks of 5 trials: pre-tDCS block, tDCS-block and post-tDCS block. In the pre-tDCS block, no tDCS was applied to all groups during the tracing-motor task. In the tDCS-block, the specific tDCS parameters were set and concurrent tDCS and tracing-motor task training were undertaken; a-tDCS priming (10 min) was next to online a-tDCS task (10 min) while c-tDCS priming (10 min) was interspersed by 10 min of rest before the online a-tDCS task (10 min) (Figure 1). In the post-tDCS block, the tracing-motor task was performed again with no tDCS after 20 min rest to assess within-day offline effects. Subjects were informed to perform the tracing-motor task as fast as possible while maintaining accuracy.

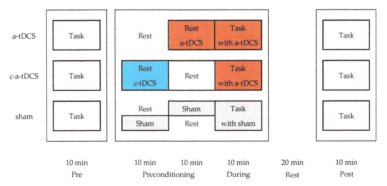

Figure 1. Schematic representation of a training day (3 blocks) for the 3 groups. The subject performed the visuo-motor task (5 trials) at three epochs interspersed by 20 min of preconditioning or delay. Pre and post times are without use of transcranial direct current stimulation (tDCS) while during depends on the specific tDCS conditions of the 3 groups exploiting different polarities (anodal: red; cathodal: blue; sham: grey) in the preconditioning phase.

All participants and one experimenter (C.D.V.) performing the tDCS applications/assessment were blind to the tDCS settings. Although tDCS is well tolerated by participants [29], a questionnaire containing rating scales of 11 unpleasant sensations compared to resting state (i.e., sitting quietly without tDCS electrodes over the head) was filled out after each stimulation sequence. This questionnaire was based on the tDCS safety guidelines proposed by Poreisz et al. [30].

2.3. Transcranial Direct Current Stimulation

A Startstim 8 tDCS system (Neuroelectrics®, Barcelona, Spain) was used to deliver constant direct currents to the left (right handers, $n = 21$) or right (left handers, $n = 4$) M1 via a 4 × 1 ring montage with HD electrodes (3.14 cm^2) applied on the skull with electrode paste (Ten20®, Weaver and Company, Aurora, CO, USA). With regard to the handedness of the participant, the active electrode was placed on the scalp overlying the dominant M1 (C3 or C4) based on the 10–20 EEG system. The 4 return electrodes surrounded the anode or cathode electrode at a centre-to-centre distance of 3.5 cm. For the anode on C3, return electrodes were placed on FC1, FC5, CP1 and CP5. For the anode on C4, return electrodes were placed on FC2, FC6, CP2 and CP4. To ensure consistency of electrodes placement throughout the multiple training sessions, the same experimenter (C.D.V.) always marked on the scalp the site of the electrodes.

In a-tDCS conditions, constant current was delivered for either 10 min or 20 min at 2 mA with a ramp up and down phases of 30 s duration. In sham, active stimulation was applied with 30 s ramp up to 2 mA, 30 s at 2 mA and 30 s ramp down (1.5 min active stimulation, [28]). For the c-a-tDCS group, c-tDCS was applied for 10 min with 30 s ramp up/down, then after a 10 min rest, a-tDCS was applied for 10 min with 30 s ramp up/down. In all testing sessions, the impedance of all electrodes was monitored at the beginning and during each period of stimulation to maintain values under 5 kΩ.

2.4. Visuo-Motor Task

The visuo-motor task was a computerized version of the circular tunnel task shown to be highly reliable over testing days [31]. Subjects were required to do circular traces as quickly as possible using a hand stylus within the boundaries of a circle of an 80 cm length and targeting the centre of 0.8 cm width (accuracy purpose) from 12.3 to 13.1 cm (see Figure 2). The index of difficulty (ID) defined by the length of circle (A) divided by the channel's width (W) was set to 100 (i.e., 80/0.8) [32]. The line tracing was recorded with a computerized tablet Wacom Intuos (gd1218U, Saitama, Japan) at the sampling frequency of 100 Hz. For data acquisition, a homemade script was created using MATLAB® (version R2012b—MathWorks, Natick, MA, USA).

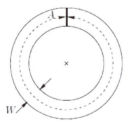

Figure 2. Representation of the circular-tracing task. A is the perimeter (dotted line) of the circle's centre (x) and W stands for the path width (continuous lines). From Accot and Zhai [31].

2.5. Data Analysis

We defined an index of performance (IP, arbitrary unit) for the task based on previous related studies [32,33] as follows:

$$IP = TED60/WVT60 \qquad (1)$$

where TED60 represents the total Euclidean distance achieved during the 60-s task and WVT60 represents the width of the virtual circular tunnel, including all the trajectories of the subject during the 60-s task.

To calculate IP, we developed a Matlab script taking in input raw data from the Wacom Intuos tablet. The first step in pre-processing raw data was calibration. For that step, we used a controlled data set and transformed the pixel indexes (X and Y positions) into Euclidean distance (in mm) from the centre of the circular tunnel. The second step consisted in re-sampling the data to obtain a fixed sampling period at 100 Hz; the interp1 function of Matlab with the "pchip" method of interpolation was used. IP was computed from the pre-treated data where TED60 was calculated by summing the Euclidean distances between 2 consecutive points for all points acquired during the motor task. WVT60 was calculated as the difference between the distance from the farthest point to the centre and the distance from the nearest point to the centre for all points. With respect to the purpose of the study, IP values and its determinants (speed and accuracy) were assessed by block of 5 trials. The speed was calculated with respect to the number of revolutions made during the 60 s. The error (accuracy) was assessed by the ratio of the number of samples outside the tunnel to the total number of samples recorded during the task.

2.6. Statistical Analysis

Values are presented as means and standard deviations except if specified. The Shapiro–Wilk test was used to examine the normal distribution of the outcomes while the sphericity assumption was tested with Mauchly's test. All data (IP, error and speed values) were subjected to repeated-measures analysis of variance (ANOVA$_{RM}$) with time (10 blocks normalized by the subtraction of B2 result as baseline, see below) as within-subject factor and polarity (3 groups: a-tDCS, c-a-tDCS and sham) as between-subject factor. A two-way ANOVA$_{RM}$ was also conducted for the subjective scalp sensation related to tDCS conditions. Where appropriate, post-hoc tests using the Bonferroni correction were applied. All statistical analyses were performed using JASP software (version 0.12.1.0, JASP, 2020, Amsterdam, The Netherlands). The level of significance was set to 0.05 for all tests. Effect size (ηp^2) values were reported for ANOVA, and effect sizes were reported with the magnitude of Hedges' g for the simple comparisons (post hoc tests) among groups for a given time (B9, B11, B12). Hedges' g is a variation of Cohen's d that corrects for biases due to small sample sizes [34] and the magnitude of Hedges' g may be interpreted using Cohen's convention as small (0.2), medium (0.5) and large (0.8).

3. Results

3.1. Subjective Scalp Sensation

All 25 participants conducted the study to the end. ANOVA$_{RM}$ indicated that no differences ($F(2,22) = 0.0199$, $p = 0.980$) were observed among the training days for the cutaneous sensation over the scalp during tDCS, indicating none of the participants were able to differentiate real tDCS from sham sessions. None of our participants reported any other tDCS application related side effects.

3.2. Changes in Motor Performance and Motor Learning Parameters

3.2.1. Baseline Training Blocks without tDCS

Over the 2 baseline training blocks without tDCS (Day 1, B1 and Day 2, B2), there were no significant differences between groups for accuracy and IP; however, speed for a-tDCS was significantly greater than c-a-tDCS ($p = 0.025$). Speed and IP increased significantly over the baseline training blocks for c-a-tDCS ($p = 0.019$ and $p = 0.029$, respectively) and a-tDCS ($p = 0.007$ and $p = 0.002$, respectively), but not for sham. Accuracy for a-tDCS decreased significantly from B1 to B2 ($p < 0.05$); while c-a-tDCS showed a tendency ($p = 0.051$) for reduced accuracy, and sham showed no changes between blocks.

Since the three groups responded differently to the baseline training, subsequent training blocks with tDCS were normalized to baseline Block 2.

3.2.2. Training Blocks with tDCS

Figure 3 shows the evolution of normalized IP values over time (Day 1, B3 to Day 3, B10, and retention Day 4, B11 and Day 18, B12) for the 3 groups. ANOVA$_{RM}$ for the IP indicated there were significant main effects of time (F(9198) = 5.380, $p < 0.001$, ηp^2 = 0.196), polarity (F(2,22) = 4.730, p = 0.020, ηp^2 = 0.148) and a significant time × polarity interaction (F(18,198) = 1.910, p = 0.017, ηp^2 = 0.302). However post-hoc analysis failed to show any between group differences. Post hoc analysis performed on the time main effect revealed only higher IP values for c-a-tDCS at B12, B11 and B10 when compared to B3 and B4. P-level and effect size values are for B3 vs. B10 (p = 0.011, g = 1.92), B3 vs. B11 ($p < 0.001$, g = 3.21), B3 vs. B12 (p = 0.012, g = 2.87), and for B4 vs. B10 (p = 0.006, g = 2.00), B4 vs. B11 ($p < 0.001$, g = 3.39), B4 vs. B12 (p = 0.007, g = 3.04).

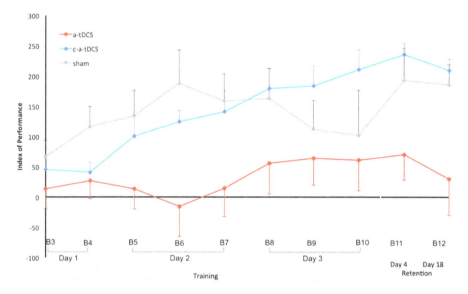

Figure 3. Evolution of the mean (and one SEM) index of performance over time (blocks—B) for each of the 3 groups. B3, B6 and B9 represent online tDCS. B4, B7 and B10 represent immediate offline. B5 and B8 represent delayed offline.

As can be seen in Figure 3, the magnitude of the difference from the start (B3) to the end of 3-days training (B10) with tDCS indicates a meaningful large increase in IP after c-a-tDCS (g = 1.92), while large increases were noted for sham (g = 0.23) and a-tDCS priming conditions (g = 0.36). In addition, the magnitude of the difference from the start (B3) to one day after the end of 3-days training (B11) indicates a meaningful large increase in IP for c-a-tDCS priming (g = 3.21), while medium increases were noted for sham (g = 1.06) and a-tDCS conditions (g = 0.49). Finally, the magnitude of the difference from the start (B3) to two weeks after the end of 3-days (B12) training indicates a meaningful large increase in IP for c-a-tDCS (g = 2.87), while medium increases was noted for sham (g = 1.39) and a-tDCS conditions (g = 0.11).

Figure 4 shows the evolution of normalized error values over time for the 3 groups. ANOVA$_{RM}$ for the error indicated a significant main effect of time (F(9198) = 11.227, $p < 0.001$, ηp^2 = 0.388), but no significant main effect of polarity (F(2,22) = 1.268, p = 0.301) or time × polarity interaction effect (F(18,198) = 1.022, p = 0.436). Post hoc analysis performed on the time main effect revealed only higher

Error values for a-tDCS at B11 and B10 when compared to B3 and B11 when compared to B5 and for sham at B3 when compared to B12, B11, B10 and B9. P-level and effect size values are for a-tDCS B3 vs. B10 ($p = 0.012$, g = 1.33), B3 vs. B11 ($p = 0.002$, g = 1.30) and for B5 vs. B11 ($p = 0.019$, g = 1.06). P-level and effect size values are for sham B3 vs. B9 ($p = 0.024$, g = 1.05), B3 vs. B10 ($p = 0.008$, g = 1.12), B3 vs. B11 ($p = 0.028$, g = 1,03) and for B3 vs. B12 ($p = 0.008$, g = 1.09).

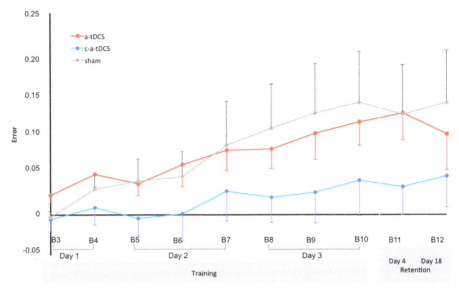

Figure 4. Evolution of mean (and one SEM) error over time (blocks—B) for each of the 3 groups. B3, B6 and B9 represent online tDCS. B3, B6 and B9 represent online tDCS. B4, B7 and B10 represent immediate offline. B5 and B8 represent delayed offline.

Figure 5 shows the evolution of normalized speed over time for the 3 groups. ANOVA$_{RM}$ for the speed indicated a significant main effect of time (F(9198) = 13.966, $p < 0.001$, ηp^2 = 0.338), but no significant main effect of polarity (F(2,22) = 0.830, $p = 0.449$) or time × polarity interaction (F(18,198) = 0.682, $p = 0.826$). Post hoc analysis performed on the time main effect revealed higher Speed values for a-tDCS at B11 and B10 when compared to B5, B4 and B3 and also for B3 when compared to B9 and B12; for c-a-tDCS at B12, B11 and B10 when compared to B5, B4 and B3 and also B9 when compared to B3; and for sham at B3 when compared to B12, B11 and B10. P-level and effect size values are for a-tDCS B3 vs. B9 ($p = 0.004$, g = 1.12), B3 vs. B10 ($p = 0.001$, g = 1.26), B3 vs. B11 ($p < 0.001$, g = 1.23), B3 vs. B12 ($p = 0.029$, g = 0.85), B4 vs. B10 ($p = 0.017$, g = 1.00), B4 vs. B10 ($p = 0.005$, g = 0.99) and for B5 vs. B10 ($p = 0.027$, g = 0.97), B5 vs. B11 ($p = 0.009$, g = 0.97). P-level and effect size values are for c-a-tDCS B3 vs. B9 ($p = 0.013$, g = 0.86), B3 vs. B10 ($p < 0.001$, g = 0.93), B3 vs. B11 ($p = 0.002$, g = 1.17), B3 vs. B12 ($p < 0.001$, g = 1.26), B4 vs. B10 ($p = 0.003$, g = 0.82), B4 vs. B11 ($p = 0.01$, g = 1.00), B4 vs. B12 ($p = 0.003$, g = 1.09), B5 vs. B10 ($p = 0.007$, g = 0.75), B5 vs. B11 ($p = 0.021$, g = 0.90) and B5 vs. B12 ($p = 0.006$, g = 0.98). P-level and effect size values are for sham B3 vs. B10 ($p = 0.029$, g = 0.90), B3 vs. B11 ($p = 0.018$, g = 1,07) and for B3 vs. B12 ($p = 0.005$, g = 1.07).

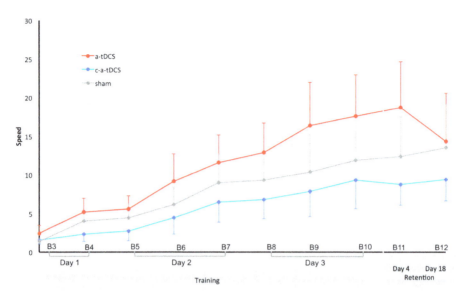

Figure 5. Evolution of of mean (and one SEM) speed over time (blocks—B) for each of the 3 groups. B3, B6 and B9 represent online tDCS. B3, B6 and B9 represent online tDCS. B4, B7 and B10 represent immediate offline. B5 and B8 represent delayed offline.

4. Discussion

The present study explored whether multiple sessions of cathodal priming and anodal tDCS (c-a-tDCS) over 3 consecutive days could further enhance motor learning and retention of an already learned visuo-motor task compared to a-tDCS or sham. The main findings of this study were that (i) multiple sessions of c-a-tDCS significantly further enhanced speed and IP above baseline training levels with a relatively minor decrease in accuracy over the 3 training days that were maintained over the 2 retention days, (ii) although the increase in IP was numerically greater for c-a-tDCS than a-tDCS or sham, a-tDCS showed a numerically greater increase in speed with concomitant reduced accuracy; while c-a-tDCS showed relatively stable accuracy with smaller increase in speed and (iii) these learning and retention performance changes for the real tDCS groups (c-a-tDCS and a-tDCS) were not significantly different from the sham group.

4.1. Influence of Cathodal Priming and Anodal tDCS on Motor Performance Retention

Our main findings with priming c-tDCS and a-tDCS are encouraging for inducing short and long-term retention. Motor performance retention was improved by adding priming c-tDCS to multiple sessions of atDCS and motor task training with a more persistent phenomenon (cf. Figure 3). These findings corroborated past results by Christova et al. [22] that reported priming c-tDCS (15 min) compared to sham a greater improvement in grooved pegboard task performance after learning with concurrent a-tDCS (1 mA, 20 min) for the non-dominant hand two weeks after. Similar to Christova et al. [22], we were not able to detect significant differences between groups 2 weeks after motor training. However, c-tDCS priming was found to be the unique condition with a significant difference from baseline with a large increase as indicated with the effect size (g = 2.87, Figure 3). In the present study, the motor performance gains 18 days after training were 22% with c-a-tDCS while a-tDCS priming and sham produced 3% and 20%, respectively. The willingness to combine priming c-tDCS and multiple sessions of a-tDCS and motor task training makes it difficult to account for the proportion of both factors in the final outcome. The lack of an experimental condition with sham priming followed by a-tDCS and motor-tracing task prevents concluding that the increase was due only to the c-tDCS priming effect. The need to have several training sessions seems to be a factor of first order, since Fujiyama et al. [23] reported for unimanual isometric force task that no significant difference between priming c-tDCS and sham persisted in a retest 24 h later.

A possible reason the sham group showed comparable learning and retention changes in circular task performance compared to the real tDCS groups may have been due to both (i) the effects of the sham group not reaching a plateau stage of learning compared to the real tDCS groups during the baseline training, and (ii) by the nature of using active sham, where there was 90 s of real stimulation applied during the training block. Therefore, we consider that the sham group in this study may not be an ideal control group to compare with the 2 tDCS groups. Nevertheless, compared to the c-a-tDCS and a-tDCS groups, the non-significant changes in performance (IP, accuracy, speed) for the sham group over the 2 baseline training blocks (B1 and B2) may have allowed greater potential for use dependent plasticity to show comparable learning and retention to that of the tDCS groups; while the 2 tDCS groups, that were working at the plateau stages of learning after the baseline training prior to tDCS training, adding tDCS to the training continued to enhance performance over the 3 days and more so for the c-a-tDCS group based on the speed–accuracy trade-off function (IP). Higher inhibitory tone at baseline, defined as a higher GABA/Glutamatergic metabolites ratio was shown to entail a greater disruptive effect of cathodal tDCS to response training gains [35]. Thus, the effects of cathodal and anodal tDCS on motor performance could be more beneficial when systems operate on suboptimal levels, e.g., regarding cortical excitability (not assessed in the present study) at baseline. However, the subtle differences in the changes in speed–accuracy trade-off (components of the IP) between c-a-tDCS (maintenance of accuracy over increasing speed) and a-tDCS (increasing speed over maintenance of accuracy) provides preliminary insights to a mechanistic modulation of performance with priming and polarity of tDCS.

The non-superiority of either priming c-tDCS or a-tDCS with motor training as compared to sham with motor training indicates that future studies are needed to control the intensity, the duration and the timing of application when manipulating priming. First, individualizing the tDCS intensity to ensure that excitability is lowered with cathodal tDCS is necessary [36]. Second, the duration of stimulation can play a role in modulating excitability since it was observed that 2×9 min without a break of c-tDCS with a conventional montage induced prolonged effects in cortical excitability changes compared to a single 9 min period [37]. However, a shorter duration of c-tDCS priming could be also more effective because an excessive and prolonged decrease in excitability may not lead to a return to the baseline during the 10 min of rest. In addition, using HD tDCS montage could induce delayed and longer lasting after-effects on motor cortex excitability as compared to conventional tDCS [13], suggesting further uncertainty in the timing of application. In our knowledge, no studies have been carried out to evaluate the optimal time to magnify the return to baseline with c-tDCS priming. Neuroimaging methods as electroencephalography or near infrared spectroscopy that can be combined with tDCS are a way to determine the optimal dosage [11,38]. Central to this endeavour is the definition of new biomarkers with such neuroimaging methods [11,39] to assess the effects of tDCS using a range of dosages in both research and translational (clinical) studies.

4.2. Impact of tDCS on a Low Learning Reserve Motor Task

The choice of a circular tracing-task with low learning reserve was voluntarily made to isolate the tDCS compared to the learning effects. While circular tracing-task based on the steering law derived from the Fitt's law [40] should have provided limited improvement in performance despite training [41], an increase in IP and speed was revealed for the c-a-tDCS and a-tDCS group 24 h after the training without tDCS (B1 vs. B2), which indicates learning has improved performance; while no changes in these performance parameters were found for sham. This could suggest that both a-tDCS and c-a-tDS groups achieved already a plateau learning (ceiling levels) after the 2 first baseline blocks of training; while the sham did not. Beyond the will to propose a task to quickly reach the relative "ceiling" levels to be in line with highly skilled individuals (e.g., elite athletes, expert operators), the important use of the upper limbs in everyday life could disrupt the neuroplastic changes. Learning is so plastic that it is vulnerable to disruption by subsequent new learning [42]. Thus, to evaluate the interest to introduce priming, the replication of study without enhancement in performance after multiple training sessions is required with the addition of priming. For example, in a visuomotor grip force tracking task with stroke patients, no difference in the improvement in upper extremity Fugl–Meyer assessment at the end of 4 weeks training with concurrent a-tDCS was revealed compared to sham [43]. Beyond the heterogeneity of the degree of recovery for the patients and the weak intensity of stimulation (0.5 mA), the shoulder–elbow Fugl–Meyer assessment sub-score improved significantly more for a-tDCS compared to sham. This shows that a-tDCS combined with the chosen task allowed improvements in specific sub-components of clinical assessments. The addition of cathodal tDCS priming could potentially, for this disease, magnify the work of rehabilitation. Since stroke affects excitatory/inhibitory balance of the lesioned hemisphere towards greater inhibition, and the addition of a cathodal priming tDCS protocol to the lesioned hemisphere could further reduce excitability and allow a greater excitatory potential during the a-tDCS and arm rehabilitation training program, a greater potential to learn to use the arm again is expected.

4.3. Methodological Considerations

Despite the novelty of the current findings, some limitations should be highlighted to recommend caution in generalizing the results. The performance variability between subjects and groups could stem from differences in interpretation of the instruction set to perform the circular task by each subject, such as choosing a strategy with higher speed and accuracy being trade-off, and better accuracy with lower speed trade-off. This heterogeneity in the strategy each subject used to perform the task most likely led to the greater variability between subjects even though the IP metric tries to account for these different speed–accuracy strategies. Giving a more precise instruction to bias speed over accuracy should be pursued in future tDCS studies of motor cortex stimulation to focus on enhancing movement speed, since this region is primarily involved in encoding the speed of movements. In the present study, the greater increase in speed for the a-tDCS group who predominantly utilized a speed bias over accuracy at the outset had the most profound increases in the speed of movement over the 3 days of training. In a clinical application of tDCS for stroke rehabilitation, Hamoudi et al. [44] has shown that 5 consecutive days of visuo-motor pinch grip training with the addition of a-tDCS led to a predominantly speed-based shift in the speed–accuracy trade-off.

Owing to varying tDCS effects due to individual differences, personalized tDCS intervention should be customized and applied. In addition, in this exploratory study, a small sample per group was enrolled. It is thus definitely needed in future studies of a larger sample size to confirm and possibly expand the current findings. This study focused on only healthy participants; therefore, it is worthwhile to explore the effects of both cathodal and anodal tDCS on motor performance and learning in patients with diminished or impaired motor function wherein ceiling effects less emerge. Whilst this investigation employed behavioural and perceptual outcomes, whether tDCS elicited a neurophysiological effect remains uncertain.

5. Conclusions

This exploratory study showed that the motor performance changes observed with c-a-tDCS condition may hold promise for short and long-term retention of an already learned motor skill. However, the lack of significant difference for the c-a-tDCS condition compared to sham limits the current interpretation on the group level. Future powered studies of larger sample size are needed to optimize the instruction set and tDCS intensity, duration and the timing of priming application on the individual level. In addition, combined neurophysiological and neuroimaging techniques are required to fully understand the mechanism of action of the priming intervention at a larger scale and therefore confirm the interest of priming before concurrent anodal tDCS and motor task training on motor performance and retention.

Author Contributions: Conceptualization, S.P., P.B., J.R. and M.M.; formal analysis, C.D.V. and P.B.; investigation, C.D.V.; data curation, C.D.V. and P.B.; writing—original draft preparation, P.B.; writing—review and editing, S.P., and M.M.; visualization, P.B.; supervision, M.M. and S.P.; project administration, S.P. All authors have read and agreed to the published version of the manuscript.

Funding: This research received no external funding.

Conflicts of Interest: The authors declare no conflict of interest.

References

1. Dissanayaka, T.; Zoghi, M.; Farrell, M.; Egan, G.F.; Jaberzadeh, S. Does transcranial electrical stimulation enhance corticospinal excitability of the motor cortex in healthy individuals? A systematic review and meta-analysis. *Eur. J. Neurosci.* **2017**. [CrossRef]
2. Saucedo Marquez, C.M.; Zhang, X.; Swinnen, S.P.; Meesen, R.; Wenderoth, N. Task-specific effect of transcranial direct current stimulation on motor learning. *Front. Hum. Neurosci.* **2013**, *7*. [CrossRef]
3. Schambra, H.M.; Abe, M.; Luckenbaugh, D.A.; Reis, J.; Krakauer, J.W.; Cohen, L.G. Probing for hemispheric specialization for motor skill learning: A transcranial direct current stimulation study. *J. Neurophysiol.* **2011**, *106*. [CrossRef] [PubMed]
4. Cuypers, K.; Leenus, D.J.F.; van den Berg, F.E.; Nitsche, M.A.; Thijs, H.; Wenderoth, N.; Meesen, R.L.J.; Kang, E.; Paik, N.; Reis, J.; et al. Is Motor Learning Mediated by tDCS Intensity? *PLoS ONE* **2013**, *8*, e67344. [CrossRef] [PubMed]
5. Reis, J.; Fischer, J.T.; Prichard, G.; Weiller, C.; Cohen, L.G.; Fritsch, B. Time- but not sleep-dependent consolidation of tDCS-enhanced visuomotor skills. *Cereb. Cortex* **2015**, *25*, 109–117. [CrossRef] [PubMed]
6. Besson, P.; Muthalib, M.; Dray, G.; Rothwell, J.; Perrey, S. Concurrent anodal transcranial direct-current stimulation and motor task to influence sensorimotor cortex activation. *Brain Res.* **2019**, *1710*, 181–187. [CrossRef] [PubMed]
7. Wiethoff, S.; Hamada, M.; Rothwell, J.C. Variability in Response to Transcranial Direct Current Stimulation of the Motor Cortex. *Brain Stimul.* **2014**, *7*, 468–475. [CrossRef] [PubMed]
8. Li, L.M.; Uehara, K.; Hanakawa, T. The contribution of interindividual factors to variability of response in transcranial direct current stimulation studies. *Front. Cell. Neurosci.* **2015**, *9*. [CrossRef]
9. Cancelli, A.; Cottone, C.; Parazzini, M.; Fiocchi, S.; Truong, D.; Bikson, M.; Tecchio, F. Transcranial Direct Current Stimulation: Personalizing the neuromodulation. In Proceedings of the 2015 37th Annual International Conference of the IEEE Engineering in Medicine and Biology Society (EMBC), Milan, Italy, 25–29 August 2015; pp. 234–237.
10. Edwards, D.; Cortes, M.; Datta, A.; Minhas, P.; Wassermann, E.M.; Bikson, M. Physiological and modeling evidence for focal transcranial electrical brain stimulation in humans: A basis for high-definition tDCS. *Neuroimage* **2013**, *74*, 266–275. [CrossRef]
11. Muthalib, M.; Besson, P.; Rothwell, J.; Perrey, S. Focal Hemodynamic Responses in the Stimulated Hemisphere During High-Definition Transcranial Direct Current Stimulation. *Neuromodulation Technol. Neural Interface* **2017**. [CrossRef] [PubMed]
12. Datta, A.; Bansal, V.; Diaz, J.; Patel, J.; Reato, D.; Bikson, M. Gyri-precise head model of transcranial direct current stimulation: Improved spatial focality using a ring electrode versus conventional rectangular pad. *Brain Stimul.* **2009**, *2*, 201–207. [CrossRef] [PubMed]
13. Kuo, H.-I.; Bikson, M.; Datta, A.; Minhas, P.; Paulus, W.; Kuo, M.-F.; Nitsche, M.A. Comparing Cortical Plasticity Induced by Conventional and High-Definition 4 × 1 Ring tDCS: A Neurophysiological Study. *Brain Stimul.* **2013**, *6*, 644–648. [CrossRef] [PubMed]
14. Stagg, C.J.; Jayaram, G.; Pastor, D.; Kincses, Z.T.; Matthews, P.M.; Johansen-Berg, H. Polarity and timing-dependent effects of transcranial direct current stimulation in explicit motor learning. *Neuropsychologia* **2011**, *49*, 800–804. [CrossRef] [PubMed]
15. Cohen Kadosh, R.; Soskic, S.; Iuculano, T.; Kanai, R.; Walsh, V. Modulating Neuronal Activity Produces Specific and Long-Lasting Changes in Numerical Competence. *Curr. Biol.* **2010**, *20*. [CrossRef]
16. Schmidt, R.A.; Lee, T.D. *Motor Control and Learning: A Behavioral Emphasis*, 5th ed.; Human Kinetics: Champaign, IL, USA, 2011.

17. Ziemann, U.; Siebner, H.R. Modifying motor learning through gating and homeostatic metaplasticity. *Brain Stimul.* **2008**, *1*, 60–66. [CrossRef]
18. Antal, A.; Nitsche, M.A.; Kincses, T.Z.; Kruse, W.; Hoffmann, K.-P.; Paulus, W. Facilitation of visuo-motor learning by transcranial direct current stimulation of the motor and extrastriate visual areas in humans. *Eur. J. Neurosci.* **2004**, *19*, 2888–2892. [CrossRef]
19. Hashemirad, F.; Zoghi, M.; Fitzgerald, P.B.; Jaberzadeh, S. The effect of anodal transcranial direct current stimulation on motor sequence learning in healthy individuals: A systematic review and meta-analysis. *Brain Cognit.* **2016**, *102*, 1–12. [CrossRef]
20. Karabanov, A.; Ziemann, U.; Hamada, M.; George, M.S.; Quartarone, A.; Classen, J.; Massimini, M.; Rothwell, J.; Siebner, H.R. Consensus Paper: Probing Homeostatic Plasticity of Human Cortex With Non-invasive Transcranial Brain Stimulation. *Brain Stimul.* **2015**, *8*, 442–454. [CrossRef]
21. Nitsche, M.A.; Paulus, W. Sustained excitability elevations induced by transcranial DC motor cortex stimulation in humans. *Neurology* **2001**, *57*, 1899–1901. [CrossRef]
22. Christova, M.; Rafolt, D.; Gallasch, E. Cumulative effects of anodal and priming cathodal tDCS on pegboard test performance and motor cortical excitability. *Behav. Brain Res.* **2015**, *287*, 27–33. [CrossRef]
23. Fujiyama, H.; Hinder, M.R.; Barzideh, A.; Van de Vijver, C.; Badache, A.C.; Manrique-C, M.N.; Reissig, P.; Zhang, X.; Levin, O.; Summers, J.J.; et al. Preconditioning tDCS facilitates subsequent tDCS effect on skill acquisition in older adults. *Neurobiol. Aging* **2017**, *51*, 31–42. [CrossRef] [PubMed]
24. Kumari, N.; Taylor, D.; Rashid, U.; Vandal, A.C.; Smith, P.F.; Signal, N. Cerebellar transcranial direct current stimulation for learning a novel split-belt treadmill task: A randomised controlled trial. *Sci Rep.* **2020**, *10*, 11853. [CrossRef] [PubMed]
25. Waters, S.; Wiestler, T.; Diedrichsen, J. Cooperation Not Competition: Bihemispheric tDCS and fMRI Show Role for Ipsilateral Hemisphere in Motor Learning. *J. Neurosci.* **2017**, *37*, 7500–7512. [CrossRef] [PubMed]
26. Oldfield, R.C. The assessment and analysis of handedness: The Edinburgh inventory. *Neuropsychologia* **1971**, *9*, 97–113. [CrossRef]
27. Bikson, M.; Grossman, P.; Thomas, C.; Zannou, A.L.; Jiang, J.; Adnan, T.; Mourdoukoutas, A.P.; Kronberg, G.; Truong, D.; Boggio, P.; et al. Safety of Transcranial Direct Current Stimulation: Evidence Based Update 2016. *Brain Stimul.* **2016**. [CrossRef] [PubMed]
28. Gandiga, P.C.; Hummel, F.C.; Cohen, L.G. Transcranial DC stimulation (tDCS): A tool for double-blind sham-controlled clinical studies in brain stimulation. *Clin. Neurophysiol.* **2006**, *117*, 845–850. [CrossRef]
29. Turski, C.A.; Kessler-Jones, A.; Hermann, B.; Hsu, D.; Jones, J.; Seeger, S.; Chappell, R.; Ikonomidou, C. Feasibility and Dose Tolerability of High Definition Transcranial Direct Current Stimulation in healthy adults. *Brain Stimul.* **2017**, *10*. [CrossRef]
30. Poreisz, C.; Boros, K.; Antal, A.; Paulus, W. Safety aspects of transcranial direct current stimulation concerning healthy subjects and patients. *Brain Res. Bull.* **2007**, *72*, 208–214. [CrossRef]
31. Accot, J.; Zhai, S. Scale effects in steering law tasks. In Proceedings of the SIGCHI Conference on Human Factors in Computing Systems, Seattle, DC, USA, 31 March–5 April 2001; ACM Press: New York, NY, USA, 2001; pp. 1–8.
32. Kulikov, S.; MacKenzie, I.S.; Stuerzlinger, W. Measuring the effective parameters of steering motions. In *CHI '05 Extended Abstracts on Human Factors in Computing Systems*; ACM Press: New York, NY, USA, 2005; p. 1569.
33. Bonnetblanc, F. Conflit vitesse-précision et loi de Fitts. *Sci. Mot.* **2008**, 63–82. [CrossRef]
34. Hedges, L.V.; Olkin, I. Acknowledgments. In *Statistical Methods for Meta-Analysis*; Academic Press: Cambridge, MA, USA, 1985; pp. 21–22. ISBN 9780080570655.
35. Filmer, H.L.; Ehrhardt, S.E.; Bollmann, S.; Mattingley, J.B.; Dux, P.E. Accounting for individual differences in the response to tDCS with baseline levels of neurochemical excitability. *Cortex* **2019**, *115*, 324–334. [CrossRef]
36. Berryhill, M.E.; Peterson, D.J.; Jones, K.T.; Stephens, J.A. Hits and misses: Leveraging tDCS to advance cognitive research. *Front. Psychol.* **2014**, *5*. [CrossRef] [PubMed]
37. Monte-Silva, K.; Kuo, M.-F.; Liebetanz, D.; Paulus, W.; Nitsche, M.A. Shaping the Optimal Repetition Interval for Cathodal Transcranial Direct Current Stimulation (tDCS). *J. Neurophysiol.* **2010**, *103*, 1735–1740. [CrossRef] [PubMed]
38. Soekadar, S.R.; Herring, J.D. Transcranial electric stimulation (tES) and NeuroImaging: The state-of-the-art, new insights and prospects in basic and clinical neuroscience. *Neuroimage* **2016**, *140*, 1–3. [CrossRef] [PubMed]

39. Herold, F.; Gronwald, T.; Scholkmann, F.; Zohdi, H.; Wyser, D.; Müller, N.G.; Hamacher, D. New Directions in Exercise Prescription: Is There a Role for Brain-Derived Parameters Obtained by Functional Near-Infrared Spectroscopy? *Brain Sci.* **2020**, *10*, 342. [CrossRef]
40. Accot, J.; Zhai, S. Performance evaluation of input devices in trajectory-based tasks. In Proceedings of the SIGCHI Conference on Human factors in Computing Systems, Pittsburgh, PA, USA, 15–20 May 1999; ACM Press: New York, NY, USA, 1999; pp. 466–472.
41. Gibbs, C.B. controller design: Interactions of controlling limbs, time-lags and gains in positional and velocity systems. *Ergonomics* **1962**, *5*, 385–402. [CrossRef]
42. Shibata, K.; Sasaki, Y.; Bang, J.W.; Walsh, E.G.; Machizawa, M.G.; Tamaki, M.; Chang, L.-H.; Watanabe, T. Overlearning hyperstabilizes a skill by rapidly making neurochemical processing inhibitory-dominant. *Nat. Neurosci.* **2017**, *20*, 470–475. [CrossRef]
43. Pavlova, E.L.; Lindberg, P.; Khan, A.; Ruschkowski, S.; Nitsche, M.A.; Borg, J. Transcranial direct current stimulation combined with visuo-motor training as treatment for chronic stroke patients. *Restor. Neurol. Neurosci.* **2017**, *35*, 307–317. [CrossRef]
44. Hamoudi, M.; Schambra, H.M.; Fritsch, B.; Schoechlin-Marx, A.; Weiller, C.; Cohen, L.G.; Reis, J. Transcranial Direct Current Stimulation Enhances Motor Skill Learning but Not Generalization in Chronic Stroke. *Neurorehabilit. Neural Repair* **2018**, *32*, 295–308. [CrossRef]

Publisher's Note: MDPI stays neutral with regard to jurisdictional claims in published maps and institutional affiliations.

© 2020 by the authors. Licensee MDPI, Basel, Switzerland. This article is an open access article distributed under the terms and conditions of the Creative Commons Attribution (CC BY) license (http://creativecommons.org/licenses/by/4.0/).

MDPI
St. Alban-Anlage 66
4052 Basel
Switzerland
Tel. +41 61 683 77 34
Fax +41 61 302 89 18
www.mdpi.com

Brain Sciences Editorial Office
E-mail: actuators@mdpi.com
www.mdpi.com/journal/brainsci